Z O O N O S E S

Recognition, Control, and Prevention

ZOONOSES

Recognition, Control, and Prevention

MARTIN E. HUGH-JONES, MRCVS, MPH, PhD

WILLIAM T. HUBBERT, DVM, MPH, PhD, Dipl. ACVPM

HARRY V. HAGSTAD, DVM, MPH, Dipl. ACVPM

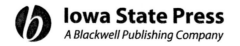

Iowa State Press
A Blackwell Publishing Company

DEDICATED TO
PAUL R. SCHURRENBERGER, DVM, MPH

He was a friend and colleague who left us before his time.
However, in his time he contributed much to our understanding of the zoonoses.

Martin E. Hugh-Jones, MRCVS, MPH, PhD, Fellow ACE, is Professor in the Department of Epidemiology and Community Health, School of Veterinary Medicine, Louisiana State University.

William T. Hubbert, DVM, MPH, PhD, Diplomate ACVPM, is Adjunct Professor in the Department of Epidemiology and Community Health, School of Veterinary Medicine, Louisiana State University.

Harry V. Hagstad, DVM, MPH, Diplomate ACVPM, Fellow ACE, is Professor Emeritus in the Department of Epidemiology and Community Health, School of Veterinary Medicine, Louisiana State University.

Iowa State Press
A Blackwell Publishing Company
2121 State Avenue
Ames, IA 50014

Orders: 1-800-862-6657   Fax: 1-515-292-3348
Office. 1-515-292-0140   Web site: www.iowastatepress.com

Authorization to photocopy items for internal or personal use, or the internal or personal use of specific clients, is granted by Iowa State Press, provided that the base fee of $.10 per copy is paid directly to the Copyright Clearance Center, 222 Rosewood Drive, Danvers, MA 01923. For those organizations that have been granted a photocopy license by CCC, a separate system of payments has been arranged. The fee code fee for users of the Transactional Reporting Service is 0-8138-1821-4/95 (hardcover); 0-8138-2542-3 (paperback) $.10.

♾ Printed on acid-free paper in the United States of America

First edition, 1995
First paperback edition, 2000

Zoonoses Recognition, Control, and Prevention replaces *Outline of the Zoonoses,* 1981 Iowa State University Press, Ames, Iowa 50014

Library of Congress Cataloging-in-Publication Data

Hugh-Jones, Martin E.
    Zoonoses: recognition, control, and prevention / Martin E. Hugh-Jones, William T. Hubbert, Harry V. Hagstad.—1st ed.
        Replaces: outline of the zoonoses / Paul R. Schnurrenberger. 1981
    Includes bibliographical references and index.
        ISBN 0-8138-1821-4 (hardcover); 0-8138-2542-3 (paperback)
        1 Zoonoses—Handbooks, manuals, etc. I Hubbert, William T. II. Hagstad, Harry V.
    III. Schnurrenberger, Paul R. Outline of the zoonoses. IV. Title.
    SF740.H84 1995
    636.0896959—DC20   95-7358

Last digit is the print number: 10 9 8 7 6 5 4

CONTENTS

v

PREFACE

When *Outline of the Zoonoses* (Schnurrenberger and Hubbert) was published in 1981, its purpose was stated as follows:

The primary purpose of this outline is to present the veterinary practitioner with an all-encompassing, concise, desk-top reference to the zoonotic diseases. In daily work, the practitioner holds the key to these diseases through accurate diagnosis and treatment of the patient and counsel to the owner on preventive and control practices. This belief in the importance of the practitioner and the primacy of preventive medicine influenced the formulation of this outline. Although designed for the veterinarian, it should be of value to physicians, nurses, public health officials, wildlife workers, and many others.

This purpose continues in *Zoonoses: Recognition, Control, and Prevention* with the updated synopses presented in Section IV.

The authors have assembled Sections I, II, and III as a result of needs identified during a collective century of professional experience. During that time, extraordinary changes have occurred in the practice of human and veterinary medicine. However, the diseases, including zoonoses, have not changed—we just understand them better. Much of our newer knowledge of the zoonoses has come from greater insight into their epidemiology and ecology. A major force for improved zoonoses prevention and control has been the introduction and application of economic analysis. Section I presents a historic background, Section II describes current principles, and Section III predicts changes we can expect in the future.

ACKNOWLEDGMENTS

The author of Chapter 6 is especially appreciative of the help of Tari Kindred, John McInerney, Roly Tinline, Alex Wandeler, and Brian Williams—the mistakes are his, the insights are theirs.

The authors appreciate the assistance of Kathleen Harrington, BS, MS, in preparation of the synopses. The authors gratefully acknowledge the expert editing advice provided by Sandra L. Hubbert, BAJ, MJ.

SECTION I

Introduction

1

INTRODUCTION TO
THE ZOONOSES

Definition

Zoonoses ("zoonosis" is singular) **are diseases the agents of which are transmitted between vertebrate animals and people.**[16,28] It is the interaction of agent, host (degree of susceptibility), and the environment they share that determines whether or not transmission of the agent will be successful, leading to infection and, ultimately, occurrence of disease. Carrier hosts, individuals infected without overt signs of disease, are important in the persistence of many zoonotic agents. Vertebrate animals are the **reservoirs** (where the agent persists in nature) of zoonoses. The agents may be transmitted either directly or indirectly by fomites or vectors. Many diseases are shared by other animals and people, but the reservoir is in the inanimate environment (soil, water), not a vertebrate animal. For example, **soil** is the reservoir for agents of systemic mycoses (e.g., *Blastomyces dermatitidis, Coccidioides immitis, Nocardia asteroides*) and many of the mycobacterioses (e.g., *Mycobacterium intracellulare, Mycobacterium kansasii*). **Water** is the reservoir for the agents of other mycobacterioses (e.g., *Mycobacterium marinum*) and free-living pathogenic amoebae such as *Naegleria fowleri*. Still other diseases clinically similar in animals and people, and once thought to be zoonotic, are now known to be the result of **endogenous infection** from the individual's own normal flora. Examples are actinomycosis (e.g., *Actinomyces bovis*—cattle, *Actinomyces israeli*—people) and disease caused by Gram-negative anaerobic organisms such as *Bacteroides melaninogenicus*.

Initial Recognition of the Agents

Clinical features for a few of the zoonoses have been recognized since early history. For example, the signs of encephalitis in dogs with rabies, ringworm in people and animals, *Mycobacterium bovis*-associated scrofula in children, glanders and tetanus in horses and humans, and epidemic urban plague (*Yersinia pestis*) have been described for many centuries.[2,4,16,23,24] Confirmation of the specific etiology for all zoonoses, however, awaited Leeuwenhoek's invention of the microscope in the late 1600s and the scientific discoveries that have followed to date.[9,19]

All major microbial and parasitic categories, from viruses to helminths, include some zoonotic agents. It is not surprising, therefore, that the larger **parasites** were the first to be examined with the primitive microscopes. In 1758, Linnaeus (the father of scientific classification) included descriptions of two cestodes (*Dipylidium caninum* and *Diphyllobothrium latum*), a trematode (*Fasciola hepatica*), and two nematodes (*Ascaris lumbricoides*, essentially identical to *A. suum*, and *Dracunculus medinensis*) in *Systema Naturae*, 10th edition. Although earlier reports exist, such as the description of *Fasciola hepatica* by Jehan de Brie in 1379 (perhaps the earliest description of a parasite), organized classification/description began with Linnaeus. By 1800, most of the cestodes had been described and, by the 1870s, so had most of the trematodes.[5,6,30] Although Bilharz had described *Schistosoma haematobium* in 1851, the zoonotic schistosomes were described a little later, *S. japonicum* in 1904, *S. mansoni* in 1907.[36] Most of the roundworm species were first described during the mid- to late 1800s, although descriptions of several *Thelazia* species first appeared between 1910 and 1930 and it was not until 1935 that *Angiostrongylus cantonensis* (rat lung worm) was first described.[13,17] From 1900 to 1910, numerous methods were described to concentrate parasite ova in feces by sedimentation, filtration, and/or flotation before microscopic examination. With only slight improvements since, these are the most widely used parasitologic methods today.[8,14] The zoonotic species of most genera of protozoa (*Babesia, Entamoeba, Giardia, Pneumocystis, Toxoplasma, Trypanosoma*) were first described between 1885 and 1915. The plasmodia of primates, however, were much later, descriptions first appearing in the 1930s to 1960s.[33] Clarification of species among the coccidia and their role as zoonoses, especially *Besnoitia, Cryptosporidium, Hammondia*, and *Sarcocystis*, has been even more recent, continuing to the present.

The **mycotic etiology** of ringworm was first described microscopically by David Gruby in the 1840s.[2] Raimond Sabouraud began using culture medium in the 1890s. The cat as reservoir of human *Microsporum canis* infection was identified in 1902. Some early descriptions of agents of systemic mycoses around 1900 suggested they were protozoa. Soil was first reported as the reservoir of a systemic mycosis, *Coccidioides immitis*, in 1932. Although the agents of the systemic mycoses are capable of producing disease when transmitted from an infected host to a susceptible host, these occurrences are uncommon, usually involving accidental inoculation of infectious material. The resulting disease is also atypical, appearing as a regional lymphangitis rather than a pneumonia and subsequent generalized infection. Inasmuch as these infections always involve transmission from an individual previously exposed to infection from an inanimate reservoir in nature, the agents of the systemic mycoses are not considered zoonotic because there is no animate reservoir. Beginning with *Coccidioides immitis* in 1932, soil has been identified as the reservoir for all of the agents of the systemic mycoses.

Although there were earlier microscopic observations of **bacterial zoonotic agents**, such as the spirochaete causing tickborne relapsing fever seen in blood (1873), it was the isolation of *Bacillus anthracis* by Robert Koch in 1877 that really opened the door to their description.[9,19] Use of aniline dyes to stain bacteria (and other organisms) in wet preparations began in the 1870s. In 1877, Koch reported the first observations of stained bacteria (*B. anthracis*) in a dried film. Hans Gram introduced decolorizing and counterstaining, i.e. the Gram stain, in 1884. Koch's early efforts at producing pure cultures involved serial dilutions in liquid medium. He introduced the first solid medium, the cut surface of a potato, in 1881. The Petri dish (glass, of course, not disposable plastic) was introduced in 1887. By 1890, most zoonotic bacteria had been described, with reports continuing to appear until 1916, when the first description of *Leptospira* was published. There was a hiatus from this time until the late 1940s (with the exception of the report of *Listeria monocytogenes* in 1924), when a few more descriptions began to emerge—*Pasteurella pneumotropica* (1948), *Yersinia enterocolitica* (1949), *Vibrio parahaemolyticus* (1953), and *Borrelia burgdorferi* (1982).[3,27,31]

Within 2 years of the initial isolation of *Pseudomonas pseudomallei* from a human patient in 1911, the agent of melioidosis had been recognized in several animal species in and around the laboratory in Rangoon. In the 1920s, only 1 of more than 20,000 wild rats examined was found infected in Saigon. It was not until the 1960s, however, that soil was identified as the true reservoir and that melioidosis was recognized as not, in fact, a zoonosis. Spread among animals and people essentially does not occur.

In 1909, Howard Ricketts described *Rickettsia rickettsii*, the agent of Rocky Mountain spotted fever.[15] Most of the remaining **zoonotic rickettsiae** were first described in the 1930s, with the agents of Queensland tick typhus (*R. australis*) and rickettsialpox (*R. akari*) first reported in 1946. The first edition of *Bergey's Manual of Determinative Bacteriology* appeared in 1923, and has become the bible of bacterial and rickettsial classification.

In 1798, Edward Jenner demonstrated that people exposed to pox material from cows were later protected against smallpox.[11] And, in 1804,

Zinke showed that normal dogs developed rabies when injected with saliva from rabid dogs. Although these were classic reports of responses to infection, they did not establish the viral nature of the agents involved. In 1898, Loeffler and Frosch passed foot-and-mouth disease serially from animal to animal using a cell-free filtrate, establishing the **filterable agent (virus)**.[37] Rabies virus isolation, as well as Negri's demonstration of the inclusion body, were first reported in 1903. This was followed by isolation of vesicular stomatitis virus, Newcastle disease virus, yellow fever virus, and louping ill virus in 1926, 1927, 1928, and 1929, respectively. Tissue culture techniques for the isolation of viruses were introduced in the late 1920s and use of the chick embryo began in 1931.

Until this time, animal virology involved infecting animals with cell-free material derived from other animals. Guinea pigs, mice, and rabbits have been standard laboratory animals since the 1800s.[35] Intracerebral injection of mice, introduced by R.A. Alexander in 1933 to produce African horse sickness vaccine, was one of the most significant innovations in virology of the time. Max Theiler, using this method, introduced the 17D yellow fever vaccine four years later. The use of ferrets in influenza studies began in the 1930s.[25] With the advent of the electron microscope in 1934, viruses could be seen and described. Most initial reports of the isolation of zoonotic viruses appeared during the 1930s.[32]

Although a lapse in reporting occurred during World War II, considerable new knowledge was acquired regarding zoonoses of military significance. Reporting picked up again during the 1950s, especially isolations of the less common arboviruses.[17] Infant (suckling) mice were already widely used to isolate arboviruses in 1948, when the technique was used in the first isolation of Coxsackie A virus.[10] In 1961, several outbreaks of human hepatitis involving prior contact with chimpanzees and other primates were first reported. Initially, these cases were referred to as simian hepatitis. Within the next decade, however, it became evident that these were undoubtedly all viral hepatitis A infections resulting from exposure to primate shedders rather than a new virus. With the exception of swine vesicular disease (1966), the most recently discovered viral zoonoses share the characteristic of high case fatality rates in people—Argentine hemorrhagic fever (1958), Bolivian hemorrhagic fever (1959), Marburg disease (1967), Lassa fever (1970), Ebola disease (1976), and Korean hemorrhagic fever (1978).[1]

The infectious etiology of cat scratch disease is only now being unraveled with presumptive evidence that the agent is a bacterium, *Rochalimaea henselae*.[26] A clinical relationship to the presence of antibody to simian immunodeficiency virus in laboratory workers has not been established.

Arthropod vectors are involved in the transmission of several zoonotic protozoan parasites, bacteria, rickettsiae, and viruses. In 1893, Smith and Kilborne first demonstrated vectorborne transmission of an infectious agent with tick transmission of *Babesia bigemina*, the agent of bovine babesiosis. Ogato, in 1896, recovered *Yersinia pestis* from rat fleas. Ross, in 1898, demonstrated avian malaria parasites in mosquitoes. In 1899, Tanaka proposed the larval red mite as a vector of scrub typhus. Reed and colleagues, in 1900, proved mosquitoborne spread of yellow fever. In 1903, Bruce and colleagues reported transmission of *Trypanosoma gambiense* by tsetse flies. In 1906, Ricketts and King independently demonstrated tick transmission of the rickettsial agent of Rocky Mountain spotted fever. By the beginning of the 1900s, the concept of vectorborne spread had been established for zoonotic members of all the major groups of infectious agents except fungi.

Application of current technology (not all of which is laboratory-based) in the recognition of agents and vectors involved in zoonotic diseases in people and animals will be presented in later chapters.

Initial Recognition of the Diseases

For many zoonoses, the risk of infection for people and animals, as well as the signs of illness, are sufficiently similar that an association between the two has been known for a long time. For instance, outbreaks of eastern and western equine encephalitis affected people and horses at the same time so often over the years that they were associated long before the agents were known. Horses, in fact, were frequently a useful sentinel before vaccination became a widespread practice. Death as a possible outcome of being bitten by a rabid dog is well known in primitive societies. Therefore, when the agents of these diseases were identified in people and animals, it was no surprise that they were the same.

In contrast, connecting disease in people, animal reservoir, and agent has required considerable effort by many investigators to solve the riddles involved. For example, David Bruce observed the agent of undulant fever in the spleen of a fatal human case on the island of Malta in 1886 and isolated it a year later.[29] It was nearly 20 years before the goat as reservoir of *Brucella melitensis* and raw goat milk as the vehicle were identified. Ten years after Bruce's discovery (1897), Bernard Bang isolated an agent of bovine abortion, *Brucella abortus*. It was another 18 years (1925) before this agent was found to also cause undulant fever or human brucellosis. The first description of an outbreak of undulant fever caused by *Br. abortus* involved college students who drank raw cow's milk in the dormitory.

Adolf Weil, in the early 1880s, was able to distinguish clinically and epidemiologically a jaundice he observed in sewer workers in Paris from other forms of jaundice. In 1907, Stimson observed the agent in the kidney of a patient believed to have died of yellow fever. In 1916, Inada and colleagues reported the isolation of the spirochaete and that field rodents were the reservoir. Unfortunately, Hideyo Noguchi confused the signs of yellow fever with those of leptospirosis and mistakenly believed that leptospires were the cause of yellow fever. He spent nearly a decade performing field trials with a vaccine he developed to protect people against yellow fever. Noguchi died of yellow fever in 1928, the year its viral agent was identified. This is an ironic example of a consequence of reporting the etiology of a disease based on insufficient evidence.

In 1912, McCoy and Chapin identified *Francisella tularensis* as the cause of a die-off in ground squirrels similar to plague in Tulare County, California. Although tularemia is widespread in the Northern Hemisphere, oddly it was nearly 30 years after it was first recognized in rodents that the first human case was reported in Tulare County. A major reason is that this locale does not harbor some of the more efficient tick vectors for spread of the agent from rodents to people.

McFadyean and Stockman first reported vibrionic abortion in sheep and cattle, caused by *Vibrio fetus*, in 1913. In 1947, more than 30 years later, Vinzent and colleagues reported the first human case of septicemic vibriosis. They attributed their success in part to the fact that they used a diagnostic laboratory that also did veterinary work. Although isolation of microaerophilic bacterial pathogens under reduced oxygen tension was a common practice in veterinary diagnostic laboratories at this time, it was later that the technique was introduced to medical laboratories. What was once called *Vibrio*, now called *Campylobacter, jejuni* was originally thought to be a commensal of animals—not being of any pathogenic significance. Since the first report by Bokkenheuser in 1970, campylobacteriosis has become recognized as a leading cause of human enteric disease. The principal reason for this increase in recognition has been a change in techniques used in diagnostic enteric bacteriology.

In 1967, the first human cases of Marburg disease were reported in Germany and Yugoslavia among researchers who had worked with the tissues of African green monkeys. Although a few human cases have been reported since in Africa, no reservoir in nature has been identified in spite of intensive searching. Ebola virus disease was first recognized in Zaire and the Sudan in 1976, the former being an extensive nosocomial outbreak. Ebola virus is morphologically identical to Marburg virus but immunologically distinct. The reservoir of Ebola virus, too, has not been identified. Lassa fever was first recognized in Nigeria in 1969 and is caused by a virus related to other viruses known to have rodent reservoirs. It was later found in the African multimammate mouse, *Mastomys natalensis*.

The status of the zoonotic protozoa changed dramatically when Rommel and Heydorn, in 1972, fed beef and pork containing sarcocysts to people, resulting in the shedding of what was for a long time previously called

Isospora hominis. What was thought to be a one-host cycle turned out to be a two-host cycle akin to taeniasis and toxoplasmosis.

Lyme disease was first described clinically in 1977 as a juvenile rheumatoid arthritis (rash and fever syndrome recognized later) in Lyme, Connecticut, following a tick bite. The agent, *Borrelia burgdorferi*, was reported in 1982. The wildlife reservoir of the spirochaete and its effects on wild and domestic animals have been described more recently.

Human cowpox infections have long been recognized in association with endemic cowpox in cattle. In 1978, the virus was isolated from pox lesions in a cat. In 1989, catpox was observed in a person at the site of a cat scratch. To date, the actual reservoir of catpox/cowpox virus is uncertain inasmuch as it is neither cats nor cows.[34]

The term **emerging microbial threat** has been used to characterize newly identified agents and newly recognized diseases in people.[20] It is likely that the agents are not newly evolved, but have existed in nature, particularly in animals. The following factors have been associated with the emergence of these threats: changing human demographics and behavior, technology and industry, economic development and land use, international travel and commerce, microbial adaptation and change, and failure of public health measures. Recognizing the presence of a disease in an animal or person, or in a flock, herd, or community, usually is much easier than recognizing the specific factors (including agent) responsible for its occurrence. Means of improving recognition of zoonoses will be presented in later chapters.

Development of Control and Prevention Strategies

Early religious laws against the eating of pork, whether or not the believers related the prohibition to risk of disease, certainly had a salutary effect in regard to risk of contracting trichinosis and cysticercosis.

During the second plague pandemic, beginning in the 1300s, quarantine (literally, 40 days) was a common practice to protect the susceptible residents of a seaport from whatever evil (plague) was being delivered to them by those on board a ship from another land (often where epidemic plague was known to exist).[24] Of course, the ship's rats died along with the crew if plague was aboard. Protecting a susceptible community by quarantine usually was not feasible for other diseases. For one thing, many of the diseases involved carriers who appeared healthy at the time of entry and who were less likely to develop with surety the severe signs of disease such as seen with plague. Therefore, they slipped in with little notice.

At one time, more than 80 major diseases of cattle flourished in East Africa because the cattle there were exposed to ruminants brought by Arab slave traders on their travels to the coast from farther west in Africa or from across the sea in Asia. Many of these diseases are zoonoses and persist today.

Boiling of milk was an early custom among some societies. Unfortunately, the custom did not always include boiling the milk to make cheese, thereby permitting spread of some of the more important milkborne agents. Commercial pasteurization of milk became widespread in developed countries during the 1920s, virtually eliminating milkborne brucellosis and tuberculosis except on the farm where there were still infected cows and milk was consumed raw, and in villages where raw milk was distributed.

Vaccine and vaccination, the words themselves being derived from vaccinia, the cowpox virus, are synonymous with protection against disease. For nearly 200 years, the vaccine was used to protect against smallpox, and the principal source of this vaccine was the lymph of calves that had been scarified with the virus. The vaccine provided an essential tool in the worldwide eradication of smallpox, so declared officially by the World Health Organization on December 9, 1979 (the last naturally occurring case was in Somalia in October 1977).[12] Zoonoses for which vaccines are widely used to protect people with high risk of exposure include plague, rabies, and yellow fever.

Glanders, a scourge of horses and people since antiquity, caused by *Pseudomonas mallei*, was eradicated from most of the world by slaughter of animals found positive to the intrapalpebral mallein test. The test was introduced in the early 1900s, and since the 1940s the only remaining endemic areas are in Asia.

A law has existed for nearly a century requiring working dogs used to shepherd livestock to be tested for tapeworms, and successfully treated if any were found before entering the United States. Since the mid-1950s, Iceland and New Zealand have had successful *Echinococcus granulosus* eradication programs based on test and treatment of dogs. *Mycobacterium bovis* is quite sensitive to several antibiotics, and drugs have been used cost-effectively to eradicate tuberculosis in cattle herds. Most national bovine tuberculosis eradication programs, however, were in existence long before these drugs were available and are based on the use of intradermal tuberculin tests and slaughter of positive animals. In the United Kingdom and New Zealand, the program has run into difficulty because of infection in wildlife.

Environmental control of arthropod vectors really came of age with the advent of DDT during World War II. Before then, fumigation was used to kill fleas within structures for plague control. Arsenicals were used to dip animals for tick control. Mosquito control involved modification of harborage, such as emptying water from receptacles to eliminate breeding sites for *Aedes aegypti* and extensive drainage programs for reduction of other vectors.

When people and their livestock lived in small, isolated communities, they shared relatively few zoonoses. The diseases were principally those for which a significant carrier state persisted in people and/or animals or the disease was sufficiently chronic, e.g., tuberculosis, to provide a continuous source of infection for new susceptibles. Times have changed. The world population has increased roughly fivefold in the last century.[18,21,22] Between 1880 and 1980, the urban percentage of the United States population increased from 28% to 74%.[7] This shift to urban living is the norm on all continents. During the period 1920 to 1980, the percentage of people actually living on farms declined from 30% to 2%. Even though much of the world is now urban, people and their possessions (food, animals) are also more mobile today. In fact, today we have a more complex picture involving relative risk of exposure to zoonotic agents and relative need for planned strategies of zoonoses control and prevention. Explanation of the underlying principles of zoonoses control and prevention, and their current applications, will be presented in later chapters.

Chronology of Events in Zoonoses Recognition, Control, and Prevention

Before 1300
Ancient descriptions of clinical observations.
Early religious dietary practices.
1300-1500
Jehan de Brie (1379) described first parasite, *Fasciola hepatica*.
Quarantining ships from foreign (plague-affected) ports began.
1501-1700
Leeuwenhoek (late 1600s) invented microscope and published first descriptions of microorganisms.
1701-1800
Linnaeus (1758) published *Systema Naturae*, 10th edition (including descriptions of five zoonotic parasites).
Jenner (1798) demonstrated that cowpox protected against smallpox.
By 1800, most cestodes had been described.
1801-1850
Zinke demonstrated rabies transmission by saliva in dogs (1804).
Gruby (1840s) described mycotic etiology of ringworm.
1851-1900
By 1870s, most trematodes had been described.
Koch (1877) isolated *Bacillus anthracis*.
Gram stain introduced (1884).
Petri dish introduced (1887).
By 1890, most zoonotic bacteria had been described.

Tick (vector) transmission of *Babesia* demonstrated (1893).

1901-1950

Rabies virus isolated and Negri body described (1903).

Goats demonstrated to be the reservoir of *Brucella melitensis* and goat milk a source of human infection (1905).

Ricketts (1909) described agent of Rocky Mountain spotted fever.

Commercial milk pasteurization introduced (1920s).

Electron microscope invented (1934).

17D yellow fever vaccine introduced (1937).

In 1930s, most zoonotic rickettsiae and viruses isolated.

Vector control with DDT introduced (1940s).

Since 1950

Marburg disease (1967), Lassa fever (1969), enteric campylobacteriosis (1970), Ebola (1976), and Lyme disease (1977) recognized.

Smallpox officially eradicated worldwide (1979).

Table 1.1. List of zoonotic agents

Agent	Disease in Humans (Class[a])
Pentastomids	
Armillifer armillatus	Pentastomid infection (U)[b]
Armillifer grandis	Pentastomid infection (U)
Armillifer moniliformis	Pentastomid infection (U)
Linguatula serrata	Pentastomid infection (U)
Nematodes	
Ancylostoma braziliense	Cutaneous larva migrans (5)
Ancylostoma caninum	Cutaneous larva migrans (5)
Angiostrongylus cantonensis	Parasitic meningo-encephalitis (5)
Angiostrongylus costaricensis	Parasitic meningo-encephalitis (5)
Anisakis marina	Anisakiasis (5)
Ascaris suum	Ascariasis (5)
Baylisascaris procyonis	Visceral larva migrans (5)
Brugia malayi	Filariasis (U)
Bunostomum phlebotomum	Cutaneous larva migrans (5)
Capillaria aerophila	Capillariasis (5)
Capillaria hepatica	Capillariasis (5)
Capillaria philippinensis	Capillariasis (5)
Dioctophyma renale	Giant kidney worm (U)
Dipetalonema perstans	Filariasis (U)
Dipetalonema streptocerca	Filariasis (U)
Dirofilaria immitis	Filariasis (U)
Dirofilaria repens	Filariasis (U)
Dirofilaria tenuis	Filariasis (U)
Dracunculus insignis	Dracunculiasis (5)
Dracunculus medinensis	Dracunculiasis (5)
Gnathostoma spinigerum	Cutaneous and visceral larva migrans (5)

Table 1.1. (*continued*)

Agent	Disease in Humans (Class[a])
Nematodes	
Haemonchus contortus	Trichostrongyliasis (U)
Loa loa	Filariasis/Loiasis (5)
Onchocerca cervicalis	Filariasis/Onchocerciasis (5)
Onchocerca volvulus	Filariasis/Onchocerciasis (5)
Ostertagia spp.	Trichostrongyliasis (U)
Strongyloides fulleborni	Strongyloidiasis (5)
Strongyloides myopotami	Strongyloidiasis (5)
Strongyloides procyonis	Strongyloidiasis (5)
Strongyloides ransomi	Strongyloidiasis (5)
Strongyloides ratti	Strongyloidiasis (5)
Strongyloides stercoralis	Strongyloidiasis (5)
Strongyloides westeri	Strongyloidiasis (5)
Thelazia californiensis	Thelaziasis (U)
Thelazia callipaeda	Thelaziasis (U)
Toxocara canis	Visceral larva migrans (5)
Toxocara cati	Visceral larva migrans (5)
Trichinella spiralis	Trichinosis (2B)
Trichostrongylus spp.	Trichostrongyliasis (U)
Uncinaria stenocephala	Cutaneous larva migrans (5)
Trematodes	
Amphimerus pseudofelineus	Opisthorchiasis (5)
Clinostomum complenatum	Clinostomiasis (U)
Clonorchis sinensis	Clonorchiasis (5)
Dicrocoelium dendriticum	Dicrocoeliasis (U)
Dicrocoelium hospes	Dicrocoeliasis (U)
Echinostoma ilocanum	Echinostomiasis (U)
Echinostoma lindoense	Echinostomiasis (U)
Echinostoma malayanum	Echinostomiasis (U)
Echinostoma revolutum	Echinostomiasis (U)
Fasciola gigantica	Fascioliasis (5)
Fasciola hepatica	Fascioliasis (5)
Fasciolopsis buski	Fasciolopsiasis (3C)
Gastrodiscoides hominis	Amphistomiasis (U)
Haplorchis pumilio	Heterophydiasis (U)
Haplorchis taichui	Heterophydiasis (U)
Haplorchis yokogawai	Heterophydiasis (U)
Heterophyes continua	Heterophydiasis (U)
Heterophyes heterophyes	Heterophydiasis (U)
Metagonimus yokogawai	Metagonimiasis (U)
Opisthorchis felineus	Opisthorchiasis (5)
Opisthorchis viverrini	Opisthorchiasis (5)
Paragonimus westermani	Paragonimiasis (5)
Schistosoma japonicum	Schistosomiasis (3C)
Schistosoma mansoni	Schistosomiasis (3C)
Cestodes	
Diphyllobothrium latum	Fish tapeworm (5)
Diphyllobothrium spp.	Sparganosis (U)
Dipylidium caninum	Dog tapeworm (U)
Echinococcus granulosus	Hydatidosis (3B)

Table 1.1. (*continued*)

Agent	Disease in Humans (Class[a])
Cestodes	
Echinococcus multilocularis	Hydatidosis (3B)
Echinococcus oligarthrus	Hydatidosis (3B)
Echinococcus vogeli	Hydatidosis (3B)
Hymenolepis diminuta	Mouse or rat tapeworm (5)
Hymenolepis nana	Dwarf tapeworm (5)
Mesocestoides lineatus	*Mesocestoides* infection (U)
Mesocestoides variabilis	*Mesocestoides* infection (U)
Raillietina spp.	Raillietiniasis (U)
Spirometra erinacei-europaei	Sparganosis (U)
Spirometra mansoni	Sparganosis (U)
Spirometra mansonoides	Sparganosis (U)
Spirometra proliferum	Sparganosis (U)
Spirometra theileri	Sparganosis (U)
Taenia hydatigena	Tapeworm-sheep/goat (U)
Taenia ovis	Tapeworm-sheep/goat (U)
Taenia saginata	Beef tapeworm (3C)
Taenia solium	Pork tapeworm (3C)
Taenia taeniaeformis	Tapeworm-rodent (U)
Protozoa	
Babesia bovis	Piroplasmosis/Babesiosis (3A)
Babesia divergens	Piroplasmosis/Babesiosis (3A)
Babesia microti	Piroplasmosis/Babesiosis (3A)
Balantidium coli	Balantidiasis (5)
Cryptosporidium parvum	Cryptosporidiosis (3B)
Entamoeba histolytica	Amebiasis (3C)
Entamoeba polecki	Amebiasis (3C)
Giardia lamblia (intestinalis)	Giardiasis (3B)
Leishmania aethiopica	Cutaneous leishmaniasis (5)
Leishmania braziliensis	American leishmaniasis (5)
Leishmania donovani	Visceral leishmaniasis (3B)
Leishmania major	Cutaneous leishmaniasis (5)
Leishmania mexicana	American leishmaniasis (5)
Leishmania tropica	Cutaneous leishmaniasis (5)
Plasmodium brazilianum	Malaria, simian (3C)
Plasmodium cynomolgi	Malaria, simian (3C)
Plasmodium eylesi	Malaria, simian (3C)
Plasmodium inui	Malaria, simian (3C)
Plasmodium knowlesi	Malaria, simian (3C)
Plasmodium simium	Malaria, simian (3C)
Plasmodium schwetzi	Malaria, simian (3C)
Pneumocystis carinii	*Pneumocystis* infection (5)
Sarcocystis hominis (bovihominis)	Sarcocystosis (U)
Sarcocystis suihominis	Sarcocystosis (U)
Toxoplasma gondii	Toxoplasmosis (3C)
Trypanosoma brucei	
var. *gambiense*	Trypanosomiasis, African (3B)
var. *rhodesiense*	Trypanosomiasis, African (3B)
Trypanosoma cruzi	Trypanosomiasis, American (3B)

Table 1.1. (*continued*)

Agent	Disease in Humans (Class[a])
Fungi	
Microsporum canis	Ringworm (4)
Trichophyton mentagrophytes	Ringworm (4)
Trichophyton verrucosum	Ringworm (4)
Gram-Negative Bacteria	
Aeromonas hydrophila	Vibriosis (4)
Brucella abortus	Brucellosis (2B)
Brucella canis	Brucellosis (2B)
Brucella melitensis	Brucellosis (2B)
Brucella suis	Brucellosis (2B)
Campylobacter fetus spp. *intestinalis*	*Campylobacter* septicemia (U)
Campylobacter jejuni	*Campylobacter* enteritis (2B)
Escherichia coli	Colibacillosis (4)
Francisella tularensis	Tularemia (3A)
Pasteurella haemolytica	Pasteurellosis (5)
Pasteurella multocida	Pasteurellosis (5)
Pasteurella pneumotropica	Pasteurellosis (5)
Pasteurella ureae	Pasteurellosis (5)
Pseudomonas mallei	Glanders (U)
Rochalimaea henselae	Cat scratch disease (5)
Salmonella arizona	Arizona infection (2B)
Salmonella spp.	Salmonellosis (2B)
Shigella boydii	Shigellosis (2B)
Shigella dysenteriae	Shigellosis (2B)
Shigella flexneri	Shigellosis (2B)
Shigella sonnei	Shigellosis (2B)
Spirillum minus	Rat bite fever (U)
Streptobacillus moniliformis	Rat bite fever (4)
Vibrio alginolyticus	Vibriosis (4)
Vibrio parahaemolyticus	Vibriosis (4)
Vibrio vulnificus	Vibriosis (4)
Yersinia enterocolitica	Yersiniosis (2B)
Yersinia pestis	Plague (1)
Yersinia pseudotuberculosis	Yersiniosis (2B)
Gram-Positive Bacteria and Actinomycetes	
Bacillus anthracis	Anthrax (2A)
Clostridium bifermentans	Clostridial histotoxic infection (U)
Clostridium botulinum	Botulism (2A)
Clostridium fallax	Clostridial histotoxic infection (U)
Clostridium histolyticum	Clostridial histotoxic infection (U)
Clostridium novyi	Clostridial histotoxic infection (U)
Clostridium perfringens	Clostridial food poisoning (4)
	Clostridial histotoxic infection (U)
Clostridium septicum	Clostridial histotoxic infection (U)
Clostridium tetani	Tetanus (2A)
Corynebacterium equi	Corynebacterial infection (U)
Corynebacterium pseudotuberculosis	Corynebacterial infection (U)
Corynebacterium pyogenes	Corynebacterial infection (U)
Corynebacterium ulcerans	Corynebacterial infection (U)
Dermatophilus congolensis	Dermatophilosis (U)

Table 1.1. (*continued*)

Agent	Disease in Humans (Class[a])
Gram-Positive Bacteria and Actinomycetes	
Erysipelothrix rhusiopathiae	Erysipeloid (U)
Listeria monocytogenes	Listeriosis (4)
Mycobacterium africanum	Tuberculosis (2B)
Mycobacterium avium	Tuberculosis (2B)
Mycobacterium bovis	Tuberculosis (2B)
Mycobacterium leprae	Leprosy (2B)
Mycobacterium tuberculosis	Tuberculosis (2B)
Staphylococcus aureus	Staphylococcosis (4)
	Staphylococcal food poisoning (4)
Streptococcus spp.	Streptococcosis (U)
Spirochaetes	
Borrelia burgdorferi	Lyme disease (3B)
Borrelia spp.	Endemic relapsing fever (3B)
Leptospira interrogans	Leptospirosis (2B)
Rickettsiales	
Chlamydia psittaci	Psittacosis (2A)
Coxiella burnetii	Q fever (3B)
Rickettsia akari	Rickettsialpox (U)
Rickettsia australis	Queensland tick typhus (3B)
Rickettsia conori	Boutonneuse fever (3B)
Rickettsia rickettsii	Rocky Mountain spotted fever (3B)
Rickettsia siberica	North Asian tick typhus (3B)
Rickettsia tsutsugamushi	Scrub typhus (3A)
Rickettsia typhi	Murine typhus (2B)

DNA Viruses

Bovine papular stomatitis (U)
Contagious ecthyma/Orf (5)
Cowpox/catpox (U)
Herpes viruses B and T   Simian herpes (U)
Monkeypox (U)
Pseudocowpox (U)

RNA Viruses

Arthropodborne (Arboviruses)
  Group A
    Eastern equine encephalomyelitis (2A)
    Venezuelan equine encephalitis (3B)
    Western equine encephalomyelitis (2A)
  Group B
    Japanese encephalitis (2A)
    Kyasanur Forest disease (3B)
    Louping ill (3B)
    Murray Valley encephalitis (2A)
    Omsk hemorrhagic fever (3B)
    Russian spring-summer encephalitis (3B)
    St. Louis encephalitis (2A)
    Wesselsbron (U)
    West Nile (3B)
    Yellow fever (1)

Table 1.1. (*continued*)

Agent	Disease in Humans (Class[a])
RNA Viruses	
Bunyamwera group (3B)	
Bwamba group (3B)	
California group (2A)	
Colorado tick fever (3B)	
Guama group (U)	
Nairobi sheep disease (3B)	
Rift Valley fever (3B)	
Simbu group (3B)	
Ebola disease (2A)	
Encephalomyocarditis (U)	
Hemorrhagic fevers	
Argentine (Junin virus) (3A)	
Bolivian (Machupo virus) (3A)	
Korean (Hantaan virus) (3A)	
Infectious hepatitis A (2A)	
Influenza (1A)	
Lassa fever (2A)	
Lymphocytic choriomeningitis (4)	
Marburg disease (2A)	
Newcastle disease (U)	
Rabies (2A)	
Reovirus (4)	
Vesicular stomatitis (3C)	

[a]Class of reportable disease. See Disease Reporting in Chapter 2 for explanation.
[b]U = unclassified.

Summary

1. Vertebrate animals (including people) are the reservoirs of zoonotic infections and the agents are transmitted directly or indirectly between them.

2. Individual identification of the agents of the zoonoses began after the invention of the microscope, starting with the larger parasites in the 1700s. Microscopic examination of the unstained agents remained virtually the only means of characterizing them until the introduction of cultural techniques and staining with aniline dyes in the latter half of the 1800s.

3. Except for a few diseases such as rabies, characterization of the host relationships of the zoonoses, particularly the modes of transmission, awaited the 20th century. This is true for all vectorborne zoonoses because it was not until the 1890s that this mode of spread was first recognized.

4. Some diseases caused by infection with zoonotic agents have been recognized clinically since early history whereas others are only now being recognized for the first time. In some instances, it is evident that the clinical

syndrome and associated agent are truly newly emerging entities. For most, however, recognition has evolved over the past century as a result of careful clinico-epidemiologic observations and innovative applications of diagnostic laboratory techniques.

5. Except for vaccination against smallpox, there were few tools to protect people and their livestock from specific diseases until the past century. Cooking meat (or not eating it), boiling milk, and avoiding exposure by quarantining immigrant people and their cattle were nonspecific protective measures used by some early societies. With recognition of the agents has come an ever-growing search for drugs to cure the diseases they cause and for vaccines to prevent them.

6. Since its introduction in the 1920s, commercial milk pasteurization has become the most effective tool in preventing brucellosis and tuberculosis (*M. bovis*) in people. Seaports where programs have been implemented to control rats and the oriental rat fleas they harbor have remained free of urban plague epidemics. Since programs to eliminate the *Aedes aegypti* mosquito have been undertaken in seaports and other susceptible areas, there have been no outbreaks of urban yellow fever. With the introduction of DDT and other chemical insecticides in the 1940s came the first highly effective means of halting outbreaks of vectorborne disease. Beginning in the 1950s, programs to immunize dogs have been effective in eliminating canine rabies.

References

1. Acha, P. N., and B. Szyfres: *Zoonoses and Communicable Diseases Common to Man and Animals,* 2nd ed. Sci. Publ. No. 503. Washington, D.C., Pan American Health Organization, 1987.
2. Ainsworth, G. C.: *Introduction to the History of Medical and Veterinary Mycology.* Cambridge, Cambridge University Press, 1986.
3. Anon.: *Zoonosis Updates from the Journal of the American Veterinary Medical Association.* Schaumburg, IL, American Veterinary Medical Association, 1990.
4. Baer, G. M.: *The Natural History of Rabies,* 2nd ed. Boca Raton, FL, CRC Press, 1991.
5. Beaver, P. C., and R. C. Jung: *Animal Agents and Vectors of Human Disease,* 5th ed. Philadelphia, Lea & Febiger, 1985.
6. Belding, D. L.: *Basic Clinical Parasitology.* New York, Appleton-Century-Crofts, 1958.
7. Bogue, D. J.: *The Population of the United States: Historical Trends and Future Projections.* New York, Free Press, 1985.
8. Cohen, S., and K. S. Warren: *Immunology of Parasitic Infections,* 2nd ed. Boston, Blackwell Scientific, 1982.
9. Collard, P.: *The Development of Microbiology.* Cambridge, Cambridge University Press, 1976.

10. Dalldorf, G., and G. M. Sickles: An unidentified, filtrable agent isolated from the feces of children with paralysis. *Science*, 108:61-62, 1948.
11. Fenner, F., and A. Gibbs: *Portraits of Viruses, A History of Virology*. Basel, S. Karger, 1988.
12. Fenner, F., D. A. Henderson, I. Arita, et al.: *Smallpox and its Eradication*, History of International Public Health, No. 6. Geneva, World Health Organization, 1988.
13. Gould, S. E.: *Trichinosis in Man and Animals*. Springfield, IL, Charles C. Thomas, 1970.
14. Hall, M. C.: *A comparative study of methods of examining feces for evidences of parasitism*, Bureau of Animal Industry Bulletin 135. Washington, D.C.: U.S. Department of Agriculture, 1911.
15. Harden, V. A.: *Rocky Mountain Spotted Fever, History of a Twentieth-Century Disease*. Baltimore, Johns Hopkins University Press, 1990.
16. Hubbert, W. T., W. F. McCulloch, and P. R. Schnurrenberger: *Diseases Transmitted from Animals to Man*, 6th ed. Springfield, IL, Charles C. Thomas, 1975.
17. Karabatsos, N.: *International Catalogue of Arboviruses*, 3rd ed. San Antonio, TX, American Society of Tropical Medicine and Hygiene, 1985.
18. Lancaster, H. O.: *Expectations of Life: A Study in the Demography, Statistics, and History of World Mortality*. New York, Springer-Verlag, 1990.
19. Lechevalier, H. A., and M. Solotorovsky: *Three Centuries of Microbiology*. New York, McGraw-Hill, 1965.
20. Lederberg, J., R. E. Shope, and S. C. Oaks, Jr.: *Emerging Infections: Microbial Threats to Health in the United States*. Washington, D.C., National Academy Press, 1992.
21. Lowry, J. H.: *World Population and Food Supply*, 2nd ed. London, Edward Arnold, 1976.
22. McKeown, T.: *The Modern Rise of Population*. New York, Academic Press, 1976.
23. Myers, J. A., and J. H. Steele: *Bovine Tuberculosis Control in Man and Animals*. St. Louis, Warren H. Green, 1969.
24. Pollitzer, R.: *Plague*, WHO Monogr. Ser. No. 22. Geneva, World Health Organization, 1954.
25. Pyle, N. J.: Use of ferrets in laboratory work and research investigations. *Am J Publ Hlth*, 30:787-796, 1940.
26. Regnery, R. L., J. G. Olson, B. A. Perkins, et al.: Serological response to *Rochalimaea henselae* antigen in suspected cat scratch disease. *Lancet*, 339 (8807):1443-1445, 1992.
27. Riemann, H., and F. L. Bryan: *Food-Borne Infections and Intoxications*, 2nd ed. New York, Academic Press, 1979.
28. Schwabe, C. W.: *Veterinary Medicine and Human Health*, 3rd ed. Baltimore, Williams & Wilkins, 1984.
29. Scott, H. H.: *A History of Tropical Medicine*, Vols. I and II. Baltimore, Williams & Wilkins, 1939.
30. Soulsby, E. J. L.: *Helminths, Arthropods and Protozoa of Domesticated Animals*, 7th ed. Philadelphia, Lea & Febiger, 1982.
31. Steele, J. H.: *Handbook Series in Zoonoses*. Sect. A: Bacterial, Rickettsial, and

Mycotic Diseases, Vols. I and II. Boca Raton, FL, CRC Press, 1979 and 1980.

32. Steele, J. H.: *Handbook Series in Zoonoses*. Sect. B: Viral Zoonoses, Vols. I and II. Boca Raton, FL, 1981.

33. Steele, J. H.: *Handbook Series in Zoonoses*. Sect. C: Parasitic Zoonoses, Vols. I, II, and III. Boca Raton, FL, 1982.

34. Vestey, J. P., D. L. Yirrell, and R. D. Aldridge: Cowpox/catpox infection. *Brit J Dermatol*, 124:74-78, 1991.

35. Wagner, J. E., and P. J. Manning: *The biology of the guinea pig*. New York, Academic Press, 1976.

36. Warren, K. S.: *Schistosomiasis, The Evolution of a Medical Literature*. Cambridge, MIT Press, 1973.

37. Waterson, A. P., and L. Wilkinson: *An introduction to the history of virology*. Cambridge, Cambridge University Press, 1978.

SECTION II

Principles

2

PRINCIPLES OF ZOONOSES RECOGNITION

Index Case

Zoonoses can create a headache for the diagnostician as well as the human patient. These headaches are **symptoms** of disease, or subjective evidence of illness that the person affected can perceive and describe to others. Affected animals have **signs** of illness, but they do not have symptoms because they cannot tell us where it hurts. Signs are that which we can some way observe in an affected person or animal. When we appropriately group these signs and symptoms, we have a **syndrome** such as Guillain-Barre syndrome or acute febrile polyneuritis associated with many infections. The first individual we recognize in a herd, household, or community who is affected with this syndrome is referred to as the **index case.**[43] This is not necessarily the same as the **proband (propositus)** or **first (primary) case** in the population. It may not even be the second or third actual case. It is simply the first case recognized. After further investigation, it may be possible to determine who (or which animal) was the first case. Serendipity has often been a critical tool in recognizing index cases of infectious disease, particularly zoonoses. An objective of efficient disease control is to increase the frequency of the index case and the first (primary) case being the same. In any event, it is important to recognize that index cases exist and that earlier, undetected, cases may have occurred. The index case often may be the "tip of the iceberg." There may be other cases clinicians have seen and treated symptomatically, and still more that were not observed by a health professional.

For any infectious disease, there is an interval of time, known as the **incubation period.**[23] It begins when the host contacts the agent and ends with onset of signs and/or symptoms of disease. This interval may be brief, as with

23

most foodborne bacterial infections for which the incubation period is less than 24 hours. In this case, it is relatively easy to relate the illness to some source of exposure. As the incubation period lengthens, more life activities occur in the interim, thereby increasing the number of events to be sorted out in relation to possible exposure. Also, memories become more hazy. The incubation period (in relation to a known or suspected time of exposure) and the syndrome presented are two elements, along with actual risk of exposure, usually found in the **definition of a case** to be counted in an outbreak.[28,66]

At the beginning of the incubation period, the susceptible host (animal or person later called a case) came in contact with a **source of infection**, and the agent was transmitted from this source. The source of infection to which the host was exposed could have been an **animal** (including a person), **arthropod vector**, or **inanimate vehicle** (e.g., milk or other food, water). For example, a person with onset of leptospiral aseptic meningitis possibly came in contact 10-12 days earlier with water contaminated by an infected animal. In this instance, the source of infection is not the **reservoir of infection**.[54] Animals (including people) are the reservoirs of zoonotic agents, i.e., animals and people are the essential elements where zoonotic agents survive and multiply in nature. Here, water was the source of infection, whereas an infected animal shedding leptospires in the urine was the reservoir that contaminated the water. The source of human exposure to rabies virus may have been the bite of an infected domestic cat, but the reservoir was most likely a bat or other infected wild mammal that earlier bit the cat. Whereas domestic dogs were a major reservoir before rabies vaccination and other control measures were introduced, domestic cats have not been a reservoir of rabies virus because cats do not maintain the virus within their own population. Cat-to-cat transmission is the exception.

The **mode of transmission** of the agent from the reservoir to the susceptible host may be **direct** or **indirect**. **Direct transmission** involves spread by intimate contact with an infected animal by such means as a bite or scratch, spray by infectious urine, inhalation of discharged respiratory droplets (from coughing or sneezing), or contact with infectious reproductive discharges. The agent may be **transmitted indirectly** by an arthropod vector (e.g., flea, mite, mosquito, sand fly, or tick), by contact with an inanimate vehicle (anything that would have been exposed to the agent and would permit survival on it or in it long enough to reach a susceptible host), or by airborne spread (droplet nuclei, dust). Foods of animal origin are the most common vehicles of zoonotic agents.[3,61] Airborne spread in which the agent may be able to survive outside the host for periods long enough to travel some distance (indoors or outdoors) is particularly important for spread of agents such as *Brucella* sp. and *Coxiella burnetii*. (See Chapter 3 for laboratory-acquired infections by airborne spread.)

Transmission of infectious agents either directly or indirectly from an infected individual to another (susceptible) individual of the same generation or earlier is referred to as **horizontal transmission**. Horizontal transmission includes the various modes of interspecies spread involved in zoonoses. When transmission occurs from one generation to the **next generation**, it is referred to as **vertical transmission**. Vertical transmission from the dam to offspring, either prenatal in utero or neonatal via colostrum, is also important in many zoonoses. Many of the zoonoses may be causes of embryonic death or abortion in livestock. Prenatal toxoplasmosis is widely recognized as a serious disease of human infants. ("**Congenital**" refers specifically to present at birth and does not indicate a mode of transmission.) Recently, the public has become aware of eggborne *Salmonella* in chickens. When the next generation of chickens is affected through the egg, it is the result of vertical transmission. Vertical transmission among arthropod vectors can occur and will be mentioned later.

Whenever a case of infectious disease occurs, clinicians have questions concerning the **probable clinical outcome (prognosis).** In addition, epidemiologists wonder who else may be affected, and where and when new cases will occur. Describing cases in relation to the **host (person or animal) affected**, the **place of occurrence**, and **time of occurrence** has long been done to provide valuable evidence for use in predicting the risk of future occurrences. **Risk factors** refer to those agent, host, and environmental characteristics that may affect (increase or decrease) the likelihood of exposure to an agent, becoming infected as a consequence, and what severity of disease (if any) may ensue.[51] Factors influencing exposure, infection, and disease are distinguishable. Typical **host characteristics** noted are age, sex, breed or race, and physiologic state (e.g., immunodeficiency).[20,59,72,75,76] **Place (spatial) factors** recorded are any associated geographic attributes, including altitude, latitude, and residence (nest).[7,8] **Time (temporal) factors** can be described in relation to any measurable period, such as day or night, summer or winter, and work or holiday.[34] Host, place, and time factors may play an important role in the risk of contracting zoonotic infections, as well as influencing the severity of disease. Characteristics such as occupation and recreation influence many zoonoses and may also be affected by host, place, and time. Time and place combined are referred to as **environment**. It is the classic interaction of host, agent, and environment that determines the outcome of exposure to an infectious agent inasmuch as the environment affects the well-being of both host and agent. Sunlight, temperature, moisture, and pH are examples of **environmental factors** that vary in regard to place and time and affect survival of infectious agents outside the host.

Various schemes have been devised to classify how people may be exposed to zoonotic agents. For example, persons at risk have been classified using the following seven professional and social groups:[2]

Group I (Agriculture): Farmers or other people in close contact with livestock and their products.

Group II (Animal-product processing and manufacture): All personnel of abattoirs and of plants processing animal products or by-products.

Group III (Forestry, outdoors): Persons frequenting wild habitats for professional or recreational reasons.

Group IV (Recreation): Persons in contact with pets or wild animals in the urban environment.

Group V (Clinics, laboratories): Health care personnel who attend patients, and health workers (including laboratory personnel) who handle specimens, corpses, or organs.

Group VI (Epidemiology): Public health professionals who do field research.

Group VII (Emergency): People affected by catastrophes, refugees, or people temporarily living in crowded or highly stressful situations.

An earlier system was based on the maintenance cycle of the zoonosis in nature, as follows:[70] (1) a **direct zoonosis** (e.g., rabies or brucellosis) that may be perpetuated in nature by a single vertebrate species; (2) a **cyclozoonosis** (e.g., taeniasis and hydatid disease) whose maintenance cycles require more than one vertebrate species; (3) a **metazoonosis** (e.g., arboviral infections and trypanosomiasis) whose cycles require both vertebrates and invertebrates; or (4) a **saprozoonosis** (e.g., visceral larva migrans) whose agent depends upon inanimate development sites as well as upon vertebrate hosts.

Risk, or probability, of exposure to zoonotic agents, and ultimately infection and disease, is not constant throughout the life cycle of the host. The basic life cycles are quite similar for most vertebrate hosts. The following life cycle will be used to illustrate the changing patterns of human risk of exposure to zoonotic agents:[46] neonate (0-28 days); infant (1-15 months); toddler (16-36 months); preschool child (3-5 years); juvenile (6-11 years); adolescent (12-17 years); young adult (18-39 years); middle years (40-59 years); old age (60+ years).

It is evident that, after the toddler period, the onset and termination of a given period in the life cycle will vary somewhat between sexes and among individuals, as well as between social groups. Therefore, the ranges depicted are arbitrary averages.

Illness observed in the **neonate** may be the result of vertical or horizontal transmission. The agent may have infected the prenatal infant by transplacental spread from the mother or by via the mother's milk.[50,84] Both are examples of vertical transmission, which is common for zoonotic agents among animal reservoirs. Therefore, risk of prenatal or neonatal infection is primarily a factor of risk of maternal infection and secondarily risk of exposure in the postnatal environment.[9] Once the **infant** begins to crawl around the house, exposure to agents associated with household pets increases. Older infants and **toddlers** are the primary age groups infected with the dog tapeworm as a result of ingesting dog or cat fleas found on the floor that are infected with *Dipylidium caninum* cysticercoids. As the toddler and **preschool child** become more active, bites and scratches from interactions with household pets become a common occurrence. Sometimes these lesions are infected with *Pasteurella multocida* or other normal oral flora of the pet.

Juveniles begin exploring the neighboring environment, particularly during the warm summer months when school is not in session. Where wooded areas are available, the explorers are likely to be at greater risk of exposure to endemic tickborne agents. Juveniles and **adolescents,** particularly in suburban and rural areas, also swim during the warm months in nearby ponds and streams that may be contaminated with leptospires and other waterborne agents from adjacent infected livestock or wildlife. These are examples of age-related recreational activities that offer increased risk of exposure to zoonotic agents.

Outdoor recreation can be a reason for increased risk of exposure to zoonotic agents among all age groups. A family event, such as a picnic, may expose everyone from infants to the elderly to an environment of increased risk. Whenever the recreation involves travel beyond the local area, the place visited and season of the year become factors in assessing risk. Camping in a park in the western United States can be of significant risk in relation to bubonic plague, whereas tularemia may be a greater risk in other regions where plague is not endemic. Hunting is a widely practiced recreation that involves exposure to wildlife and their environment, and poses potential risk of foodborne exposure. There may be contact with the animal's ectoparasites, as well as infected tissues when dressing the carcass. Exposure may be seasonal, depending on legal restrictions on hunting. International travel, whether for business and/or recreation, introduces additional geographically related risk factors, particularly exposure to arboviruses with restricted regional distribution. Foods of animal origin are the most important single factor in risk of exposure to zoonoses worldwide. Their source, handling, storage, and preparation all affect safety.[13] This source of exposure is important whether we travel or eat at home. Travel may introduce risk of exposure to exotic foodborne agents as well as exotic foods.

Occupation-related activities associated with zoonoses begin to increase significantly during the juvenile years and continue through most of the **adult years.** Children not only help in "doing the chores" on the farm, but also help in nonagricultural employment such as in pet stores, dog kennels, and veterinary hospitals. Adolescents often seek part-time jobs in all these facilities. Adults seek such careers as livestock or poultry producer, abattoir worker, fish handler, zoo employee, wildlife biologist, veterinarian, and biomedical researcher, all of which present increased occupational risk of exposure to zoonotic agents.[24,42,48] The zoonoses of concern will depend on the animal species associated with their employment.

The very young and very old are recognized to be at greater risk of severe disease (including zoonoses) because of reduced immunocompetency, but these two groups may be at reduced risk of exposure to environmental hazards such as arthropodborne agents because they spend less time outdoors. With the advent of the acquired immunodeficiency syndrome (AIDS), and use of immunosuppressive drugs, immunodeficiency has become a major predisposing factor in the occurrence of zoonoses. For example, *Pneumocystis carinii* pneumonia is a major problem among AIDS-infected individuals. It is these characteristics we look for in the history of each case (patient) to alert us to a pattern of factors associated with zoonotic disease.

The risk of exposure, infection, or disease in relation to various risk factors can be expressed quantitatively as **risk rates** such as **relative risk** or **attributable risk**.[21,32,40,49,60,65,73,80] (See Table 2-1.) **Relative risk** compares the rate of occurrence among those with (exposed to) the factor to the rate among those without (not exposed to) the factor.[19,81] (**Odds ratio** provides information similar to relative risk except the former is calculated using data obtained from a sample of a larger population rather than from a complete enumeration of a herd or neighborhood.) **Attributable risk** is a measure of the benefit that will be derived from removing a known risk or the excess occurrence attributable to its presence.

In this era of public concern regarding risk of disease associated with exposure to infectious and noninfectious agents, the terminology used in communicating risk among scientists, and between scientists and the public, becomes increasingly important. The following set of terms has been devised by the National Research Council to aid in making key distinctions:[56]

Table 2-1. Risk relative to exposure

	Occurred	Did Not Occur	
Exposed to Factor (EF)	A	B	A + B
Not Exposed to Factor	C	D	C + D
	A + C	B + D	N = A + B + C + D

A/A+B = rate of occurrence among those with the factor.
C/C+D = rate of occurrence among those without the factor.
Relative Risk (RR) = (A/A+B) / (C/C+D).
Attributable Risk (AR) = (A/A+B) − (C/C+D).

Hazard: An act or phenomenon posing potential harm to some person(s) or animal(s). The magnitude of the hazard is the amount of harm that might result, including the seriousness and the number of people (and/or animals) exposed.

Risk: Adds to the hazard and its magnitude the probability that the potential harm or undesirable consequence will be realized.

Risk assessment: The characterization of potential adverse effects of exposures to hazards; includes estimates of risk and of uncertainties in measurements, analytical techniques, and interpretive models. Quantitative risk assessment characterizes the risk in numerical representations.

Risk control assessment: Characterization of alternative interventions to reduce or eliminate the hazard and/or unwanted consequences; considers technological feasibility, costs and benefits, and legal requirements or restrictions.

Risk management: The evaluation of alternative risk control actions, selection among them (including doing nothing), and their implementation. The responsible individual or office (risk manager) sometimes oversees preparation of risk assessments, risk control assessments, and risk messages. Risk management may or may not be open to outside individuals or organizations.

Risk communication: An interactive process of exchange of information and opinion among individuals, groups, and institutions; often involves multiple messages about the nature of risk or expressing concerns, opinions, or reactions to risk messages or to legal and institutional arrangements for risk management.

Risk message: A written, verbal, or visual statement containing information about risk; may or may not include advice about risk reduction behavior. A formal risk message is a structured written, audio, or visual package developed with the express purpose of presenting information about risk.

In the next section, **Surveillance,** data needed for risk assessment will be described. Hazard characteristics such as attack rate and case fatality rate are described later in the chapter, under **Epidemic/Outbreak.** Risk varies depending upon such factors as potential for exposure to the agent, whether the disease is endemic or exotic, and the factors involved in initiation of an epidemic. Risk control assessment, risk management, and risk communication are tools used in disease control and prevention, the principles of which will be presented in Chapter 4.

Surveillance

Effective programs of infectious disease control and prevention need information that is accurate and timely about the presence and extent of the disease and about changes that may be occurring as a result of natural factors or planned interventions. This need is particularly true for zoonoses inasmuch as the information is usually required in relation to both animal and human populations involved. **Disease surveillance** is the overall activity specifically planned to detect disease in populations, measure its extent, identify needed interventions, and evaluate the impact of any intervention.[1,30,37,77,78] The design of the surveillance will depend on the diseases of concern and the population at risk.[17,52,62,74,79] It can be as limited in scope as that involved in a disease control program for a cattle feedlot. (If the activity is limited to disease detection and does not include measurement of the success of the control program, it is referred to as **disease monitoring.**) Surveillance can be as complex as the international surveillance for a disease such as Venezuelan equine encephalomyelitis affecting both horses and humans. Organized surveillance is always active, such as the periodic collection of blood from a sample of the cattle population to test for serologic evidence of brucellosis, or the pre-scheduled review of human tetanus case statistics as an indicator of the status of immunization in the population.

The reservoir hosts of zoonoses have already been defined as "where the agent persists in nature." The design of surveillance to detect infection in potential host populations will depend on the life cycle of the agent. For parasites with a multi-host life cycle, reservoirs are generally **primary,** or **definitive hosts,** in which the parasite attains maturity or passes its sexual stage. The parasite is in a larval, or asexual, state in **secondary,** or **intermediate hosts**. For example, people are the definitive host and cattle are the intermediate host for the beef tapeworm, *Taenia saginata*. People and cattle both are essential to persistence of this parasite (both are reservoirs), but examination of beef muscle at slaughter is the usual (easier) way in which we look for evidence of its presence in a reservoir population.

In the life cycle of an infectious agent, it is passage of infection from the infected host to the susceptible host that is critical to its persistence. Therefore, the **carrier of infection** is critical to maintenance of the agent. The carrier may be a **healthy** or **asymptomatic (subclinical) carrier** for whom no clinical signs are evident throughout the course of infection. On the other hand, the carrier may be an **incubationary** or **convalescent carrier** who harbors the agent for a period before or after clinical illness. The carrier state may be temporary or chronic in duration. Although a carrier harbors the agent, the role of the carrier in the spread of the agent depends on the mode of transmission involved. First, the agent must be in an infective state if the carrier is to be a source of infection. This is particularly important for parasites that undergo changes within the host, maturing from a noninfective stage to an infective stage. For arthropodborne infections, this introduces the **period of infectivity,** when the vector can become infected from feeding on blood or other fluids/tissues. For diseases such as beef tapeworm, people must eat the bovine host. When the agent is spread by direct transmission, the carrier must be in a **shedder state** so that the agent is actually being excreted in a body fluid such as saliva, genital secretions, milk, nasal secretions, feces, or urine. If shedding by carriers is a major factor in the spread of an agent of concern, surveillance to determine risk of exposure to the agent in the population must involve some means of estimating the shedder rate.

Contact between domestic animals and people, whether occupational or in the home, is relatively easy to anticipate. The **home range** of domestic animals, i.e., the area traversed routinely in their daily activities, is well defined when under human constraint.[10] Some domestic animals, such as dogs and cats, are **free-ranging** at least part of the day, i.e., without immediate human supervision on public property or on private property with immediate unrestrained access to public property. The distance they stray within their home range is related principally to their food sources. These animals may be owned, or at least harbored and fed, by people. They also may be **feral**, living entirely outside of human harborage and not depending directly on people for food.

For many zoonoses, however, free-living vertebrate species are involved. The habitat where they live may be urban or rural (**sylvatic** refers to woods and pastures). Some of these species, such as roof rats (*Rattus rattus*) are **domiciliated**, living in and being dependent on human habitats. When these species are maintenance hosts for zoonotic agents, their habitat becomes the location in which the agents are found. This area can be quite small. For example, the home range of some sylvatic rodents that are maintenance hosts for plague is less than 100 m. One entire area where infected rodents are found may be no larger than 10 times the home range of one rodent, i.e., a few hundred square meters. This area of infected maintenance hosts is referred to as a **natural focus, nidus, or niche of infection**.[7,45] Infection may persist for many years in such natural foci without overt evidence of disease. Typically, these maintenance hosts are resistant to disease with these agents and, therefore, no signs of death or illness are observed to be associated with them. It is when species that are susceptible to these diseases intrude upon this niche that outbreaks of disease ensue. When domestic rats **commingle** with plague-infected field mice, die-offs in the rats occur that may spread to produce an outbreak of urban plague. Intrusions by people into the rain forest niche of "jungle" yellow fever have been the beginnings of outbreaks of "urban" yellow fever.

Surveillance methods for vectors of arthropodborne agents depend greatly on the vectors involved (fleas, mites, ticks, conenose bugs, mosquitoes, gnats, flies, sandflies).[31] Certain principles apply to all, however, in considering the vector potential of the arthropod. For example, some arthropods such as fleas are **nest-dwelling (commensal)** and active throughout the year, whereas others such as mosquitoes and ticks are **field-dwelling (campestrine)** and are active only during the warmer months. The arthropod may be involved simply in the mechanical carriage of the agent from infected host to susceptible host (**mechanical vector**). With the possible exception of tabanids, mechanical vectors play a secondary role in the spread of infectious agents. On the other hand, the agent may multiply in the vector and/or undergo some developmental change (**biological vector**).

If the agent must undergo a change from a noninfective to an infective state in the vector, the time required to reach the infective state is referred to as the **extrinsic incubation period**. In some vectors, the agent is passed to the next generation via the egg (**transovarial** or vertical **transmission**), whereas in other arthropods it may only be passed from one stage to another of the same generation in its life cycle (**transstadial transmission**). These differences are significant in relation to the role of the arthropod in maintaining the agent outside the vertebrate host, as well as anticipating when and where it may contact susceptible hosts. Although the arthropod may play an essential role as a vector in maintaining infection, and vertical transmission may occur, the vertebrate host is still the ultimate reservoir without which infection will not persist indefinitely.

Susceptible animal hosts are sometimes used as **sentinels** to detect the presence of infections (infectious agents) when other means are less sensitive or more costly.[55] For example, they may be placed in contact with suspected carrier animals to detect shedding of the agent when the most sensitive laboratory methods may require analysis of tissues difficult to collect from the living animal. This method has been used to detect foot-and-mouth disease (FMD) virus in animals to be imported from FMD-endemic countries. Sentinel animals have been used extensively to detect arbovirus activity by confining animals susceptible to infection (e.g., chickens or hamsters) in areas where viruses are suspected to be circulating among mosquito vectors and wild bird reservoirs. Specimens are collected periodically from the sentinels and tested for presence of virus or serum antibodies. In the past, horses were considered sentinels for such viruses as eastern equine encephalomyelitis (EEE). Although unvaccinated horses are quite sensitive to infection with EEE, they are not a sensitive indicator of EEE activity within the reservoir because, first of all, the mosquitoes primarily involved in infecting wild birds do not feed on horses. Secondly, the wild birds involved are migratory and, for horses and humans to be exposed, birds with virus and mosquito species that feed on both birds and mammals need to be active in the area at the same time. Because these events do not happen with precise regularity, surveillance with sentinel animals has been used to determine when control of mosquito vectors that infect humans (and horses) is indicated.

Although horses are affected clinically by EEE, they are a **dead-end host** in regard to virus transmission inasmuch as the viremia produced by EEE in horses is not sufficient to infect additional mosquitoes. Whenever situations arise in which the virus is transmitted to vertebrate hosts other than the reservoir (wild birds for EEE), and the virus multiplies sufficiently to infect other mosquitoes (vectors), these animals (or humans) are referred to as **amplifying hosts** (domestic pheasants for EEE) because they may participate in increasing spread of the agent. Amplifying hosts are usually only of importance during epidemic situations. Surveillance for zoonotic agents among wildlife reservoirs may be further complicated by seasonal reproductive patterns among these hosts. This results in a seasonal increase in the number of susceptible animals (immature individuals not yet exposed). New technology is rapidly improving the precision and timeliness of surveillance data gathering. For example, since **remote sensing** by satellite images became available in the 1970s, studies of mosquito habitat have allowed accurate predictions of mosquito vector populations in relation to occurrence of outbreaks of arbovirus infection.[47]

Epidemic/Outbreak

Whenever the number of cases of illness, or frequency of infection, in a locality exceeds the **expected (endemic) number,** we have an **epidemic.** An **outbreak** is a group or cluster of cases that may or may not exceed the expected number. If one case of canine rabies occurs in Australia or Hawaii, locally it would be considered an epidemic because the expected number is zero inasmuch as these areas are rabies-free. Actually, the first case may have been imported and therefore a second, **local** case resulting from **local** transmission would be needed to have an epidemic. In contrast to endemic areas where rabies occurs regularly, i.e. is maintained continuously in the local population, rabies is an **exotic or foreign disease** in Australia and Hawaii. Outbreaks of some diseases occur **sporadically,** such as vesicular stomatitis (VS) in the United States. The occurrence of such diseases, although expected, cannot be predicted. One or more years may pass between **sporadic outbreaks** of VS, whereas in endemic areas of Central America they are an annual event. The widespread, international occurrence of epidemic disease is referred to as a **pandemic.** Urban plague and yellow fever are two zoonoses well known for their historic pandemics, spreading from seaport to seaport.

Historically, vital statistics, such as death records, have been useful in retrospective studies of epidemic disease. More recently, they have been applied to quantify the current status. For example, **excess pneumonia mortality** has been used in predicting the occurrence of influenza epidemics and measuring their severity.[71] Calculations involve (a) determination of a secular trend and its extrapolation, (b) estimation of seasonal variation, and (c) distinction between epidemiologically significant departures from expected weekly mortality and random variation from endemic levels. In Figure 2-1, illustrating U.S. influenza epidemics during 1957-1960, the **epidemic threshold** line was placed at a distance of 1.64 standard deviations above the normal incidence trend line. Experience had shown this distance to be useful for distinguishing epidemic increase from random variation.

If more than one case of a zoonosis is to occur, an important risk factor is the **communicable period** of the initial infected host (which may be the primary case or carrier). This is the interval during which the agent may be transferred directly or indirectly from an infected host to a susceptible host. For example, the observation period established for biting animals suspected of being infected with rabies virus is based on our knowledge of how long virus is shed during the **prodromal** (early onset of signs) **period**. This is the critical communicable period in the spread of rabies. For many zoonotic agents, it is the period when they are shed by the carrier host in milk, urine, or other body fluids that is of prime concern. In the case of vectorborne agents, it is the infective period of the arthropod that is the relevant communicable period. A **contact** is an individual who has been in association with an infected individual (direct transmission) or has been in a locale

Fig. 2-1. Weekly pneumonia-influenza deaths in 108 cities of the United States.

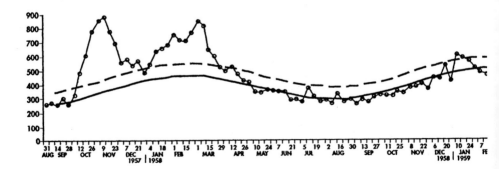

(environment) where exposure to the agent is likely to occur (indirect transmission).

An epidemic may have a **common source**, such as a food contaminated with *Salmonella* sp. If the food was consumed during a single meal, the period of exposure would have been brief, resulting in a **point source** of exposure. On the other hand, direct or indirect exposure to a primary case may result in the **propagation** of secondary cases. **Secondary cases** are those that occur within an accepted incubation period after exposure to a primary case. The **serial interval** is the interval between initiation of new cases.[35] Depending on the maximum period of infectiousness, it can be equal to, shorter than, or longer than the incubation period. The serial interval may be longer when there is convalescent shedding or vectorborne spread. It may be shorter if there is shedding (infectious state) before the onset of signs. An epidemic with this chronologic pattern is referred to as a **propagative epidemic** and may involve a series of cycles. It is not uncommon for agents with fecal-oral spread, such as *Salmonella* sp., to result in combinations of common source and propagative epidemics.

Quantitative expressions, i.e., rates, provide objective means of evaluating the impact of epidemics on populations affected. The **attack rate** is the number of individuals affected among those at risk. Comparing attack rates in relation to various foods eaten is an important tool in the investigation of foodborne outbreaks. In a propagative epidemic, the **secondary**

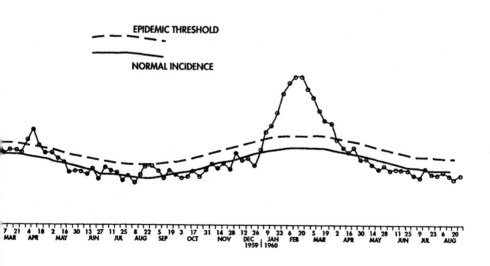

attack rate is the number of individuals affected among those who were in contact with the primary case (or carrier) at a previous time equivalent to the accepted incubation period. The **incidence rate** is the number of new cases occurring during a specified period (often a year) in relation to the number in the population at risk (susceptibles potentially exposed). Changes in incidence rates indicate whether an epidemic is increasing or decreasing in intensity. **Morbidity (illness)** and **mortality (death) rates** are incidence rates reflecting the respective numbers occurring in the total population during the period specified. In contrast, the **prevalence rate** is the number of actual cases (or infected) in relation to the population at risk at a specific time (**point prevalence**) or during a specified time period (**period prevalence**). Serologic surveys for evidence of infection typically provide (point) prevalence data. For chronic diseases such as tuberculosis, it is more difficult to determine the number of new cases, particularly among older populations; therefore, tuberculosis statistics are more likely to be prevalence data. The **case fatality rate** is a particularly important indicator of the severity of an epidemic. It is the number who die among those affected. Dramatic differences in case fatality rate are usually noted between epidemics of bubonic and pneumonic plague as well as between outbreaks of eastern and western equine encephalitis.

Attack Rate = number of individuals affected/population at risk

Secondary Attack Rate = number of individuals affected/number who were in contact with primary case

Incidence Rate = number of new cases during period /population at risk

Morbidity Rate = number becoming ill/total population

Mortality Rate = number dying/total population

Prevalence Rate = number of actual cases/population at risk

Case Fatality Rate = number dying/number diseased (usually associated with a specific outbreak)

Outbreak Investigation

Outbreak investigation involves all those activities needed to identify the immediate source of the agent and its mode of transmission to the susceptibles at risk.[12,36,44,57] This is the information essential for effective control. Outbreak investigation begins with recognition of the possibility that the index case may not be a sporadic singular occurrence. The index case may be one of a group of cases clustered in relation to time and/or space. It is, therefore, important to develop an effective means of facilitating this initial recognition as early as possible. Outbreak investigations are usually **cross-sectional,** or **point-in-time, data-gathering** activities in contrast to disease surveillance, or **longitudinal data gathering**. The **data** gathered in an outbreak investigation are referred to as **retrospective** because the events have already occurred, whereas surveillance data are **prospective** because the study is designed to collect data from now until some time in the future. Use of serum banks for long-term retrospective studies of the occurrence of infection in a population is an exception to surveillance data being prospective.[53] There is also greater urgency associated with an outbreak investigation than with surveillance, e.g., a clinical examination of a febrile patient vs an annual physical examination of a healthy individual.

Most outbreaks of zoonoses in people have an **epidemic curve** consistent with a common source, regardless of mode of transmission, because secondary cases from human-to-human transmission occur infrequently. Foodborne zoonotic pathogens are the major exception. With these, the typical first curve represents a point source (food) and then a smaller more protracted curve of secondary cases resulting from exposure to persons (or food they prepared) infected from the initial source. Therefore, much of the outbreak investigation will involve **case finding** (patients with similar clinical history) and tracing the cases to some common source of infection. How we identify what the patients share in their immediate history, beginning with the index case, affects both case finding and source identification. If the index case is an adult, the likely source might be related to occupation, residence, or recreation. If occupational, co-workers should be affected, but household contacts and neighbors (not related to the workplace) should not. Also, the occupation should have some increased risk of exposure to animals, directly or indirectly, if animals are the source. Details of outbreak investigation will be presented in later chapters.

Disease Reporting

A **system of case reporting** is a critical tool in infectious disease surveillance.[25,26,58] An effective chain of reporting usually begins with the health professional who observes the individual patient and reports this observation to the local health agency. The chain of reporting may continue to the state, national, and international level depending on the disease. For example, plague and yellow fever are two zoonoses for which reporting of human cases by national public health authorities to the World Health Organization is required. The national animal health agency of contracting countries also may be required to report to the Office International des Epizooties the occurrence in animals of certain zoonoses such as anthrax and rabies.

A disease is referred to as **reportable (notifiable)** when there is a legal requirement that the attending health professional, diagnostic laboratory, hospital administrator, or other entity report any observations to the appropriate health agency.[14,16,22,29,38,63,69,82,85] For a zoonosis such as brucellosis, this usually means that veterinarians are required to report observed animals to the local (or state) animal health agency and physicians are required to report observed human patients to the public health agency. Every state in the United States requires reporting of one or more zoonoses in animals or humans to the appropriate health agency.[68] Interestingly, no zoonosis, including such diseases of concern as brucellosis and rabies, is required to be reported by all states for either animals or humans.

The only valid reason for requiring diseases to be reported is that some action may be needed based on the information obtained.[18,27] Therefore, reporting is not required for all diseases. For the notifiable diseases, how they are to be reported depends on the urgency of the action. In some instances, reporting may be required if infection or disease is suspected, whereas for others it is only needed if laboratory confirmation has been received. Also, the timeliness of reporting required may differ from immediately via telephone or fax to weekly (or less often) by mail. The American Public Health Association (APHA)[11] has published the following system of classifying human diseases (derived from the World Health Organization classification scheme) according to the benefit to be derived from reporting:

Class 1: Case Report Universally Required by International Health Regulations (IHR) or as a Disease under Surveillance by WHO.
  1A. Diseases subject to IHR, i.e. the internationally quarantinable diseases—e.g. plague, yellow fever
  1B. Diseases under surveillance by WHO—e.g. louseborne typhus (uncertain role of flying squirrel in maintenance of agent, *Rickettsia prowazekii*)
Class 2: Case Report Regularly Required Whenever the Disease Occurs.
  1A. Two subclasses based on relative urgency for investigation of contacts and source of infection, or for starting control measures.
  2A. Case report to local health authority by telephone, telegraph, or other rapid means. These are forwarded to next superior jurisdiction weekly by mail, except that first recognized case in an area or first case outside the limits of known affected local area is reported by telephone or telegraph—e.g. botulism
  2B. Case report by most practical means; forwarded to next superior jurisdiction as a collective report, weekly by mail—e.g. brucellosis
Class 3: Selectively Reportable in Recognized Endemic Areas. In many states and countries, diseases of this class are not reportable. Reporting may be prescribed in particular regions, states, or countries by reason of undue frequency or severity. Subclasses 3A and 3B are primarily useful

under conditions of established endemicity as a means of leading toward prompt control measures and to judge the effectiveness of control programs. The main purpose of 3C is to stimulate control measures or to acquire essential epidemiologic data.

3A. Case report by telephone, telegraph, or other rapid means in specified areas where the disease ranks in importance with Class 2A; not reportable in many countries—e.g. tularemia and scrub typhus

3B. Case report by most practicable means; forwarded to next superior jurisdiction as a collective report by mail weekly or monthly; not reportable in many countries—e.g. Rocky Mountain spotted fever

3C. Collective report weekly by mail to local health authority; forwarded to next superior jurisdiction by mail weekly, monthly, quarterly, or sometimes annually—e.g. fasciolopsiasis

Class 4: Obligatory Report of Epidemics—No Case Report Required. Prompt report of outbreaks of particular public health importance by telephone, telegraph, or other rapid means; forwarded to next superior jurisdiction by telephone or telegraph. Pertinent data include number of cases, time frame, approximate population involved, and apparent mode of spread—e.g. staphylococcal food poisoning, unidentified syndrome.

Class 5: Official Report Not Ordinarily Justifiable. Diseases of this class are of two general kinds: those typically sporadic and uncommon, often not directly transmissible among vertebrate hosts; or of such epidemiologic nature as to offer no special practical measures for control (common cold).

A list of 166 zoonotic agents (65 parasites, 2 fungi, 57 bacteria and rickettsiae, 41 viruses, and 1 uncertain) is presented in Chapter 1 with the reporting class using the APHA system for human zoonoses indicated for each. Table 2-2 is a summary by agent group and class of reportable disease.

It is evident that, for 48% of the zoonoses, reporting of the disease in humans is not considered justifiable (Class 5) or has not even been classified (U). For another 7%, no case reports are required (Class 4). Therefore, reporting of individual human cases is not required (not considered justifiable) for more than half of the zoonoses. When diseases are infrequent, underreporting occurs.

In Class 4 of the APHA reporting system, an epidemic of an unidentified syndrome is to be reported. There are no guidelines, however, as to the syndromes that should be candidates for reporting. Health professionals clearly prefer an "agent orientation" when preparing lists of reportable diseases rather than listing the predominant signs or syndromes associated with diseases caused by the agents of concern. On the other hand, two of the most remarkable programs of communicable disease eradication depended

Table 2-2. Agent groups and classes of reportable diseases

Agent Group	|	Reportable Disease Class									
	1	1A	2A	2B	3A	3B	3C	4	5	U*	Total
Pentastomids										2	2
Nematodes			1						15	5	21
Trematodes							3		6	6	15
Cestodes						3	2		3	5	13
Protozoa				1		5	3		4	1	14
Fungi								2			2
Bacteria											
Gram-Negative	1			10	1			3	3	5	23
Gram-Positive			3	3				4	2	10	22
Spirochaetes				1		2					3
Rickettsiales			1	1	1	5				1	9
Viruses											
DNA									1	5	6
RNA	1	1	11		3	12	1	2		4	35
Uncertain										1	1
Total	2	1	15	16	6	27	9	11	35	44	166

*U = unclassified.

largely on reports of signs and/or syndromes for evidence of their progress and ultimate success. In the worldwide smallpox eradication program, absence of observable lesions for a defined period was the principal indicator that an area was smallpox-free. During the period 1950-1965, the Peoples' Republic of China eradicated socially transmitted disease (all of the four diseases then recognized and referred to as venereal diseases) from one-fourth of the world's population by strategic use of mass therapy and surveillance for signs associated with these diseases.[33] Both programs emphasized careful observation in the field and prompt reporting.

Although laboratory confirmation often is essential to an etiologic diagnosis, this additional step may be a deterrent to early recognition of potentially serious outbreaks of disease. Attending physicians are often more likely to recognize (and report) a syndrome such as (aseptic) meningitis in a patient than they are to report an etiologic diagnosis requiring prior collection, storage, and shipment of acute and convalescent sera or demonstration of the agent. Similarly, veterinarians are more likely to report occurrences of abortion in cattle than to report an etiologic diagnosis of one of the many diseases (including several zoonoses) that could be the cause. However, both physicians and veterinarians are usually expected to report suspected or confirmed cases of an etiologic diagnosis even though that diagnosis may be far down the list of etiologies they perceive to be considered significant in the initial differential diagnosis. Observations by lay personnel can be a valuable aid in recognizing the presence of disease so that it is brought to the attention of the health professional. For example, there was high diagnostic agreement between feedlot personnel and veterinarians in the recognition of lower (87.6%) and upper (97.7%) respiratory tract disease in cattle.[67] Although suggested for use by nonmedical workers in reporting possible infectious diseases during a major disaster,[4] Table 2-3 lists **symptom-syndrome characteristics** that could be equally useful as a checklist for human disease-reporting decisions by all health professionals.

Problems associated with case reporting occur at every stage. At the beginning, there may be **underreporting** by the attending clinician.[5,15,41] Many reasons have been put forth, but some of the more common are (1) Didn't know how to report, (2) Didn't know the disease was reportable, (3) Reporting was too time consuming, (4) Didn't know I had to report.[39] A

Table 2-3. Checklist for reportable human diseases

Syndrome	Characteristics
Febrile systemic disease	Sudden or progressive onset with or without rash, fever, headache, myalgias; with or without gastrointestinal symptoms; no source
Febrile rash	Fever with systemic symptoms; generalized eruption or localized; nonhemorrhagic
Hemorrhagic fever	Fever and systemic symptoms; second phase after 3–5 days with cutaneous bleeding or petechiae, internal or mucosal bleeding, jaundice; with or without shock syndrome
Febrile lymphadenopathy	Fever with systemic symptoms; suppurative or nonsuppurative, localized or generalized
Febrile neurologic disease	Occasional onset with fever and systemic symptoms; meningitic signs, encephalitis, paralysis
Febrile respiratory	Fatigue; cough, thoracic pain, tract disease dyspnea; sputum
Febrile gastrointestinal	Systemic symptoms may be mild or absent; nausea, disease vomiting, cramps; diarrhea with or without blood or mucus; occasional neurologic signs; food poisoning may be present without fever
Febrile icterus	Initial phase as per first syndrome but may be only later jaundiced; if hemorrhagic, see third syndrome
Afebrile disease	Some signs or symptoms of preceding diseases but without fever

common explanation for not reporting given by both physicians and veterinarians is that reporting violates physician-patient/veterinarian-client confidentiality.[64] Regardless of the stated reason for not reporting, there must be a reason for reporting that is accepted by the clinician and patient/client before any (government-based) reporting system will be most effective. It is a common practice to regularly distribute in tabular form a summary of the data received. Although such reports provide feedback to the reporting health professionals in the community, they do not stimulate enthusiastic reporting.[83] Whenever questions of timely interest to those reporting (e.g., questions related to observation of a new syndrome or response to a new therapy) are combined with a narrative summary explaining some recent event (e.g., outbreak of new syndrome) in the locality, interest in the reports and response rates tend to be higher.

Differences between governmental jurisdictions in their systems of disease reporting, such as in regard to definitions for a case, how a case is to be counted, and sources of data used, make analyses at the national level and between time periods very difficult. Surveillance studies, e.g., routine contact of clinicians by telephone or mail, have demonstrated that some underreporting occurs with passive reporting systems. A major question is, to what extent are the cases that are reported representative of all those at risk in the population? For zoonoses that are not reportable, this problem is even greater inasmuch as we are entirely dependent upon laboratory-based studies with investigators who have a particular local interest. Therefore, reported geographic distribution and other population parameters may be entirely misleading. A classic example is the early study of Rocky Mountain spotted fever limited to the Rocky Mountains, a disease with considerably greater frequency in other geographic areas.

There is no multi-tiered scheme for reporting zoonoses in animals beginning with the attending veterinarian comparable to the APHA system for people beginning with the attending physician. Most animal health agencies have animal disease-reporting requirements. Unfortunately, however, the disease lists presented have not been developed with a clear indication of why the disease is to be reported in relation to future action needed. Typically, the **rapidity of reporting** required (telephone vs mail) and whether or not the etiology must first be confirmed are not indicated. Fever and early death (high case fatality rate) in weaned pigs could be the result of African swine fever, hog cholera, or salmonellosis. Because prompt action is important to control of all these diseases, reporting should be by telephone when an outbreak is first observed. In contrast, a confirmed case of eastern equine encephalitis in a horse in an endemic area could be reported by mail because no immediate action is required related to the specific case. The information is added to the database indicating the level of immunization against encephalitis among horses in the area.

The International Office of Epizootics (OIE) has developed a Disease Code List, distinguishing diseases in domestic animals in relation to their relative socioeconomic and public health consequences.[6] The diseases on that list of public health consequence are zoonoses and all are grouped into Lists A, B, and C, defined as follows:

List A: Communicable diseases that have the potential for very serious and rapid spread, irrespective of national borders; are of serious socioeconomic or public health consequence; and are of major importance in the international trade of livestock and livestock products. Reports are submitted to the OIE as often as necessary to comply with Articles of the International Zoo-Sanitary Code (ISC). Examples: Newcastle disease, Rift Valley fever, and vesicular stomatitis.

List B: Communicable diseases that are considered to be of socioeconomic and/or public health importance within countries and are significant in the international trade of livestock and livestock products. Reports are normally submitted once a year, although more-frequent reporting may in some cases be necessary to comply with Articles of the ISC. Examples: African trypanosomiasis, anthrax, bovine tuberculosis, brucellosis, campylobacteriosis, cysticercosis, dermatophilosis, echinococcosis/hydatidosis, equine encephalomyelitis, glanders, Japanese encephalitis, leishmaniasis, leptospirosis, Nairobi sheep disease, pasteurellosis, psittacosis, Q fever, rabies, rodent tularemia, and trichinosis.

List C: Communicable diseases with important economic influence at individual production level. Examples: blackleg, botulism, other clostridial infections, coccidiosis, contagious pustular dermatitis (contagious ecthyma), listeriosis, liver fluke, salmonellosis, swine erysipelas, and toxoplasmosis.

You will note that some of the diseases on List C, such as salmonellosis, are considered to be serious human health hazards by public health authorities, whereas they are considered by animal health authorities to be less of a threat to animal production. These differences can be a factor in establishing agreement among government agencies on zoonoses control priorities.

Summary

1. When a clinical syndrome involving a zoonotic agent in people or other animals is first recognized in a community or herd, it is the index case that stimulates further investigation, usually including the initial etiologic diagnosis (See Chapter 3).

2. The clinical onset is at the end of an incubation period that began with exposure to the agent, the source of which may have been a vertebrate animal, an arthropod vector, or an inanimate vehicle (e.g. food).

3. Infection as a result of contact with an infected animal maintenance host represents a direct mode of transmission of a zoonotic agent from the reservoir, whereas infection as a result of contact with a vector or vehicle is an indirect mode. Transmission may be horizontal, between members of the same generation, or vertical, from one generation to the next.

4. Factors affecting risk of infection involve interaction of characteristics of agent, host, and environment (time and place).

5. Surveillance involves longitudinal data gathering and is planned to detect infection/disease in populations, measure its extent, identify needed interventions, and evaluate the impact of any intervention.

6. An epidemic occurs whenever the number of cases exceeds the expected (endemic) number, whereas in an outbreak the number of cases may or may not exceed the expected number. The epidemic or outbreak may be as a result of exposure to a common source or it may be propagative, in which secondary cases occur as a result of direct or indirect exposure to a primary case.

7. Outbreak investigations involve cross-sectional data-gathering to provide the information essential for effective control, i.e., the immediate source of the agent and its mode of transmission to the susceptibles at risk. Much of outbreak investigation involves case finding, i.e., patients with a similar clinical history.

8. Although health professionals are not required to report most of the 166 zoonoses observed to any animal health or public health agency, plague and yellow fever are legally reportable to the World Health Organization.

9. The only valid reason for requiring a disease to be reported is that some action may be needed based on the information obtained. How the information is to be used is especially important in deciding the rapidity of reporting required (telephone vs mail) and whether or not the etiology must first be confirmed.

References

1. Abrutyn, E., and G. H. Talbot: Surveillance strategies: A primer. *Infect Control*, 8:459-464, 1987.
2. Acha, P. N., and B. Szyfres: *Zoonoses and Communicable Diseases Common to Man and Animals*, 2nd ed. Sci. Publ. No. 503. Washington, D.C. Pan American Health Organization, 1987.
3. Acuff, G. R., R. A. Albanese, C. A. Batt, et al.: Implications of biotechnology, risk assessment, and communications for the safety of foods of animal origin. *J*

Am Vet Med Assoc, 199:1714-1721, 1991.

4. Aghababian, R. V., and J. Teuscher: Infectious diseases following major disasters. *Ann Emerg Med*, 21:362-367, 1992.

5. Alter, M. J., A. Mares, S. C. Hadler, et al.: The effect of underreporting on the apparent incidence and epidemiology of acute viral hepatitis. *Am J Epidemiol*, 125:133-139, 1987.

6. Anon.: *International Zoo-Sanitary Code (International Animal Health Code)*, 5th ed. Paris, Office International des Epizooties, 1986.

7. Audy, J. R.: The localization of disease with special reference to the zoonoses. *Trans Roy Soc Trop Med Hyg*, 52:308-328, 1958.

8. Audy, J. R.: Medical ecology in relation to geography. *Brit J Clin Pract*, 12:102-110, 1958.

9. Bartlett, A. V., M. E. Paz de Bocaletti, and M. A. Bocaletti: Neonatal and early postneonatal morbidity and mortality in a rural Guatemalan community: the importance of infectious diseases and their management. *Pediatr Infect Dis J*, 0:752-757, 1991.

10. Beck, A. M.: *The Ecology of Stray Dogs*. Baltimore, York Press, 1973.

11. Benenson, A. S. (ed.): *Control of Communicable Diseases in Man*, 14th ed. Washington, D.C., American Public Health Association, 1985.

12. Bryan, F. L. (chrmn.): *Procedures to Investigate Foodborne Illness*, 4th ed. rev. Ames, IA, International Association of Milk, Food and Environmental Sanitarians, Inc., 1988.

13. Bryan, F. L.: Risks of practices, procedures and processes that lead to outbreaks of foodborne diseases. *J Food Prot*, 51:663-673, 1988.

14. Budnick, L. D., and E. Bell: Disease reporting by physicians in New York City. *Bull NY Acad Med*, 64:422-429, 1988.

15. Campos-Outcalt, D., R. England, and B. Porter: Reporting of communicable diseases by university physicians. *Public Health Rep*, 106:579-583, 1991.

16. Chorba, T. L., R. L. Berkelman, S. K. Safford, et al.: Mandatory reporting of infectious diseases by clinicians. *J Am Med Assoc*, 262:3018-3026, 1989.

17. Chungue, E., J. P. Boutin, and J. Roux: Dengue surveillance in French Polynesia: An attempt to use the excess number of laboratory requests for confirmation of dengue diagnosis as an indicator of dengue activity. *Eur J Epidemiol*, 7:616-620, 1991.

18. Dickinson, J. A.: Notification of disease, worthwhile or not? *Austral Fam Physician*, 20:772, 774-775, 777, 780, 1991.

19. Dohoo, I. R., and D. Waltner-Toews: Interpreting clinical research, Part III. Observational studies and interpretation of results. *Compend Contin Educ Pract Vet*, 7:S605-S610, S612, S616, 1985.

20. Fang, F. C., and J. Fierer: Human infection with *Salmonella dublin*. *Medicine*, 70:198-207, 1991.

21. Feinstein, A. R.: *Clinical Epidemiology: The Architecture of Clinical Research*. Philadelphia, W. B. Saunders, 1985.

22. Fox, D. M.: From TB to AIDS: Value conflicts in reporting disease. *Hastings Center Rep*, 16(6):Suppl. 11-16, 1986.

23. Fox, J. P., C. E. Hall, and L. R. Elveback: *Epidemiology: Man and Disease*. New York, Macmillan, 1970.

24. Frame, J. D., W. R. Lange, and D. L. Frankenfield: Mortality trends of American missionaries in Africa, 1945-1985. *Am J Trop Med Hyg*, 46:686-690, 1992.
25. Frank, G. R., M. D. Salman, and D. W. MacVean: Use of a disease reporting system in a large beef feedlot. *J Am Vet Med Assoc*, 192:1063-1067, 1988.
26. Gardner, I.: Techniques of reporting disease outbreak investigations. *Vet Clin No Amer: Food Anim Pract*, 4(1):109-125, 1988.
27. Gateley, K.: Communicable disease reporting: Why? *J Tenn Med Assoc*, 83:512-513, 1990.
28. Giesecke, J.: Some remarks on definition and validity of terms used in models for infectious disease spread. *Math Biosci*, 107:149-153, 1991.
29. Hall, W. N.: A report on Michigan's new Lyme disease reporting requirement. *Michigan Med*, 89:45, 1990.
30. Halperin, W., and E. L. Baker, eds.: *Public Health Surveillance*. New York, Van Nostrand Reinhold, 1992.
31. Harwood, R. F., and M. T. James: *Entomology in Human and Animal Health*, 7th ed. New York, Macmillan, 1979.
32. Hennekens, C. H., and J. E. Buring: *Epidemiology in Medicine*. Boston, Little, Brown, 1987.
33. Ho, K.-C.: Epidemiologic methodology as used in China. *J Rheumatol Suppl*, 10:82-85, 1983.
34. Hope-Simpson, R. E.: The role of season in the epidemiology of influenza. *J Hyg Camb*, 86:35-47, 1981.
35. Hugh-Jones, M. E., and R. R. Tinline: Studies on the 1967-68 foot-and-mouth disease epidemic: incubation period and herd serial interval. *J Hyg Camb*, 77:141-153, 1976.
36. International Association of Milk, Food and Environmental Sanitarians, Inc.: *Procedures to Investigate Arthropod-borne and Rodent-borne Illness*. Ames, IA, 1983.
37. Kirsch, T. D.: Local area monitoring (LAM). *Wld Hlth Statist Quart*, 41:19-25, 1988.
38. Kirsch, T., and R. Shesser: A survey of emergency department communicable disease reporting practices. *J Emerg Med*, 9:211-214, 1991.
39. Konowitz, P. M., G. A. Petrossian, and D. N. Rose: The underreporting of disease and physicians' knowledge of reporting requirements. *Public Health Rep*, 99:31-35, 1984.
40. Kramer, M. S.: *Clinical Epidemiology and Biostatistics*. New York, Springer-Verlag, 1988.
41. Ktsanes, V. K., D. W. Lawrence, K. Kelso, et al.: Survey of Louisiana physicians on communicable disease reporting. *J La State Med Soc*, 143:27-28, 30-31, 1991.
42. Lange, W. R., D. L. Frankenfield, J. Carico, et al.: Deaths among members of the Public Health Service Commissioned Corps, 1965-89. *Public Health Rep*, 107:160-166, 1992.
43. Last, J. M.: *A Dictionary of Epidemiology*, 2nd ed. New York, Oxford University Press, 1988.
44. Lessard, P. R., and B. D. Perry (eds.): Investigation of disease outbreaks and impaired productivity. *Veterinary Clinics of North America: Food Animal Practice*,

Vol. 4, No. 1, 1988.

45. Levine, N. D. (ed.): *Natural Nidality of Transmissible Diseases*. Urbana, IL, University of Illinois Press, 1966.

46. Lidz, T.: *The Person: His and Her Development Throughout the Life Cycle*. New York, Basic Books, 1983.

47. Linthicum, K. J., C. L. Bailey, C. J. Tucker, et al.: Application of polar-orbiting, meteorological satellite data to detect flooding of Rift Valley fever virus vector mosquito habitats in Kenya. *Med Vet Entomol*, 4:433-438, 1990.

48. Martin, R. J., T. Habtemariam, and P. R. Schnurrenberger: The health characteristics of veterinarians in Illinois. *Int J Zoon*, 8:63-71, 1981.

49. Martin, S. W., A. H. Meek, and P. Willeberg: *Veterinary Epidemiology: Principles and Methods*. Ames, IA, Iowa State University Press, 1987.

50. Meeuwisse, G. W.: Immunological considerations on breast vs. formula feeding. *Klin Padiat*, 197:322-325, 1985.

51. Miller, D. G.: Preventive medicine by risk factor analysis. *J Am Med Assoc*, 222:312-316, 1972.

52. Moore, P. S., B. D. Plikaytis, G. A. Bolan, et al.: Detection of meningitis epidemics in Africa: A population-based analysis. *Int J Epidemiol*, 21:155-162, 1992.

53. Moorhouse, P. D., and M. E. Hugh-Jones: Serum banks. *Vet Bull*, 51:277-290, 1981.

54. Muul, I.: Mammalian ecology and epidemiology of zoonoses. *Science*, 170:1275-1279, 1970.

55. National Research Council: *Animals as Sentinels of Environmental Health Hazards*. Washington, D.C., National Academy Press, 1991.

56. National Research Council: *Improving Risk Communication*. Washington, D.C., National Academy Press, 1989.

57. Palmer, S. R.: Epidemiology in search of infectious diseases: methods in outbreak investigation. *J Epidemiol Comm Health*, 43:311-314, 1989.

58. Payne, J. N.: The introduction of a computerized system for notification and improved analysis of infectious diseases in Sheffield. *J Publ Health Med*, 14:62-67, 1992.

59. Powles, J.: Changes in disease patterns and related social trends. *Soc Sci Med*, 35:377-387, 1992.

60. Putt, S. N. H., A. P. M. Shaw, A. J. Woods, et al.: *ILCA Manual No. 3: Veterinary epidemiology and economics in Africa*. Addis Ababa, Ethiopia, International Livestock Centre for Africa, 1987.

61. Riemann, H., and F. L. Bryan: *Food-Borne Infections and Intoxications*, 2nd ed. San Diego, Academic Press, 1979.

62. Rosenberg, J., and L. H. Clever: Medical surveillance of infectious disease endpoints. *Occup Med*, 5:583-605, 1990.

63. Rushworth, R. L., S. M. Bell, G. L. Rubin, et al.: Improving surveillance of infectious diseases in New South Wales. *Med J Aust*, 154:828-831, 1991.

64. Ryan, C. P.: Informing health officials of reportable diseases. *J Am Vet Med Assoc*, 197:962-963, 1990.

65. Sackett, D. L., R. B. Haynes, G. H. Guyatt, et al.: *Clinical Epidemiology: A Basic Science for Clinical Medicine*, 2nd ed. Boston, Little, Brown, 1991.

66. Sacks, J. J.: Utilization of case definitions and laboratory reporting in the surveillance of notifiable communicable diseases in the United States. *Am J Public Health*, 75:1420-1422, 1985.
67. Salman, M. D., G. R. Frank, D. W. MacVean, et al.: Validation of disease diagnoses reported to the National Animal Health Monitoring System from a large Colorado beef feedlot. *J Am Vet Med Assoc*, 192:1069-1073, 1988.
68. Schnurrenberger, P. R., and W. T. Hubbert: Reporting of zoonotic diseases. *Am J Epidemiol*, 112:23-31, 1980.
69. Schramm, M. M., R. L. Vogt, and M. Mamolen: The surveillance of communicable disease in Vermont: Who reports? *Public Health Rep*, 106:95-97, 1991.
70. Schwabe, C. W.: *Veterinary Medicine and Human Health*, 3rd ed. Baltimore, Williams & Wilkins, 1984.
71. Serfling, R. E.: Methods for current statistical analysis of excess pneumonia-influenza deaths. *Public Health Rep*, 78:494-506, 1963.
72. Shofer, F. S., W. T. London, P. Lyons, et al.: Adverse effect of splenectomy on the survival of patients with more than one kidney transplant. *Transplantation*, 42:473-478, 1986.
73. Smith, R. D.: *Veterinary Clinical Epidemiology: A Problem-Oriented Approach.* Stoneham, MA, Butterworth-Heinemann, 1991.
74. Snacken, R., J. Lion, V. Van Casteren, et al.: Five years of sentinel surveillance of acute respiratory infections (1985-1990): The benefits of an influenza early warning system. *Eur J Epidemiol*, 8:485-490, 1992.
75. Sumaya, C. V.: Major infectious diseases causing excess morbidity in the Hispanic population. *Arch Intern Med*, 151:1513-1520, 1991.
76. Syrjanen, J., V. V. Valtonen, M. Iivanainen, et al.: Preceding infection as an important risk factor for ischaemic brain infarction in young and middle aged patients. *Brit Med J*, 296:1156-1160, 1988.
77. Thacker, S. B., K. Choi, and P. S. Brachman: The surveillance of infectious diseases. *J Am Med Assoc*, 249:1181-1185, 1983.
78. Thacker, S. B., and R. L. Berkelman: Public health surveillance in the United States. *Epidemiol Rev*, 10:164-190, 1988.
79. Thacker, S. B., S. Redmond, R. B. Rothenberg, et al.: A controlled trial of disease surveillance strategies. *Am J Prev Med*, 2:345-350, 1986.
80. Thrusfield, M.: *Veterinary Epidemiology*. London, Butterworths, 1986.
81. Tillett, H. E.: Statistical analysis of case-control studies of communicable diseases. *Int J Epidemiol*, 15:126-133, 1986.
82. Watkins, M., S. Lapham, and W. Hoy: Use of a medical center's computerized health care database for notifiable disease surveillance. *Am J Public Health*, 81:637-639, 1991.
83. Weiss, B. P., M. A. Strassburg, and S. L. Fannin: Improving disease reporting in Los Angeles County: Trial and results. *Public Health Rep*, 103:415-421, 1988.
84. Wilson, C. B.: Immunologic basis for increased susceptibility of the neonate to infection. *J Pediatr*, 108:1-12, 1986.
85. Wood, C.: Notifiable disease reporting in Kansas. *Kansas Med*, 89:314-317, 1988.

3

ROLE OF THE LABORATORY IN ZOONOSES RECOGNITION

Laboratory Purposes

The **clinical laboratory** is there to assist the attending physician or veterinarian in answering questions involving diagnosis, therapy, or prognosis of a patient. Laboratory test results may help to confirm or rule out a diagnosis.[20,30,48,54,55,91,92,96,97,105,113,118] Periodic testing may provide data essential to evaluating the progress of therapy. Laboratory tests may be needed to detect the existence and measure the severity of a condition not detectable clinically by physical examination and thus aid in rendering a more precise prognosis. In addition, laboratory tests are valuable in screening clinically healthy patients for evidence of subclinical (without visible signs or symptoms) disease. In the private practice of human or veterinary medicine, these services are generally available from laboratories in the office, hospital, or local, private laboratory.

These local, private laboratories meet the usual needs of clinicians and patients. They also handle most of the specimens from patients affected by zoonotic agents. Examining fecal specimens for parasite ova or larvae is a routine procedure performed worldwide.[11,94] Bacteria are detected in clinical specimens by a host of direct procedures as well as culture, and their in vitro sensitivity to antibiotics determined. Seldom, in the management of individual patients, is it necessary to go beyond this capability. The basic purpose of the **clinical laboratory** is to assist in **patient management**. As long as the therapy is successful, identifying the genus, species, or other characteristics of the agent not evident from data needed in management of the patient is an unjustifiable expense to the human patient or veterinary client. Even routine blood culture of children with febrile illness cannot be justified as a management strategy.[60] In some instances, identification of the agent is helpful in reaching a prognosis and determining the probability of relapse/recurrence. However, prevention of **nosocomial infections** from exposure to patients hospitalized with communicable diseases does not require identification of the agent involved before preventive measures are introduced. **Hospital infection control** practices should be routine.[13,58]

Although institutional clinical laboratories may have ancillary activities such as research and teaching presumed to be important, it is really only when the therapy of the individual patient fails to achieve the anticipated result that additional laboratory capability actually may be called upon. Often, this need is identified from patient history in association with clinical course. For example, a severe viral infection in a patient with a history of recent foreign travel will need more precise diagnosis, particularly if a hyperimmune serum may be available for specific treatment. In other words, more appropriate laboratory analysis may result from either preplanned clinical examination or from the failure of patient response to routine therapy.

The need for expanded support also may be evident from the patient history when similar illness is reported in others associated with the patient. This is when the **local (state/regional) animal health or public health laboratory** usually becomes involved.[8,21,27,29,31,35,39,46,47,56,63,67,88,110,116,117] The problem has expanded from routine patient management to one of specialized need or community concern. In developing countries, these laboratories perform most, if not all, of the functions described earlier for private clinical laboratories in the diagnosis of animal and human infectious diseases.[81]

When the local animal health or public health laboratory becomes involved, the services available become more specialized, usually emphasizing a limited group of diseases, and the focus shifts from the individual to the herd or community. For example, a unit may be involved solely in mass serologic testing for a specific disease such as bovine brucellosis or in examining animal brains for rabies. Typically, these laboratories provide the interface between the private sector and public facilities at the state and national levels. They may offer animal necropsy services or assist the coroner's office in examining tissues from human autopsies. In some areas, the animal health and public health laboratories are combined, thus making more efficient use of available laboratory expertise and other resources. Whereas the clinical laboratory is there to serve the attending clinician, the epidemiologist involved in population studies is a major user of the animal health/public health laboratory. In the more populous states, there may be several local laboratories with one or more reference laboratories at the state level providing more specialized services such as testing sera for arboviral antibodies. A major function of the state laboratory is support of disease control and surveillance programs directed by the state agency. Another important function should be development and implementation of improved systems of laboratory diagnosis and communication.

National animal health and public health laboratories provide support to national programs. In the United States, for example, the U.S. Department of Agriculture (USDA), Animal and Plant Health Inspection Service (APHIS), operates the National Veterinary Services Laboratories (NVSL). These laboratories provide support to national and international animal disease control and eradication programs. Major divisions of the NVSL include diagnostic bacteriology, diagnostic virology, pathobiology, and foreign animal disease diagnostic services. Although the work of the laboratories emphasizes diseases of economic concern to livestock and poultry production, areas of emphasis also include such endemic zoonotic diseases as salmonellosis, leptospirosis, brucellosis, and bovine tuberculosis. In the pathobiology laboratory, for example, granulomatous lesions of cattle found at slaughter by federal inspectors are routinely examined for confirmatory evidence of *Mycobacterium bovis* infection.

The U.S. Department of Health and Human Services, as part of the Centers for Disease Control, operates the National Center for Infectious Diseases (NCID), which provides national leadership in the investigation and diagnosis of infectious diseases of public health significance. Within NCID, laboratories with major involvement in zoonoses include enteric (e.g., *Salmonella, Campylobacter*), respiratory (e.g., chlamydiosis), parasitic, vectorborne (e.g., arboviruses, bacterial zoonoses), meningitis and special pathogens (e.g., *Listeria, Leptospira, Brucella*, anthrax, relapsing fever), mycotic diseases, and viral and rickettsial diseases (e.g., hepatitis, poxviruses, rabies, rickettsiae). Various national organizational structures exist in countries worldwide to meet their particular diagnostic requirements.

Internationally, the World Health Organization (WHO) has two regional zoonoses centers: the Mediterranean Zoonoses Control Centre, Athens, Greece; and the Pan American Institute for Food Protection and Zoonoses, Martinez, Argentina. The latter, operated by the Pan American Health Organization, was originally the Pan American Zoonoses Center (CEPANZO), opened in 1956. These facilities provide reference laboratory, research, and teaching services for the countries in the respective regions. In addition, the WHO has designated numerous Collaborating Centres (usually university or national government laboratories) around the world, recognizing them for specific expertise and contributions to studies of zoonoses. The Food and Agriculture Organization (FAO) of the United Nations has identified several FAO Reference Laboratories worldwide to provide expert assistance in the diagnosis of specific communicable diseases of animals, some of which are zoonotic.[12] Numerous joint FAO/WHO Collaborating Centres offer specific consultative services such as serotyping of specific zoonotic agents.

Hazards in the Laboratory

We all recognize that certain physical, chemical, and biological hazards are included in every biomedical laboratory.[19,28,74,82,93,111] Many of the more serious **biohazards** are zoonotic agents.[2,32,50,64,76,79,98,100,120,121] Exposure of laboratory personnel can involve a combination of physical and biological hazards when, for instance, one is injected with infectious material when an errant needle misses the laboratory mouse and enters the palm of the hand.[115] Needle sticks are a common occurrence. It is essential to have well-trained individuals performing every step in which a hazard exists using procedures designed to prevent mishap. Just because we work with infectious agents, it does not mean we inevitably must become infected with them from exposure in the laboratory.

In 1974, the National Institutes of Health published a summary of nearly 6,000 **laboratory-acquired infections** reported worldwide.[7] The eight most frequently reported infections were:

Infection	Number Infected
Typhoid	293
Brucellosis	276
Tuberculosis	217
Q fever	214
Infectious hepatitis	182
Tularemia	133
Soviet hemorrhagic fever	113
Venezuelan equine encephalitis	107

Among the eight infections, five (or six if *M. bovis* is included with *M. tuberculosis* as a possible tuberculosis agent[6]) involve zoonotic agents. An epidemic of laboratory-acquired infection was reported in nine instances, seven of which involved zoonotic agents.

Infection	Year	Number Infected
Psittacosis	1930	11
Brucellosis	1938	94
Q fever	1940	15
Murine typhus	1942	6
Q fever	1946	47
Coccidioidomycosis	1950	13
Histoplasmosis	1955	18
Venezuelan equine encephalitis	1959	24
Tularemia	1961	5

The overall case fatality rate among the 6,000 cases was 4%, with the highest (7.3%) among viral infections and the lowest (no fatalities) among cases of parasitic infection. Although 70% of the 6,000 infected individuals recovered completely, infection in 26% of those clinically affected resulted in some permanent disability. At least one fatal case of laboratory-acquired Chagas disease (not included in the above summary of parasitic infections) has been reported.[18]

In a review of 3,700 laboratory-acquired infections, a specific cause or event resulting in the infection was identified in approximately 20% of the cases.[18] Among these, the following were the five most-frequently recognized causes:

Cause	Percent of Infections
Oral aspiration through pipettes	4.7
Accidental syringe inoculation	4.0
Animal bites	1.4
Spray from syringes	1.2
Centrifuge accidents	0.8

It is likely that most of the 80% for which the cause was classified as "unknown" involved exposure to an infectious aerosol generated by some procedure. When multiple individuals share a laboratory, it is not uncommon for the person or persons infected to be unaware of the activity of another that can result in creation of an aerosol.[61]

Although veterinarians occasionally are exposed to *B. anthracis* when they cut themselves while performing a necropsy and later develop an anthrax eschar at the wound site, these infections seldom are reported as laboratory-acquired because the necropsy was not performed in the laboratory. Similarly, persons who have been injected with equine-origin rabies immune serum because of exposure to rabies virus in the laboratory and who later develop painful and debilitating arthus reactions are not counted among the laboratory-acquired infections.

The U.S. Public Health Service and the USDA jointly established a system of **classifying etiologic agents based on hazard** to provide minimal safety standards.[83] Similar systems have been established in other countries. The system includes four **biosafety levels for infectious agents** as well as four **biosafety levels for infected vertebrate animals** based on increasing hazard. In addition, the USDA maintains a list of foreign animal pathogens (some of which are zoonotic, e.g., louping ill and Rift Valley fever viruses) excluded from the United States because of hazard to domestic livestock and/or poultry.

Biosafety Levels for Infectious Agents

Level 1: Practices, safety equipment, and facilities are appropriate for undergraduate and secondary educational training and teaching laboratories and for other facilities in which work is done with defined and characterized strains of viable microorganisms not known to cause disease in healthy adult humans. *Bacillus subtilis, Naegleria gruberi,* and infectious canine hepatitis virus are representative of those microorganisms meeting these criteria. Many agents not ordinarily associated with disease processes in humans are, however, opportunistic pathogens and may cause infection in the young, the aged, and in immunodeficient or immunosuppressed individuals. Vaccine strains that have undergone multiple in vivo passages should not be considered avirulent simply because they are vaccine strains.

Level 2: Practices, equipment, and facilities are applicable to clinical, diagnostic, teaching, and other facilities in which work is done with the broad spectrum of indigenous moderate-risk agents present in the community and associated with human disease of varying severity. With good microbiologic techniques, these agents can be used safely in activities conducted on the open bench, provided the potential for producing aerosols is low. Hepatitis B virus, the salmonellae, and *Toxoplasma* spp. are representative of microorganisms assigned to this containment level. Primary hazards to personnel working with these agents may include accidental autoinoculation, ingestion, and skin or mucous membrane exposure to infectious materials. Procedures with high aerosol potential that may increase the risk of exposure of personnel must be conducted in primary containment equipment or devices.

Level 3: Practices, safety equipment, and facilities are applicable to clinical, diagnostic, teaching, research, or production facilities in which work is done with indigenous or exotic agents where the potential for infection by aerosols is real and the disease may have serious or lethal consequences. Autoinoculation and ingestion also represent primary hazards to personnel working with these agents. Examples of such agents for which Biosafety Level 3 safeguards are generally recommended include *Mycobacterium tuberculosis,* St. Louis encephalitis virus, and *Coxiella burnetii.*

Level 4: Practices, safety equipment, and facilities are applicable to work with dangerous and exotic agents that pose a high individual risk of life-threatening disease. All manipulations of potentially infectious diagnostic materials, isolates, and naturally or experimentally infected animals pose a high risk of exposure and infection to laboratory personnel. Lassa fever virus is representative of the microorganisms assigned to Level 4.

Biosafety Levels for Infected Vertebrate Animals

The recommendations describe four combinations of practices, safety equipment, and facilities for experiments on animals infected with agents that are known or believed to produce infections in humans (Table 3-1).

Although the classification system places considerable emphasis on physical containment in the laboratory for the more hazardous agents (Levels 3 and 4), most zoonotic agents are in Level 2. For these agents, prevention of laboratory-acquired infection primarily involves proper performance of safe procedures by trained personnel. For example, mouth pipetting should never be performed and must be replaced by equally efficient and considerably safer pipetting with the aid of a mechanical

Table 3-1. Biosafety recommendations

Level	Practices	Safety Equipment	Facilities
1	Standard animal care and management	None	Basic
2	Laboratory coats, decontamination of all infectious wastes and animal cages before washing, limited access, protective gloves and hazard warning signs as indicated	Partial containment and/or personal protective devices used for activities and manipulations of agents or infected animals	Basic
3	Level 2 practices plus special laboratory clothing, controlled access	Partial containment and/or personal protective devices used for *all* activities and manipulations of agents or infected animals	Containment
4	Level 3 practices plus enter through clothes change room where street clothing is removed and laboratory clothing is put on, shower on exit, all wastes are decontaminated before removal from the facility	Maximum containment (i.e., Class III biological safety cabinet or partial containment in combination with full-body, air-supplied positive-pressure personal suit) used for all procedures and activities	Maximum containment

dispenser. Specific procedures for balancing centrifuges should be posted and reviewed with each person using the equipment. Only LUER-LOK-type syringes and needles should be used with infectious material and an alcohol pledget should be placed around the stopper when removing the needle from a vaccine bottle. This simple procedure is particularly important in preventing exposure to *Br. abortus* strain 19 vaccine, which has been responsible for many laboratory-acquired infections. Autoclaving and chemical decontamination are other routine procedures that can, when not performed properly, present hazards in the laboratory.

Specimens for the Laboratory

For many who have collected specimens in the field or processed them in the laboratory, perhaps the most important lesson learned was to **anticipate needs**. Liberal application of the old adage PLAN AHEAD will help keep clinicians, epidemiologists, microbiologists, parasitologists, and pathologists happy. When tissues are routinely submitted in formalin, do not expect a report to include the genus and species of the infectious agent isolated. Not all viruses survive freezing well. Therefore, some tissues may need to be shipped on "wet" ice rather than on carbon dioxide. If specimens are to be collected in areas remote (beyond walking distance) from the hospital or laboratory, be sure to take all the items needed to collect and transport the tissue or fluid in the condition required for appropriate examination in the laboratory. The best way to assure success is to discuss your needs with all concerned before you start. One of the most common problems, and one easily avoided by advance communication, is incorrectly estimating the number of specimens that can be collected or processed in a given time period by the personnel available. A sudden major increase in a laboratory's volume of work upsets routines and may temporarily reduce quality of output if the change was not anticipated. It is also important to anticipate the information needed regarding the circumstances of the specimen collection (i.e., species, age, sex, location, etc.) so that a form outlining the data needed can be devised in advance to aid recording at the site. Because more and more laboratories are using electronic recording of information as well as reporting of results, it is important that the form be consistent with the data needs of the laboratory.

Several factors influence the decision regarding **which specimens to collect** for the detection of zoonotic agents. Most important is whether the individual host is healthy or diseased. Blood is most often a primary source of the agent during an acute febrile illness, whereas it seldom is in a healthy carrier. Among the zoonoses, significant differences also may exist between species in relation to organ systems affected and portals of exit for a given agent. For example, blood or sputum would be primary sources of *Coxiella burnetii* in a person ill with Q fever, whereas uterine fluids expelled at parturition would be the primary source in a healthy carrier cow or ewe. Such species differences are the rule among parasitic zoonoses with multihost life cycles. For many zoonoses, particularly viral and rickettsial, isolation of the agent is not required for patient management or to reach a confirmatory etiologic diagnosis. Results of serologic tests using acute and convalescent sera will provide the information needed without exposing laboratory personnel to risk of infection associated with unnecessary isolation procedures.

Because of the resources immediately at hand, **collecting a specimen** from a hospitalized patient is rather straightforward once the specimen needed has been determined. Blood and cerebrospinal fluid usually present the greatest array of choices with untreated tubes for clot, tubes with anticoagulant, and tubes with culture medium. Most other specimens, such as feces, urine, or sputum, usually can await the brief trip to the laboratory before further processing begins. This is often not the case with field-based studies involving animals[99] or ambulatory persons in the community. Isolating the agent in question, such as fragile *Leptospira* spp. from urine of carrier animals or people, will require immediate inoculation of the urine into a specialized medium for greatest success. Various transport media have been developed to enhance isolation of some agents when there will be a prolonged period before the specimen arrives in the laboratory. For some agents, such as anaerobic bacteria, inoculation of the culture medium at the moment the specimen is collected will significantly enhance recovery rates. Specialized techniques, such as adsorbing blood on filter paper for transport, are available for collecting specimens of the minute quantities available from small mammals, arthropods, and birds, particularly if they are to be tagged and released alive. If potential arthropod vectors are to be collected, there are specialized procedures for handling them, both for identifying the vector and the agent.

Shipment of potentially infected tissues or fluids from the field to the laboratory, as well as cultures of infectious agents from one laboratory to another, requires careful planning and compliance with certain regulations (Fig. 3-1). Internal and external containers should be durable to prevent breakage and leakproof. In fact, postal authorities and private transport companies have specific safety requirements for shipment of infectious materials. All containers should be clearly labeled, including the species, disease suspected, and tissue or fluid. A permit from the national animal health authorities is usually required to receive shipments of potentially infectious material of animal origin or cultures of zoonotic agents, particularly for international shipment. If refrigeration is needed, an appropriate refrigerant in a quantity that will last for the duration of the shipment must

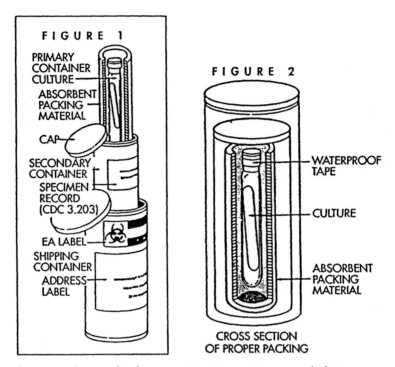

The Interstate Shipment of Etiologic Agents (42 CFR, Part 72) was revised July 21, 1980, to provide for packaging and labeling requirements for etiologic agents and certain other materials shipped in Interstate traffic.

Figures 1 and 2 diagram the packaging and labeling of etiologic agents in volumes of less than 50 ml. in accordance with the provisions of subparagraph 72.3 (a) of the cited regulation. Figure 3 illustrates the color and size of the label, described in subparagraph 72.3 (d) (1 -5) of the regulations, which shall be affixed to all shipments of etiologic agents.

For further information on any provision of this regulation contact:

Centers for Disease Control
Attn: Biohazards Control Officer
1600 Clifton Road
Atlanta, Georgia 30333

Telephone: 404/329-3883
          FTS-236-3883

FIGURE   3

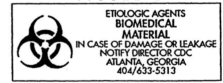

Fig. 3-1. Packaging and labeling of etiologic agents.

be included in suitable packaging. This means watertight for wet ice, but *not* airtight for dry ice, as it expands and may cause explosion if placed in an improper container. Although wet ice is freely available, dry ice is sometimes hard to find in the field. Good sources are ice cream factories and companies producing liquid nitrogen or oxygen. If frozen specimens are to be shipped for isolation of viruses or other agents, it is often useful to send duplicates in case further studies (e.g., different cell lines) are needed. Try to send the shipment so it will arrive on a weekday during regular working hours; avoid shipment on Fridays or on the eve of holidays. In any event, notify the receiving laboratory of the time and method of shipment so its arrival can be anticipated. Place all accompanying documents (printed or otherwise legible) in a separate watertight envelope so they will arrive in readable condition.

Space for specimen storage is often a problem in a busy laboratory. When a volume of specimens arrives that is greater than that routinely anticipated, interim storage before processing can be a problem. This is particularly true for frozen specimens, making prior arrangements essential. In some instances, it may be necessary to temporarily rent freezer space. If significant numbers of fixed tissues in blocks or lyophilized cultures are to be stored, it is well to plan for the space needed. A carefully planned system of serum storage can be an especially valuable tool in any diagnostic laboratory. The clinical laboratory may need to store **acute phase sera** from patients until the **convalescent sera** are received. If the **paired sera** are to be sent to another laboratory for testing, then an aliquot of each should be kept until the results are available and a final diagnosis has been reached. This is important because of occasional loss in transit or mistakes in the laboratory involving test performance or data recording. **Serum banks** are structured collections of sera from animals or humans representing some particular population, usually collected over time and identified/catalogued by time, place, and host.[77] These have been established in many laboratories around the world to provide a unique resource for retrospective studies of infectious and noninfectious conditions.[53,57,106,122] A serum bank can be especially useful in long-term studies of zoonotic agents if the sampling has been planned to include sera from representatives of subsets among the population according to species, age, sex, vaccination history, location, date of serum collection, and any other characteristic of interest.

Laboratory Tests

For many years, the Negri body was considered to be a **pathognomonic**, i.e., specific without any false-positive results, microscopic **lesion** on which a **confirmatory etiologic diagnosis** of rabies could be established. This diagnosis required observation of the lesion by direct microscopic examination of brain obtained after death of the patient. A **presumptive etiologic diagnosis** of plague meningitis can be established by examination of cerebrospinal fluid stained by the Gram method (if a short, bipolar, Gram-negative rod is seen). Both are well-known tests useful in the detection of infectious agents involving direct microscopic examination of tissues or fluids. Today, there is a great array of laboratory tests to aid in reaching either a confirmatory or presumptive etiologic diagnosis of infection with zoonotic agents. The central issue is selection of those tests that we know will give us the answer we need.

Identification of a specific zoonotic agent in a body tissue or fluid confirms **infection** with that agent. Additional signs (and/or symptoms in people) are needed to establish the presence of **disease**. A significant change in serum antibody titer to an antigen specific for an agent likewise confirms that the infection occurred. It does not confirm that the infection persists. Both clinicians and epidemiologists, when considering the diagnosis of zoonoses, are interested in tests that aid in the presumptive or confirmatory etiologic diagnosis of infection rather than disease. Clinicians already have observed signs such as fever, pneumonia, CNS disturbance, diarrhea, or abortion, all associated with zoonotic diseases in animals and people. The clinical concern is to direct therapy toward a relatively specific etiology. Similarly, the epidemiologist is asking, What is the etiology of this outbreak? Is this individual a healthy carrier (and shedder) of the agent? The clinical concern often has a perceived greater sense of urgency in seeking immediate answers that may be satisfied with presumptive diagnoses, and most of the time they meet the need (e.g., Gram-negative rod vs Gram-positive coccus). The need of the epidemiologist may be no less urgent, however, in the face of a possible outbreak of a disease with a high attack rate and a high case fatality rate.

For most zoonoses, the clinical pattern of response to infection, beginning with the incubation period, and progressing through the course of illness to recovery or death, is well documented. Graphs of the typical immune response in relation to clinical course are common in textbooks of medicine. In cases of trichinosis after eating undercooked pork, for example, it is even possible to estimate the concentration of *Trichinella spiralis* in the pork and the quantity of pork consumed in relation to the severity of disease. It is also possible, with a given severity of disease (clinical syndrome), to anticipate the numbers of trichinae to be seen in the direct microscopic examination of the muscle biopsy used to confirm the diagnosis. This type of information, i.e., the concentration of the agent in relation to tissue or fluid and time after exposure, is needed to predict the likelihood of confirming infection. For example, the interval during the prodromal period when rabies virus can be found in the saliva of infected animals is a question that has received exceptionally intense study.[22,62,86,114] Answers to questions of this sort are crucial to understanding exposure to most zoonotic agents.

The Gram stain and other long-standing laboratory methods have provided rapid results from the examination of tissues and fluids. Now, advances in **biotechnology**[15,24,25,33,40,43,49,65,66,69,102,107,112] such as **monoclonal antibodies** are adding greatly to the diagnostic capabilities needed by clinicians and epidemiologists. With fluorescein conjugated monoclonals, we have highly sensitive and specific tools to make direct examination of sputum and other materials for identification of agents such as *Brucella, Chlamydia, Coxiella, Francisella, Toxoplasma,* and *Yersinia.* Monoclonals now permit differentiation of host-related strains of rabies virus, thus allowing greater insight into the likely source, e.g., bat vs fox. Electron microscopy combined with **immunoassay techniques** offer rapid means of virus detection that avoid the hazards of culture as well as increasing ability to detect some agents that are difficult to culture. Commercially produced **enzyme-linked immunosorbent assay (ELISA)** kits are widely available for several zoonoses. The ELISA offers a highly sensitive and specific rapid tool for detecting antibody.[10,14,23,78] Extremely sensitive molecular probes utilizing the **polymerase chain reaction (PCR)** can detect, for example, less than five *Borrelia burgdorferi* in the urine of patients with Lyme disease.[45] A persistent problem is the lack of **standardized procedures** for performance of tests, including new ones, and interpretation of the results so that findings can be compared between tests and between laboratories. The Office International des Epizooties (OIE) has published lists of diagnostic tests with interpretations of results recommended by international experts for the diagnosis of animal diseases on its Lists A and B (See Chapter 2).[108] Tests for diseases on List C have not yet been published by OIE. The tests are designated in one of the following three categories:

Prescribed: Tests that are required by the *International Animal Health Code* for the screening of animals before they are moved internationally.

Alternative: Tests that are suitable for the diagnosis of disease within a local setting and can also be used in the import/export of animals after bilateral negotiation.

Other: Tests that may also be of some practical value in local situations or may still be in a state of development.

To assure accuracy in reaching a confirmatory etiologic diagnosis of a current infection, a test is needed that is **sensitive** and **specific**.[1,41,44,59,68,75,84,85,87,103,109] The **sensitivity of the test** refers to the frequency in which it is positive when the infection is present. The **specificity of the test** refers to the frequency in which it is negative when the infection is absent. These can be expressed quantitatively (Table 3-2).

If A = 100 and C = 0, then the sensitivity of the test would be

Table 3-2. Sensitivity and specificity of diagnostic tests

	Infection		
Test	Present	Absent	Total
Positive	True + (A) *Positive*	False + (B) *Positive*	(A + B) Test Positive
Negative	False − (C) *Negative*	True − (D) *Negative*	(C + D) Test Negative
	(A + C) Total Infected	(B + D) Total Not Infected	(A + B + C + D) Total Tested

Sensitivity = A/[A + C] = true positive/total infected
Specificity = D/[B + D] = true negative/total not infected

100/[100 + 0] or 100%. If D = 100 and B = 0, then the specificity of the test would be 100/[100 + 0] or 100%. This would be a marvelous test, detecting all those who are infected and none of those who are not. Such a test would be the ultimate **reference test** or **"gold standard"** with which to compare the sensitivity and specificity of every other test in its ability to detect the infection in question.

Unless the sensitivity and specificity of a test equal 100%, an inverse relationship exists between the two. Usually, the specificity and sensitivity of a test do not change. However, if one is increased, the other must simultaneously decrease. As the **cut-off point** for a "positive" titer is redefined, a shift in the number of false-positive and false-negative animals occurs. For example, a shift in the definition of "positive" titers to include all infected individuals (i.e., 100% sensitivity) will increase the number of uninfected individuals that will now become "false positives" and thus reduce the specificity. The test has not changed, merely the way the results are being interpreted (Fig. 3-2).

For most tests, the results are a continuous variable, i.e., there is no single positive or negative value. It is for this reason that cut-off points are selected. The **receiver-operating-characteristic (ROC) curve (or relative operating characteristics curve)** is a method of graphically depicting the impact on diagnosis of selecting a given cut-off point on which to make decisions based on a single test.[9,72,73,101,119] The proportion of positive tests among all who are actually infected, the true-positive (TP) ratio (A/A+C), is plotted on the Y-axis and the proportion of positive tests among all who are not infected, the false-positive (FP) ratio (B/B+D), is plotted on the X-axis. When these values are plotted, a curve is produced extending from the lower left-hand corner (highest specificity) to the upper right-hand corner (highest sensitivity). **The measure of accuracy** is the proportion (A) of the

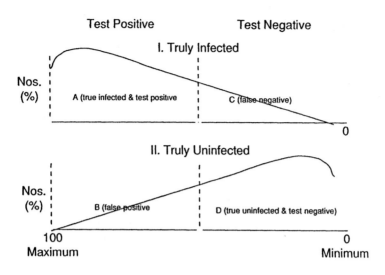

**Fig. 3-2. Interpretation of test results vs cut-off
point.**

area of the graph beneath the curve. When A = 0.5 and the curve is a
straight line between the diagonals, the results can be achieved by chance
alone, i.e., the true-positive and false-positive proportions are equal. When
A = 1.0, on the other hand, the TP ratio = 1.0 and the FP ratio = 0,
resulting in perfect discrimination. The location on the curve where a cut-off
point, or decision threshold, is selected is referred to as the **operating
position**. As an example, the published[52] results of complement fixation (CF)
and Rivanol tests for *Br. abortus* performed on sera of adult-vaccinated cows
were plotted on the ROC curve (Fig. 3-3). Isolation of field strain or Strain
19 *Br. abortus* from milk was used as the "gold standard." It is evident that
in both tests the cut-off point can be increased 2-3 dilutions with little effect
on sensitivity with a concurrent significant decrease in false positives.
Various statistical analyses to determine test discrimination (e.g., the
probability that a test will be "more abnormal" in an infected individual than
a normal one) can be applied to the ROC curve.[9,101]

The **biological reasons for false-positive and false-negative test results**
in relation to actual presence or absence of infection are associated with the
agent, host, and test itself. Many agents share antigens that result in
serologic cross-reactivity, e.g., *Yersinia pestis* vs *Yersinia pseudotuberculosis* 1B,
Brucella abortus vs *Yersinia enterocolitica* serotype 9, and *Leptospira* serovars.
The detectable host response depends on stage of infection (e.g., anergy in
chronic cases) as well as such factors as age (e.g., prenatal), species, and
carrier state (often little or no detectable antibody). The test may not detect
the antibody class (IgG, IgM, or IgA in secretions) present or it may be

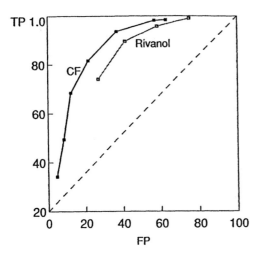

Fig. 3-3. Receiver-operating-characteristic (ROC) curves comparing two serologic tests for bovine brucellosis.

insufficiently sensitive to detect the antibody concentration present. Tests using biological reagents such as red blood cells may have false-positive results (e.g., hemagglutination) from the presence of normal antibody in the test serum unless adequate controls are included. Of course, technical errors during performance or interpretation of the test also may contribute to false results.

The **validity** of a test refers to how well it performs in relation to the "gold standard." This is comparable to always finding the pathognomonic lesion for rabies (Negri body) when it is there (and reporting it as positive) and never confusing it with a CNS lesion caused by some virus other than rabies (always reporting these latter cases as negative). Of course, this method does not always detect rabies infection inasmuch as a discernible inclusion body is not always present (false negative) and some of the brains with Negri bodies are fluorescent antibody negative (false positive). In this example, therefore, the specificity of the test may be less than 100% (some of those reported as negative may be infected with rabies) and the sensitivity is also likely to be less than 100% (a few of the infected will not be detected). The sensitivity and specificity of the intradermal tuberculin test to detect infection among 172 cattle, the entire population of three infected herds, presents a real world example.[36] The "gold standard" in this instance was the histopathologic and cultural examination of lymph nodes as well as any lesions collected from all animals at slaughter.[80]

In Table 3-3, the sensitivity of the test to detect infection was 58/61 or

Table 3-3. Sensitivity and specificity of an intradermal tuberculin test on 172 cattle

Test Result	Disease Status		Total
	Positive	Negative	
Positive	58	42	100
Negative	3	69	72
Total	61	111	172

95%, whereas the specificity was 69/111 or 62%. Although only 5% (3/61) of the infected failed to be detected, 38% (42/111) of them were falsely reported as infected. Since we know how many were actually infected without evident lesions or were anergic, the validity of the test is in relation to infection as well as disease.

In the above examples, **"true" sensitivity and specificity** were calculated because a "true"-positive and "true"-negative infection or disease status was likely based on the extensive postmortem gross, cultural, and histopathologic examination. The validity of the test was measured because a "gold standard" existed and was used. More often, the sensitivity of a test (particularly serologic tests) will be presented in relation to the sensitivity of another test. In addition, serologic tests usually measure antibody, a host response to infection, and not the infection itself.[3,37,70,71] These test comparisons measure **"relative" sensitivity** and **"relative" specificity**, referring to the results of one test relative to the other to detect some secondary indicator of infection such as antibody. The 2×2 table would be similar to those presented earlier (Table 3-4).

The resulting calculations then indicate the relative sensitivity of the comparative test to detect the antibody in question, when it was detected by the reference test, and the relative specificity of the comparative test to not detect antibody when the reference test did not. If the reference test is poor, the comparative test can appear to be an excellent choice **in comparison** and still be worthless in its ability to detect infection. There are many studies of the comparative sensitivity of brucellosis serologic tests, but few have actually compared serologic tests with isolation results to determine sensitivity and specificity of the tests.

Table 3-4. Comparison of one test relative to another

Comparative Test Results	Reference Test Results	
	Positive	Negative
Positive	True + (A)	False + (B)
Negative	False − (C)	True − (D)

Laboratory tests for the zoonoses are used primarily to determine if the individual is infected or not. In other words, we want to know how well the test is able to predict infection. If there is evidence of disease and a history suggesting exposure to the agent, then success is more likely because we have this additional suggestive evidence. But, what if there is no history of recent exposure, and you want to know if this healthy individual may be a carrier? This is the typical situation when a cow is tested with the tuberculin test or with a serologic test for brucellosis. The **predictive value** of a test depends on the frequency of the infection in the population. A **positive predictive value** is the proportion of individuals with a positive test who are actually infected. It can be considered as the number of tests that must be performed to find an infected individual. On the other hand, a **negative predictive value** is the proportion of individuals with a negative test who are actually not infected. These can be expressed quantitatively as follows (refer to earlier 2×2 tables for symbols):

Positive predictive value = A/[A+B] = true positive/total test positive

Negative predictive value = D/[C+D] = true negative/total test negative

If the prevalence is 100%, any negative test result is false, whereas if the prevalence is 0%, any positive test is false. Using the data for the tuberculin test presented earlier (61/172, or 35.5% actually diseased), the positive predictive value would be 58/[58+42], or 58%, whereas the negative predictive value would be 69/[3+69], or 96%. Only half of those that tested tuberculin positive were in fact infected, whereas virtually all those that tested tuberculin negative were healthy. What if a tuberculin test of the same sensitivity and specificity was applied to a population with an infection (sic disease) rate of 0.1%, or 100 infected/100,000 cattle (such as would be similar to bovine tuberculosis in the United States)? In Table 3-5 with the sensitivity of 95%, 95 out of 100 truly infected cattle actually would be tested as "positive"; whereas with the specificity of 62%, 61,938 out of 99,900 truly uninfected cattle would be tested as "negative." Then the positive predictive value would be 95/38,057, or only 0.25%, and the negative predictive value would be 61,938/61,943, or 99.9%.

Table 3-5. Results from test with 95% sensitivity and 62% specificity used on cattle with 0.1% infection rate

Test Result	"Disease" Status		Total
	Positive	Negative	
Positive	95 (A)	37,962 (B)	38,057
Negative	5 (C)	61,938 (D)	61,943
Total	100	99,900	100,000

At this point, it is clear that a test such as the tuberculin test in the above example is of limited value in large-scale searches when the prevalence of infection is low. It will still be of some use in testing known infected herds or herds in contact with them, i.e., where a higher probability of infection exists. Traditionally, an inexpensive screening test with a high sensitivity (e.g., 95%) and a good specificity (e.g., >80%) has been used to identify animals probably infected. The *Brucella* card test is an excellent example of such a screening test with a 95.2% sensitivity and a 98.5% specificity.

Subsequently, a more expensive second test, with high specificity, can be used to identify the probably truly infected among the more limited numbers of first-test-positive animals. This keeps to a minimum the cost of slaughtering false positives, although a few infected (false-negative) animals may be missed. Eventually, these too will be identified when the herd is retested. As an example, suppose two tests are used on a population with 1% prevalence of infection (Table 3-6). The first test has 95.2% sensitivity, 98.5% specificity, and costs $1.35/test. The second test has 97.5% sensitivity, 99.0% specificity, and costs $8.00/test.

With two tests, 93/100 infected animals were identified, whereas only two false positives were slaughtered. For an additional cost of $2,744 to perform second testing, 341 false positives were not slaughtered, which amounted to considerable savings to the producers as well as increased believability of the program.

The real-world situation is often somewhere between the two extremes presented. In other words, more would be known than an estimate of the national prevalence and less than the necropsy results for the entire herd after it had been tested. For example, the herd would be tested because a tuberculous lesion had been found earlier at slaughter in a cow from the herd, or the herd was adjacent to a known infected herd. All these factors

Table 3-6. Results from sequential tests of varying sensitivity and specificity on animals with a 1.0% infection rate

Test Result	"Infection" Status		Total
	Positive	Negative	
(Results of First Test of 10,000 Animals)			
Positive	95	248	343*
Negative	5	9,752	9,757
Total	100	9,900	10,000
(Results of Second Test of 343 First-Test-Positive Animals)*			
Positive	93	2	95
Negative	2	246	248
Total	95	248	343

would increase the likelihood that the herd was infected. In addition to the prevalence of infection in the population to be tested, predictive values are influenced by the sensitivity and specificity of the test. Therefore, these factors must also be considered in decisions involving test selection.[38,104] There is no one answer that fits all situations involving test selection.

It should be evident that the likelihood of failing to detect infection in a population decreases as the number of individuals tested increases. This is the reasoning behind herd tests for tuberculosis and other zoonoses—to assure that at least one infected individual in the group will be detected. The risk is assuming that, as a result of a single test, we know precisely which individuals are infected and which are not. These tests are usually valuable tools in epidemiologic investigations, i.e., they provide population estimates such as evidence of herd infection. The **standards for interpretation** of the tests are arbitrary in that a cutoff point has been established, indicating when the test is positive that infection has occurred. We get into trouble when these results are translated to mean that this animal with the positive test is, with absolute certainty, still infected now, and the other animal with the negative test is not.

To make decisions regarding the presence of infection in individuals usually requires repeated application of the same test to the same animal (similar to paired, acute, and convalescent sera from a patient) or application of multiple tests. For example, use of cultural procedures (or at least direct examination of tissue or fluid) may be needed to confirm presumptive serologic evidence that infection (and shedding) is present.[42] A **general strategy for testing** low-prevalence populations would involve either (1) initial application of an inexpensive, highly sensitive screening test followed with a highly specific confirmatory test of the screen test-positive individuals, or (2) using one test that is both highly sensitive and highly specific. The latter strategy is often more expensive but may be justified, especially in terminal stages of disease eradication. **Break-even curves** and other means of estimating risk are sometimes used to aid in making decisions.[34]

Another measure of a test is its **efficiency**, which is the frequency with which the test is correct. It is also dependent on the frequency of infection in the population and can be expressed quantitatively as follows:

$$\text{Test efficiency} = [A+D]/[A+B+C+D] = \text{true positive} + \text{true negative/total tested}$$

Using the tuberculin test model, test efficiency would be 127/172, or 74% (at 35.5% prevalence). Whereas, at a prevalence of 0.1%, it would be 62,033/ 100,000, or 62% of the time the test was correct.

Laboratory Evaluation

Finding the "user friendly" laboratory that is competent to perform the tests needed with the results available when they are needed may take some time. The farther away the laboratory from the clinician or epidemiologist who collected the specimens, i.e., beyond the individual's span of control, the more important it is to determine at the outset how the system works.[51] This is particularly true if the tests needed are not performed routinely in the local laboratory where personal contact can be established and maintained. Whenever special needs can be anticipated, it is advantageous to make contact beforehand to assure that all goes as expected when the need arises. A common example is knowing in advance what to do with the animal head when rabies is suspected, to avoid any delay in receiving a report. This is especially important when human exposure is involved and the answer is needed to decide on post-exposure treatment. One recommendation is to submit a specimen (e.g., head of dog that died of suspected distemper) initially to "test the system."

It is usually a good idea to divide specimens into two or more aliquots at the time of collection, and this is especially true when evaluating laboratory performance. Duplicate aliquots with different identification can be submitted. At least one additional aliquot should be withheld in the event the original shipment goes astray or if further testing/validation by the first or another laboratory is needed. If two or more laboratories are available, aliquots can be sent to each. Without standardization of test performance between laboratories, however, confusion can result from trying to make sense of different results obtained on tests of the same samples. In addition, several "known" test specimens discretely packaged and labeled to avoid detection and processing bias can be included. Just as this procedure is useful in initial identification of a satisfactory laboratory, it can be repeated whenever a change in performance quality is suspected.

Although effective communication is an essential element in the diagnostic process, which includes communication between clinician and laboratory, it is only a part of what is required to get the needed answer. The laboratory needs an adequate staff of trained people with sufficient physical facilities to perform according to acceptable standards. Acceptable **standards of performance**, or quality control standards, are not generally available for diagnostic laboratories to assure valid test results, and the quality of work varies within and between laboratories. Standard protocols for the performance and interpretation of specific tests are published. This does not equate to evaluating the **competency** of a laboratory to perform the tests. For example, when veterinarians submit fecal specimens to a laboratory where parasitologic examination of specimens from animals is not routine, they often receive spurious results.

In the United States, the first efforts to compare competencies between laboratories were done in the early 1930s, when the USPHS Communicable Disease Center (CDC) began evaluating ability to perform serologic tests for syphilis.[16] Mainly voluntary technical proficiency surveys of clinical and public health laboratories grew thereafter through the 1960s. Unknown specimens (including microbiologic and parasitologic) were distributed principally by mail. In 1934, the USDA initiated a national bovine brucellosis eradication program based on serologic testing and slaughter of seropositive (reactor) cattle. (Actually, Uniform Methods and Rules were first published in 1947.) A network of state-federal cooperative laboratories was established to perform the testing.[95] Laboratory personnel, whether state or federal, were trained by the USDA, and a system of USDA-administered check testing was begun that continues today. In the 1970s, the College of American Pathologists (CAP) took the lead in proficiency testing, after CDC reduced its activity in this area.[26] The CAP actually began a voluntary laboratory accreditation program in 1962. Since then, the CAP has accredited more than 4,300 laboratories. Federal obligatory standards are being developed as a result of the Clinical Laboratory Improvement Amendments (CLIA) of 1988.[17] The American Association of Veterinary Laboratory Diagnosticians (AAVLD) has developed a voluntary program for the accreditation of veterinary medical diagnostic laboratories.[4] As of 1991, 32 laboratories had been accredited nationwide.[5] Although there has been considerable activity and interest in the area, with the exception of the USDA program for bovine brucellosis serology, a generally accepted and utilized national system of evaluating performance of animal health and public health laboratories is not yet available in the United States.

Virtually every country in the world and its major political subdivisions require physicians and veterinarians to report cases of certain human and animal diseases. Many of these diseases are zoonotic, including plague and yellow fever, for which there are international **requirements for reporting** to the World Health Organization. In the United States, for example, there are 51 political subdivisions (states). Among them, as many as 53 zoonoses in people are considered reportable by a public health agency and as many as 33 zoonoses in animals are considered reportable by an agricultural (animal health) agency.[89] For most of these diseases, laboratory assistance is needed to be able to report a confirmatory, rather than presumptive, etiologic diagnosis. However, the laboratory assistance available to meet these needs may vary greatly among the state agencies involved. In a 1977 survey, the number of reportable diseases for which laboratory assistance was available among public health agencies varied from 8 to 51, and among agricultural agencies it varied from 1 to 44.[90] For some zoonoses considered reportable, therefore, even at the state level only a presumptive etiologic diagnosis is possible. Absence of reports is not presumptive of absence of disease.

Although infections do not recognize political boundaries, diseases often appear to do so.

Summary

1. The role of clinical laboratories emphasizes support for individual patient management whereas animal health and public health laboratories place greater emphasis on recognition of diseases in animal and human populations. These differences in principal purpose are reflected in the relatively greater capability of the latter laboratories to confirm etiologic diagnoses of zoonoses.

2. Most of the laboratory-acquired infections among biomedical laboratory personnel involve zoonotic agents. Appropriate precautions are essential to avoid the hazard of these often serious, occasionally life-threatening, diseases.

3. The specimen submitted is the usual, and generally most critical, connection between the clinician or epidemiologist and the laboratory. The material required to answer the diagnostic questions asked and the appropriate conditions for its transport should be established in advance by careful planning and communication among all concerned to avoid sometimes considerable fruitless effort.

4. The perfect test, or "gold standard," would always confirm an etiologic diagnosis when the infection is present, i.e., 100% sensitive, and never indicate the presence of infection when there is none, i.e., 100% specific. In addition, it would be rapid, inexpensive, and easy to perform.

5. Because of biological reasons involving agent, host, and test, at least a few false-positive and false-negative test results always occur. In addition, the predictive value of a test will vary depending on the frequency of the infection in the population.

6. As a result of the imperfections inherent in testing, strategies have been developed to gain the greatest recognition of those actually infected while keeping to a minimum the numbers falsely identified as infected. Frequently, this involves application of multiple tests applied in sequence, the first being highly sensitive to identify all actually infected and the second being highly specific to eliminate those who are not infected.

7. The value of laboratory tests depends, in part, on the skill of the individuals performing the tests. To obtain consistently accurate test results, a dependable laboratory is required. Initial selection and periodic evaluation of the laboratory should be done with care to assure its suitability to perform the tests needed.

References

1. Ades, A. E.: Evaluating the sensitivity and predictive value of tests of recent infection: toxoplasmosis in pregnancy. *Epidemiol Infect*, 107:527-535, 1991.
2. Al-Aska, A. K., and A. H. Chagla: Laboratory-acquired brucellosis. *J Hosp Infect*, 14:69-71, 1989.
3. Alton, G. G., J. Maw, B. A. Rogerson, et al.: The serological diagnosis of bovine brucellosis: An evaluation of the complement fixation, serum agglutination, and Rose Bengal tests. *Austral Vet J*, 51:57-63, 1975.
4. American Association of Veterinary Laboratory Diagnosticians, Inc.: *Essential Requirements for an Accredited Veterinary Medical Diagnostic Laboratory*, November, 1989.
5. American Association of Veterinary Laboratory Diagnosticians, Inc.: *Newsletter*, January, 1992.
6. American Thoracic Society: Diagnostic standards and classification of tuberculosis. *Am Rev Resp Dis*, 142:725-735, 1990.
7. Anon.: *National Institutes of Health Biohazards Safety Guide*. Washington, D.C., U.S. Government Printing Office, 1974.
8. Balows, A., W. J. Hausler, Jr., M. Ohashi, et al.: *Laboratory Diagnosis of Infectious Diseases, Principles and Practice, Volume I, Bacterial, Mycotic, and Parasitic Diseases*. New York, Springer-Verlag, 1988.
9. Beck, J. R., and E. K. Schultz: The use of relative operating characteristic (ROC) curves in test performance evaluation. *Arch Pathol Lab Med*, 110:13-20, 1986.
10. Behymer, D. E., H. P. Riemann, W. Utterback, et al.: Mass screening of cattle sera against 14 infectious disease agents, using an ELISA system for monitoring health in livestock. *Am J Vet Res*, 52:1699-1705, 1991.
11. Belding, D. L.: *Basic Clinical Parasitology*. New York, Appleton-Century-Crofts, 1958.
12. Bellver-Gallent, M., and V. R. Welte: *Animal Health Yearbook*, FAO Anim Prod Hlth Ser. No. 30. Rome, Food and Agriculture Organization of the United Nations, 1990.
13. Bennett, J. V., and P. S. Brachman: *Hospital Infections*, 3rd ed. Boston, Little, Brown, 1992.
14. Berends, B. R., J. F. M. Smeets, A. H. M. Harbers, et al.: Investigations with enzyme-linked immunosorbent assays for *Trichinella spiralis* and *Toxoplasma gondii* in the Dutch 'Integrated Quality Control for finishing pigs' research project. *Vet Q*, 13:190-198, 1991.
15. Blackwell, J. M.: Leishmaniasis epidemiology: all down to the DNA. *Parasitol*, 104:S19-S34, 1992.
16. Boone, D. J.: Evaluating laboratory performance: Historical and governmental perspectives. *Arch Pathol Lab Med*, 112:354-356, 1988.
17. Boone, D. J.: Literature review of research related to the Clinical Laboratory Improvement Amendments of 1988. *Arch Pathol Lab Med*, 116:681-693, 1992.
18. Brener, Z.: Laboratory-acquired Chagas disease: comment. *Trans R Soc Trop Med Hyg*, 81:527, 1987.

19. Brody, M. D.: AVMA guide for veterinary medical waste management. *J Am Vet Med Assoc*, 195:440-452, 1989.
20. Cannon, H. J., Jr., E. S. Goetz, A. C. Hamoudi, et al.: Rapid screening and microbiologic processing of pediatric urine specimens. *Diagn Microbiol Infect Dis*, 4:11-17, 1986.
21. Carter, G. R., and J. R. Cole, Jr.: *Diagnostic Procedures in Veterinary Bacteriology and Mycology*, 5th ed. New York, Academic Press, 1990.
22. Charlton, K. M., W. A. Webster, G. A. Casey, et al.: Recent advances in rabies diagnosis and research. *Can Vet J*, 27:85-89, 1986.
23. Christenson, V. D., and D. H. White: Evaluation of four commercially available ELISA assays for the serologic diagnosis of Lyme disease. *J Clin Lab Anal*, 5:340-343, 1991.
24. Clayman, M. D., A. Raymond, D. Colen, et al.: The *Limulus* amebocyte lysate assay. *Arch Intern Med*, 147:337-340, 1987.
25. Cohen, S., and K. S. Warren: *Immunology of Parasitic Infections*, 2nd ed. Boston, Blackwell Scientific, 1982.
26. College of American Pathologists: *Laboratory Accreditation Program*.
27. Collins, C. H., and J. M. Grange: *Isolation and Identification of Micro-organisms of Medical and Veterinary Importance*, Soc. Appl. Bacteriol. Tech. Ser. No. 21. New York, Academic Press, 1985.
28. Collins, C. H., E. G. Hartley, and R. Pilsworth: *The Prevention of Laboratory Acquired Infection*, Publ. Hlth. Lab. Serv. Monogr. Ser. No. 6. London, Her Majesty's Stationery Office, 1974.
29. Committee on Foreign Animal Diseases: *Foreign Animal Diseases*, 5th ed. Richmond, VA, United States Animal Health Association, 1992.
30. Coonrod, J. D., L. J. Kunz, and M. J. Ferraro: *The Direct Detection of Microorganisms in Clinical Samples*. New York, Academic Press, 1983.
31. Cottral, G. E.: *Manual of Standardized Methods for Veterinary Microbiology*. Ithaca, NY, Cornell University Press, 1978.
32. Cracea, E.: Q fever epidemiology in Romania. *Zbl Bakt Hyg A*, 267:7-9, 1987.
33. Cutler, S. J., and D. J. M. Wright: Evaluation of three commercial tests for Lyme disease. *Diag Microbiol Infect Dis*, 13:271-272, 1990.
34. Dargatz, D. A., and M. D. Salman: The use of break-even curves in decision making. *Compend Contin Ed Pract Vet*, 12:1347-1351, 1990.
35. Davies, E. T.: *Manual of Veterinary Investigation Laboratory Techniques*, Ref. Book 362, 2nd ed. Pinner, UK, Ministry of Agriculture, Fisheries and Food, 1978.
36. Dodd, K.: Estimation of the sensitivity, specificity and predictive value of the intradermal tuberculin test. *Irish Vet J*, 32:87-89, 1978.
37. Dohoo, I. R., P. F. Wright, G. M. Ruckerbauer, et al.: A comparison of five serological tests for bovine brucellosis. *Can J Vet Res*, 50:485-493, 1986.
38. Dominguez, A., J. Canela, and L. Salleras: Inclusion of laboratory test results in the surveillance of infectious diseases. *Int J Epidemiol*, 20:290-292, 1991.
39. Duncan, J. R., and K. W. Prasse: *Veterinary Laboratory Medicine*, 2nd ed. Ames, IA, Iowa State University Press, 1986.
40. Fawcett, P. T., K. M. Gibney, C. D. Rose, et al.: Adsorption with a soluble *E. coli* antigen fraction improves the specificity of ELISA tests for Lyme disease.

J Rheumatol, 18:705-708, 1991.

41. Feinstein, A. R.: *Clinical Epidemiology: The Architecture of Clinical Research.* Philadelphia, W. B. Saunders Co., 1985.

42. Feresu, S. B.: Isolation of *Leptospira interrogans* from kidneys of Zimbabwe beef cattle. *Vet Rec*, 130:446-448, 1992.

43. Gambino, R.: Diagnostic tests for Lyme disease. *J Am Med Assoc*, 264:692, 1990.

44. Glickman, L., P. Schantz, R. Dombroske, et al.: Evaluation of serodiagnostic tests for visceral larva migrans. *Am J Trop Med Hyg*, 27:492-498, 1978.

45. Goodman, J. L., P. Jurkovich, J. M. Kramber, et al.: Molecular detection of persistent *Borrelia burgdorferi* in the urine of patients with active Lyme disease. *Infect Immun*, 59:269-278, 1991.

46. Greenberg, A. E., L. S. Clesceri, and A. D. Eaton: *Standard Methods for the Examination of Water and Wastewater*, 18th ed. Washington, D.C., American Public Health Association, 1992.

47. Greenberg, A. E., and D. A. Hunt: *Laboratory Procedures for the Examination of Seawater and Shellfish*, 5th ed. Washington, D.C., American Public Health Association, 1984.

48. Henry, J. B.: *Clinical Diagnosis and Management by Laboratory Methods*, 16th ed. Philadelphia, W. B. Saunders, 1979.

49. Hill, W. E., and S. P. Keasler: Identification of foodborne pathogens by nucleic acid hybridization. *Int J Food Microbiol*, 12:67-75, 1991.

50. Hofflin, J. M., R. H. Sadler, F. G. Araujo, et al.: Laboratory-acquired Chagas disease. *Trans R Soc Trop Med Hyg*, 81:437-440, 1987.

51. Hubbert, W. T.: Leptospirosis in California. *Publ Hlth Rep*, 82:429-433, 1967.

52. Huber, J. D., and P. Nicoletti: Comparison of the results of card, Rivanol, complement-fixation, and milk ring tests with the isolation rate of *Brucella abortus* from cattle. *Am J Vet Res*, 47:1529-1531, 1986.

53. Hugh-Jones, M. E.: Utilization of a working serum bank. *Proceedings 4th International Symposium on Veterinary Epidemiology & Economics*, pp. 179-182. Singapore, Singapore Veterinary Assoc., 1986.

54. Isada, N. B., and J. H. Grossman III: A rapid screening test for the diagnosis of endocervical group B streptococci in pregnancy: Microbiologic results and clinical outcome. *Obstet Gynecol*, 70:139-141, 1987.

55. Jorgensen, J. H.: Clinical situations in which rapid methods may best be applied. *Diagn Microbiol Infect Dis*, 3:3S-7S, 1985.

56. Kaplan, M. M., and H. Koprowski: *Laboratory Techniques in Rabies*, 3rd ed., WHO Monogr. Ser. No. 23. Geneva, World Health Organization, 1973.

57. Kellar, J. A.: Canada's bovine serum bank—a practical approach. *Third International Symposium on Veterinary Epidemiology and Economics*, pp. 38-43. Edwardsville, KS, Veterinary Medicine Publ. Co., 1983.

58. Koontz, F. P.: A review of traditional resistance surveillance methodologies and infection control. *Diagn Microbiol Infect Dis*, 15:43S-47S, 1992.

59. Kramer, M. S.: *Clinical Epidemiology and Biostatistics*, 2nd ed. New York, Springer-Verlag, 1991.

60. Kramer, M. S., D. A. Lane, and E. L. Mills: Should blood cultures be obtained in the evaluation of young febrile children without evident focus of bacterial

infection? A decision analysis of diagnostic management strategies. *Pediatrics*, 84:18-27, 1989.

61. Kruse, R. H., W. H. Puckett, and J. H. Richardson: Biological safety cabinetry. *Clin Microbiol Rev*, 4:207-241, 1991.
62. Larghi, O. P., E. Gonzalez L., and J. R. Held: Evaluation of the corneal test as a laboratory method for rabies diagnosis. *Appl Microbiol*, 25:187-189, 1973.
63. Lennette, E. H., P. Halonen, and F. A. Murphy: *Laboratory Diagnosis of Infectious Diseases, Principles and Practice, Volume II, Viral, Rickettsial, and Chlamydial Diseases.* New York, Springer-Verlag, 1988.
64. Lloyd, G., and N. Jones: Infection of laboratory workers with hantavirus acquired from immunocytomas propagated in laboratory rats. *J Infect*, 12:117-125, 1986.
65. Luger, S. W., and E. Krauss: Serologic tests for Lyme disease. Interlaboratory variability. *Arch Intern Med*, 150:761-763, 1990.
66. Magnarelli, L. A.: Quality of Lyme disease tests. *J Am Med Assoc*, 262:3464-3465, 1989.
67. Marshall, R. T.: *Standard Methods for the Examination of Dairy Products*, 16th ed. Washington, D.C., American Public Health Association, 1992.
68. Martin, S. W., A. H. Meek, and P. Willeberg: *Veterinary Epidemiology: Principles and Methods.* Ames, IA, Iowa State University Press, 1987.
69. Mayer, L. W.: Use of plasmid profiles in epidemiologic surveillance of disease outbreaks and in tracing the transmission of antibiotic resistance. *Clin Microbiol Rev*, 1:228-243, 1988.
70. McDiarmid, S. C., and J. S. Hellstrom: An intradermal test for the diagnosis of brucellosis in extensively managed cattle herds. *Prev Vet Med*, 4:361-369, 1987.
71. McDiarmid, S. C., and J. S. Hellstrom: Surveillance for brucellosis using a skin test of low sensitivity. *Acta Vet Scand*, Suppl 84:209-211, 1988.
72. McNeil, B. J., and S. J. Adelstein: Determining the value of diagnostic and screening tests. *J Nucl Med*, 17:439-448, 1976.
73. McNeil, B. J., E. Keeler, and S. J. Adelstein: Primer on certain elements of medical decision making. *N Engl J Med*, 293:211-215, 1975.
74. Miller, C. D., J. R. Songer, and J. F. Sullivan: A twenty-five year review of laboratory-acquired human infections at the National Animal Disease Center. *Am Ind Hyg Assoc J*, 48:271-275, 1987.
75. Monfort, J. D., and G. Y. Miller: Evaluation and application of diagnostic tests in food animal practice. *Compend Contin Ed Pract Vet*, 12:1182-1190, 1990.
76. Montes, J., M. A. Rodriguez, T. Martin, and F. Martin: Laboratory-acquired meningitis caused by *Brucella abortus* Strain 19. *J Infect Dis*, 154:915-916, 1986.
77. Moorhouse, P. D., and M. E. Hugh-Jones: Serum banks. *Vet Bull*, 51:277-290, 1981.
78. More, S. J., and D. B. Copeman: A highly specific and sensitive monoclonal antibody-based ELISA for the detection of circulating antigen in bancroftian filariasis. *Trop Med Parasitol*, 41:403-406, 1990.
79. Muller, H. E.: Laboratory-acquired mycobacterial infection. *Lancet*, 2(8606): 331, 1988.
80. O'Reilly, L. M., and B. N. MacClancy: A comparison of the accuracy of a

human and a bovine tuberculin PPD for testing cattle with a comparative-cervical test. *Irish Vet J*, 29:63- 70, 1975.

81. Poedjomartono, S., and D. H. A. Unruh: The development of laboratory supported disease investigation system in developing countries: The Indonesian experience. *Proceedings 4th International Symposium on Veterinary Epidemiology & Economics*, pp. 189-192, Singapore, Singapore Veterinary Assoc., 1986.

82. Rayburn, S. R.: *The Foundations of Laboratory Safety, A Guide for the Biomedical Laboratory*. New York, Springer-Verlag, 1990.

83. Richardson, J. H., and W. E. Barkley (eds.): *Biosafety in Microbiological and Biomedical Laboratories*, 2nd ed., HHS Publ. No. (NIH) 88-8395. Washington, D.C., U.S. Government Printing Office, 1988.

84. Robertson, T. G.: Diagnosis of bovine tuberculosis. 1- The evaluation of tuberculin tests. *N Z Vet J*, 11:6-10, 1963.

85. Rock, R. C.: Interpreting laboratory tests: A basic approach. *Geriatrics*, 39:49-50, 53-54, 1984.

86. Rudd, R. J., and C. V. Trimarchi: Development and evaluation of an in vitro virus isolation procedure as a replacement for the mouse inoculation test in rabies diagnosis. *J Clin Microbiol*, 27:2522-2528, 1989.

87. Sackett, D. L., R. B. Haynes, G. H. Guyatt, et al.: *Clinical Epidemiology: A Basic Science for Clinical Medicine*, 2nd ed. Boston, Little, Brown and Co., 1991.

88. Schmidt, N. J., and R. W. Emmons: *Diagnostic Procedures for Viral, Rickettsial, and Chlamydial Infections*, 6th ed. Washington, D.C., American Public Health Association, 1989.

89. Schnurrenberger, P. R., and W. T. Hubbert: Reporting of zoonotic diseases. *Am J Epidemiol*, 112:23-31, 1980.

90. Schnurrenberger, P. R., and W. T. Hubbert: Correlation between laboratory services and reporting requirements for selected zoonoses. *Publ Hlth Rep*, 96:162-165, 1981.

91. Schnurrenberger, P. R., and W. T. Hubbert: *Outline of the Zoonoses*. Ames, IA, Iowa State University Press, 1982.

92. Silverman, J. F.: *Guides to Clinical Aspiration Biopsy, Infectious and Inflammatory Diseases and Other Nonneoplastic Disorders*. New York, Igaku-Shoin, 1991.

93. Simmons, M. L.: *Biohazards and Zoonotic Problems of Primate Procurement, Quarantine, and Research*, DHEW Publ. No. (NIH) 76-890. Frederick, MD, Litton Bionetics, 1976.

94. Sloss, M. W., and R. L. Kemp: *Veterinary Clinical Parasitology*, 5th ed. Ames, IA, Iowa State University Press, 1978.

95. Smith, R. W. (chr.): *A Review of the Cooperative State-Federal Brucellosis Eradication Program*. Washington, D.C., U.S. Department of Agriculture, January 1964.

96. Spence, M. R.: A rapid screening test for the diagnosis of endocervical group B streptococci in pregnancy: Microbiologic results and clinical outcome (letter). *Obstet Gynecol*, 71:284, 1988.

97. Staneck, J. L.: Screening tests and "rapid" identification. Is anybody out there listening? *Diagn Microbiol Infect Dis*, 3:51S-57S, 1985.

98. Steckelberg, J. M., C. L. Terrell, and R. S. Edson: Laboratory-acquired

Salmonella typhimurium enteritis: Association with erythema nodosum and reactive arthritis. *Am J Med*, 85:705-707, 1988.

99. Strafuss, A. C.: *Necropsy Procedures and Basic Diagnostic Methods for Practicing Veterinarians.* Springfield, IL, Charles C. Thomas, 1988.

100. Swann, A. I., C. L. Garby, P. R. Schnurrenberger, et al.: Safety aspects in preparing suspensions of field strains of *Brucella abortus* for serological identification. *Vet Rec*, 109:254-255, 1981.

101. Swets, J. A.: Measuring the accuracy of diagnostic systems. *Science*, 240:1285-1293, 1988.

102. Thorne, G. M.: Diagnosis of infectious diarrheal diseases. *Infect Dis Clin North Am*, 2:747-774, 1988.

103. Thrusfield, M.: *Veterinary Epidemiology.* London, Butterworths, 1986.

104. Thurmond, M. C., J. P. Picanso, and S. K. Hietala: Prospective serology and analysis in diagnosis of dairy cow abortion. *J Vet Diagn Invest*, 2:274-282, 1990.

105. Tilkian, S. M., M. B. Conover, and A. G. Tilkian: *Clinical implications of laboratory tests.* St. Louis, C. V. Mosby, 1979.

106. Timbs, D. V.: The New Zealand national bovine serum bank. *Proceedings of the Second International Symposium on Veterinary Epidemiology and Economics*, pp 76-80. Canberra, Australian Government Publishing Service, 1980.

107. Tokue, Y., S. Shoji, K. Satoh, et al.: Comparison of a polymerase chain reaction assay and a conventional microbiologic method for detection of methicillin-resistant *Staphylococcus aureus. Antimicrob Agents Chemother*, 36:6-9, 1992.

108. Truszczynski, M., J. Pearson, and S. Edwards: *Manual of Standards for Diagnostic Tests and Vaccines*, for Lists A and B diseases of mammals, birds and bees, 2nd ed. Paris, Office International des Epizooties, 1992.

109. Tyler, J. W., and J. S. Cullor: Titers, tests, and trisms: Rational interpretation of diagnostic serologic testing. *J Am Vet Med Assoc*, 194:1550-1558, 1989.

110. Vanderzant, C., and D. F. Splittstoesser, eds.: *Compendium of Methods for the Microbiological Examination of Foods*, 3rd ed. Washington, D.C., American Public Health Association, 1992.

111. Vesley, D., and H. M. Hartmann: Laboratory-acquired infections and injuries in clinical laboratories: A 1986 survey. *Am J Publ Hlth*, 78:1213-1215, 1988.

112. Walls, K. W., and P. M. Schantz: *Immunodiagnosis of Parasitic Diseases*, Vol. 1, Helminthic Diseases. New York, Academic Press, 1986.

113. Wang, E., and H. Richardson: A rapid method for detection of group B streptococcal colonization: Testing at the bedside. *Obstet Gynecol*, 76:882-885, 1990.

114. Webster, W. A.: A tissue culture infection test in routine rabies diagnosis. *Can J Vet Res*, 51:367-369, 1987.

115. Wedum, A. G., W. E. Barkley, and A. Hellman: Handling of infectious agents. *J Am Vet Med Assoc*, 161:1557-1567, 1972.

116. Wentworth, B. B.: *Diagnostic Procedures for Bacterial Infections*, 7th ed. Washington, D.C., American Public Health Association, 1987.

117. Wentworth, B. B.: *Diagnostic Procedures for Mycotic and Parasitic Infections*, 7th ed. Washington, D.C., American Public Health Association, 1988.

118. Wilson, M., and J. B. McAuley: Laboratory diagnosis of toxoplasmosis. *Clin*

Lab Med, 11:923-939, 1991.

119. Wisecarver, J. L., M. C. Haven, and R. S. Markin: A macro-driven Lotus 1-2-3™ template for calculating and plotting receiver-operator characteristic curves for clinical laboratory tests. *Comput Biol Med,* 20:121-127, 1990.

120. Wong, T. W., Y. C. Chan, E. H. Yap, et al.: Serological evidence of hantavirus infection in laboratory rats and personnel. *Int J Epidemiol,* 17:887-890, 1988.

121. Woo, J. H., J. Y. Cho, Y. S.Kim, et al.: A case of laboratory-acquired murine typhus. *Korean J Intern Med,* 5:118-122, 1990.

122. Young, P., N. Hunt, I. Ibrahim, et al.: Establishment of a national serum bank in Indonesia. In: *Veterinary Viral Diseases: Their Significance in South-East Asia and the Western Pacific,* A.J. Della-Porta, ed. Sydney, Academic Press Australia, 1985, pp. 581-584.

4

PRINCIPLES OF
ZOONOSES CONTROL
AND PREVENTION

Prevention, Control, and Eradication

The world's population at the beginning of the 14th-century plague epidemic is estimated to have been only 100 million people, yet Europe had 25 million deaths resulting from plague in that century. Today, plague is not endemic in Europe. By means of calfhood vaccination and slaughter of reactor adult cattle, the prevalence of bovine brucellosis in the United States has decreased dramatically, and in countries such as Denmark it has been eradicated. As the reservoir of infection in domestic animals decreased, human exposure and the number of human cases of brucellosis also decreased.[65,115] Since World War II the annual incidence of rabies among domestic animals in the United States has declined primarily as a result of reduction in canine rabies brought about by immunization campaigns. From these examples, it is obvious that great strides have been made in the control of zoonotic diseases in the developed nations.[1,56,112] This chapter describes the techniques for accomplishing prevention, control, and eradication.[4,10,68,99]

There is an important distinction among the terms "prevention," "control," and "eradication." **Prevention** is defined as inhibiting the introduction of a disease agent into an area, a specific population group, or an individual. **Control** efforts consist of steps taken to reduce a disease problem to a tolerable level and maintain it at that level. The term "control" is more appropriate when a given infectious disease agent is already present. For example, an arboviral infection may be endemic in a wildlife reservoir in an area where eradication is not feasible, but its impact may be greatly reduced in people and domestic animals by vector control and immunization programs. Mastitis is impossible to completely prevent, even in the best managed dairy herds, but a good control program will greatly reduce the number of clinical as well as subclinical cases.[89]

Prevention and control are sometimes referred to as "primary prevention" and "secondary prevention." **Primary prevention** is aimed at maintaining a healthy population, i.e., preventing the occurrence of disease. **Secondary prevention** attempts to minimize damage after disease has occurred. Rehabilitation, after both primary and secondary prevention have failed, is sometimes referred to as **"tertiary prevention."**[100] An important economic aspect of disease control and prevention programs is that, as one progresses from primary through secondary to tertiary prevention, the cost increases per unit of population.

Eradication is the final step in a disease control program. It consists of the elimination of a disease-producing agent from a defined population or geographic area. The first serious proposal to eradicate an infectious disease (smallpox) was presented in 1767 by a Dr. Maty in a paper entitled "The Advantages of Early Inoculation."[19] To achieve eradication of a disease-producing agent from an area or population, it is necessary to obstruct transmission until endemicity (including carriers) ceases, and prevent the reestablishment of the agent from imported sources of infection.[35,52,76] The disease may be eliminated (brucellosis from a herd of cows; tuberculosis from herds in a political subdivision) yet remain a threat to animals in that population as a result of travel of susceptible animals out of the area or import of infected animals or animal products. *Brucella melitensis*, for example, has not been reported from the United States goat population for more than 50 years, but people along the Mexico/United States border have been infected with the organism. During the period 1982 through 1986, 67% of human cases in the United States were linked to the ingestion of cheese that had been made from unpasteurized goat milk and brought across the border from Mexico.[104,116]

There is a distinction between total eradication and practical eradication. **Total eradication** means that the disease agent has been completely removed from the area of concern. On a worldwide basis, smallpox is the only disease agent that has been totally eradicated.[38,39] **Practical eradication** refers to the elimination of the organism from the reservoirs of importance to humans or their domestic animals, rather than total eradication from the region. For example, practical eradication of canine rabies has been accomplished in the United States, whereas eradication of rabies from the wildlife reservoir has not been achieved. A frequent limitation of attempting total eradication is economic. In test-and-slaughter programs, for instance, the initial cost of identifying infected individuals is low on a per animal basis when the prevalence is high. As the program progresses, and the prevalence decreases, the effort and time required to identify the remaining infected animals increases exponentially without careful planning.

Practical eradication also has limitations. A primary limitation, as mentioned above with rabies, is the lack of effective methods for eradicating agents from wildlife reservoirs, especially when the reservoir consists of multiple species. Attempting to eliminate vectorborne agents when the vector utilizes wildlife hosts is another example of the limitations of practical eradication. It may not be difficult to remove mosquitoes in areas populated primarily by humans, but the task often becomes difficult (and expensive) when the ecologic niche of the vector is among wildlife. Sometimes the term **"disease free"** is used to describe an area in which the incidence or prevalence of a particular disease of interest has dropped below a certain level—usually an identified goal in a control program. This term was used by the U.S. Department of Agriculture in its brucellosis eradication program. An area was designated brucellosis free when the known herd infection rate dropped below 1.0%. (This terminology has been replaced by a "Free, A, B, or C" classification scale, each denoting different levels of herd infection.)[83,107,110]

The basic principles of zoonoses control and prevention programs are focused upon breaking the chain of transmission at its epidemiologically weakest link. Three factors are involved: the reservoir, transmission from the reservoir to the susceptible host, and the susceptible host. These principles are described in the following sections.

Reservoir Neutralization

The ultimate source of zoonotic infection is the infected reservoir host. Whenever infection in the reservoir can be reduced or eradicated, other sources of infection progressively become less significant or disappear. Three methods used to neutralize the reservoir are (1) removing infected individuals, (2) rendering infected individuals "non-shedders," and (3) manipulating the environment. Increasing host resistance, which will be described later as a separate control method, also can neutralize a reservoir if the number of infected animals is reduced, such as that which happened with smallpox vaccination of humans and rabies immunization of dogs.

Removal of infected individuals can be accomplished in two ways: (1) test and slaughter, and (2) mass therapy.

Infection may be removed from a herd by **testing and slaughtering** those found to be infected. This method has been successfully used to control bovine brucellosis and tuberculosis as well as equine dourine and glanders. To be effective, a sufficiently sensitive and specific test is required, i.e., all infected animals need to be detected by the test if all infection is to be erased without removing large numbers of false-positive animals. When such a test is not available, it may be necessary to use a less-sensitive test, such as clinical diagnosis, on which to base a decision. Even before initial recognition of the agent, bovine pleuropneumonia, foot-and-mouth disease, and scrapie could be differentiated clinically and eradicated. Adequate history and individual identification of each animal tested must be provided to properly interpret test results and assure recognition of reactors. When using serologic tests, it is important to realize that the term "reactor" is not absolute. With bovine brucellosis, for example, an agglutination titer of 1/100 would be a positive finding for a non-vaccinated cow. If a cow that had been calfhood vaccinated with *Brucella abortus* strain 19 had the same titer, it would be classed as "suspect" because the vaccine may produce an elevation in titer. This is a problem particularly in animals vaccinated as adults. Once animals have been identified as infected, stringent controls are necessary to ensure their prompt removal unless they can be rendered safe by treatment or isolation. Two factors that affect the decision to use test and slaughter are expense and the method of transmission. This method has been most effective with agents spread by direct transmission and in which a limited number of reservoir species are involved. The high cost to government and industry has prevented its use in many countries.

Often, with highly prevalent infectious diseases, the initial approach has been to increase host resistance by immunization (such as with bovine brucellosis) to decrease the reservoir before instituting test and slaughter. With foot-and-mouth disease, slaughtered animals were buried or burned, thus increasing the cost by loss of salvageable carcasses. The longer a program is needed to reach its desired goals, the greater the cost of administration. The bovine brucellosis and tuberculosis eradication programs in the United States are examples of lengthy and, therefore, expensive programs. Loss of breeding stock may destroy a valuable gene pool, as occurred with the destruction of prized Suffolk sheep flocks affected with scrapie. Slaughter of affected animals will be ineffective if an inanimate reservoir exists. Also, the efficiency of slaughter decreases as the host range of interspecies transmission increases, particularly if wildlife are included. If the agent is vectorborne, it is usually more economical to control the vector than to eliminate the infection in the vertebrate reservoir, particularly if the reservoir is a wildlife species. Specific-pathogen-free (SPF) programs, such as have been developed in swine herds and laboratory animal colonies, also are examples of reservoir neutralization to prevent disease.

Examples of control programs that use test and slaughter to remove infected individuals are those developed for bovine brucellosis, bovine tuberculosis, and avian pullorum disease. In the brucellosis control program, the "card test" (an agglutination test), which is very sensitive (but not extremely specific), is used to identify infected animals. Animals that "card test" positive are then retested for brucellosis antibody using a more specific test like the rivanol, complement fixation, or Particle Concentration Fluorescence Immunoassay (PCFIA) test.[107] For the brucellosis test to be effective, it is necessary that accurate immunization records be available for the correct interpretation of test results.

In the tuberculosis program, a skin test is used, similar to the Mantoux test for humans. This test cross-reacts with other mycobacteria and with infections and conditions that produce connective tissue or granulomatous responses.[114] Efficiency of this test is greater when the prevalence of *M. bovis* infection is high, i.e., a lower percentage of false positives will result. As the prevalence decreases, the proportion of cows with no visible lesions at slaughter will increase. Test sensitivity will vary with injection site, the number of units of the antigen (PPD) used, and stage of infection (anergy).

To control pullorum disease in poultry, an agglutination test is used to detect infected birds.

Examples of diseases that have been eradicated from many countries using the test-and-slaughter method are equine dourine and glanders. In the dourine eradication program, a complement fixation test was used to detect horses infected with *Trypanosoma equiperdum*. For detection of horses infected with *Pseudomonas mallei*, the causative agent of glanders, the mallein skin test was utilized.

A second method for neutralizing the reservoir by removing infected individuals is **mass therapy**. Mass therapy is usually restricted to a local situation in which all potentially infected animals or people are treated without first testing them to identify infected individuals. In certain situations, particularly with endemic diseases in the less-developed portions of the world where diagnostic resources may be minimal, treatment without prior screening may reduce the cost factor 2 to 6 times.[17] The cost effectiveness of mass therapy as a control method increases as the prevalence of infection in the population increases. For example, it is 10 times more cost effective if, at the beginning of treatment, 100% are infected rather than 10%. For control purposes, the treatment must eliminate infection in carriers, not just cure clinical illness. Risks associated with mass therapy, particularly if improperly done, are the development of resistant strains of infectious agents and adverse side effects.

The antibiotic treatment of parakeets imported into the United States, to prevent human psittacosis, and the prevention of echinococcosis by treating all dogs in a given geographic area, to break the dog-sheep cycle, are examples of mass therapy of animal reservoirs.[8,18,72,84,86]

Many of the problems associated with internal parasites of humans are being reduced by mass therapy. Diethylcarbamazine is being used to combat loiasis,[84] and ivermectin is being used to combat onchocerciasis.[108] Combined with vector control, mass therapy has reduced the incidence of schistosomiasis and African trypanosomiasis.[49,77] Using syndrome surveillance as a measure of success, China has reported the eradication of venereal disease (pre-AIDS) through mass therapy.[55,96,97]

Environmental manipulation is a method of reservoir neutralization designed to break the chain of transmission between the portal of exit of the infected (shedder) host and the susceptible host by reducing survival of the agent in vectors or vehicles (food, water, soil, vegetation). The environment of concern is wherever the agent may be found outside the vertebrate host. A limitation is that it is a local measure, effective only in the immediate area where the controls are actually instituted. Various parasite control strategies that provide examples of this approach are proper fecal waste disposal (acting on the portal of exit), disinfection of fecal wastes, and pasture rotation to decrease exposure of susceptible hosts (portal of entry).[47] Provision of adequate toilet facilities, coupled with education and supervision to ensure their use, will prevent the spread of *Taenia saginata* from feedlot employees to cattle. If facilities are not convenient, employees may use haystacks, feed bunks, or other locations, which can result in contamination of cattle feed.[60] The use of fermentation lagoons to destroy agents transmitted by the fecal-oral route has proven very successful. Recently, composting, using aerobic, thermophilic bacteria, has been introduced as a cost-effective method for reducing the viability of infective organisms contained in organic wastes.[79] If human waste is to be used for fertilization of pastures, it is important to first provide proper sewage treatment to prevent transmission of viable parasite ova before the effluent is applied to pastures.

Snail intermediate hosts of flukes require water to complete their life cycle. Therefore, to augment the seasonal use of flukicides, fencing ponds to prevent access by livestock and creating effective drainage are examples of how the environment may be changed to control infection. If the source of water is essential for maintaining livestock, molluscicides may be used to kill the snails.

Pasture rotation has long been used to reduce exposure to gastrointestinal nematodes. The time required to produce a significant reduction in the numbers of infective larvae will vary, depending upon the species. In warm climates (with little kill by cold or freezing), the interval may be so long that it may be necessary to alternate pasture use with row crop cultivation, or alternate host species on the pasture, e.g., cattle vs horses.

Environmental manipulation may also be used to control vectors of disease agents. The efficiency of this control method depends upon the life cycle of the vector. In some situations, disruption of the vector's habitat (breeding sites or resting places) has been successful, but in many instances, a direct attack upon the vector is more effective. Insecticides may be applied to animals by dipping, dusting, spraying, or the use of collars, tags, or (for small mammal reservoirs) insecticide-baited boxes. This approach, however, may have disadvantages. An agent such as *Babesia bigemina*, which uses only a one-host tick as its vector, is much more vulnerable to attack than an agent utilizing a two- or three-host tick vector. Another disadvantage of this method is that arthropods develop resistance to pesticides, necessitating constant monitoring to assure effectiveness, and alternating chemicals if resistance develops. Wide-scale spraying, such as is done by crop dusters or during major outbreaks of mosquitoborne disease, has the added disadvantage of possible destruction of beneficial arthropods or, with some chemicals, illness among domestic animals or humans. The effectiveness of preventing mosquitoborne encephalitides by using mosquito reduction programs to neutralize the reservoir will vary. During an epidemic of Venezuelan equine encephalomyelitis, for example, newly infected horses serve as highly viremic, amplifying hosts, capable of infecting not only thousands of mosquitoes per horse, but also biting flies, which can then serve as mechanical vectors. Mosquito reduction programs, which are seldom 100% effective, will not halt the outbreak. Concurrent vaccination of horses is required to prevent their infection (and death) and subsequent infection of more mosquitoes.

Introduction of sterilized males, which has been very effective in eradicating screwworms, depends upon the life cycle and breeding pattern of the arthropod. This method would not be as effective in controlling screwworms if the proportion of nonirradiated males was high or if the female flies bred with more than one male. Biological control, using natural predators or pathogens of vectors, has been used with some success to reduce mosquito populations. Examples are introduction of *Gambusia* fish to consume mosquito larvae and use of a competitor snail, *Marisa cornuarietis*, to drive out *Australorbis* spp. snails, an intermediate host of schistosomes. This technique, however, is dependent upon the population density of the vector and has ecologic limitations.[27,67,82,113]

A contributing factor to the rabies problem in some Latin American nations has been the presence of open dumps that provide food sources and harborage for stray dogs.[9,98] Proper landfill operations, coupled with scavenger control programs, can alter the environment to reduce this problem. In some situations, the environmental manipulation is done on a small scale as, for example, when a rodent eradication program is instituted around a feed mill to remove the source of fecal contamination of feed with infectious agents such as salmonellae.

Environmental manipulation is used extensively when the immediate source of infection is inanimate. To be precise, this may be referred to as **vehicle manipulation**. It is used in water purification, pasteurization, food (human and animal) preservation, and disinfection.

Purification of drinking water has become so commonplace in developed societies that the role of water as a source of microbiologic contamination is sometimes overlooked. In any outbreak investigation involving enteric pathogens, drinking water must be considered as a source, even in communities with water purification systems. Water, for example, is consistently implicated as the source of most *Giardia* infections originating in the United States. Whereas the vegetative form of protozoan parasites is easily destroyed by chlorination, the cyst stage is not, and cities that get their water from rivers or lakes often are not required to use sand filtration, which will remove these cysts. A similar situation exists with *Taenia* wherever numerous human shedders occur and inadequately treated sewage effluent is used on pastures. Although water and sewage treatment may be adequate for protection against enteric bacterial pathogens, additional precautions may be needed with some zoonotic parasites that involve sewage and waterborne spread in endemic areas. Boiling water or using iodine (which will kill the encysted stage of protozoa) for water disinfection while traveling may be the only safe alternative, particularly for individuals with lowered resistance. The use of sewage for fertilizing pastures can present risks from toxic chemicals (heavy metals, etc.) as well as from infectious (parasitic) agents and, therefore, is not generally recommended.

Pasteurization, developed initially to stop fermentation of wine, has been used to control milkborne tuberculosis transmission as well as to extend somewhat the shelf life of milk. It has progressed from the effective, but slow, long-time holding process, through short-time, high-temperature systems, to today's ultra-high-temperature procedure, which only requires a few seconds to achieve desired results. The key to success in this procedure is the relationship between temperature and time. The older, slow method used a temperature of 61.7°C/143°F for 30 minutes to destroy tubercle bacilli. Later it was increased to 62.8°C/145°F to destroy *Coxiella burneti*. Ultrapasteurization takes only 2 seconds but requires a temperature of 138°C/280°F. There is an axiom that any mechanical system is only as good as its operator. During the last few years, *Listeria monocytogenes* outbreaks have been traced back to inadequately pasteurized milk. Furthermore, the availability of pasteurization systems in a community does not guarantee that all milk or milk products consumed will have passed through these systems. In spite of ample evidence linking the consumption of raw milk with foodborne disease, it is, like bootleg liquor, usually available for those who want it and, in many areas, *legally* so.

Disease agents in food can be controlled by several procedures, including application of heat or cold, dehydration, irradiation, and treatment with preservative chemicals.[58] The application of heat, as it is used in modern canning techniques, is the most common way of ensuring the mass distribution of safe food. Unlike pasteurization, which is designed only to remove pathogens, the canning procedure, when done properly, sterilizes the food, i.e., ensures destruction of all microbial contaminants. Because of this, countries where foot-and-mouth disease is endemic can legally ship canned meat products to the United States. The canning process uses destruction of nontoxic, putrefactive clostridia as the standard to ensure that the highly toxigenic, but less heat tolerant, *Clostridium botulinum* is destroyed.

Low temperatures provide an excellent means of preserving food, and very low temperatures (freezing), using a time-temperature relationship, is used as a method for destroying the cysts of *Taenia saginata* in beef, *Trichinella spiralis* in pork, and *Anisakis* larvae in fish. Although low temperature is a very effective method for food preservation, it is also an Achilles heel. Most foodborne disease outbreaks reported in the United States are the result of a breakdown in the cold chain somewhere along the distribution path.

Dehydration is effective in preserving food because it reduces enzymatic activity within cells, thereby retarding autolytic changes, and decreases the moisture content, producing an unfavorable environment for bacterial growth and survival.

As early as 1921, a U.S. patent was issued for using X rays to destroy trichinae in pork. Acceptance of irradiation as a method of food preservation has been slow because of public fear that irradiated food might be carcinogenic or present other hazards. Also, the food industry has been reluctant to use irradiation because doing so might be interpreted by the public as a mechanism to market contaminated meat. Another complication is the fact that in some countries, such as the United States, irradiation of food has been subject to restrictive governmental regulations. Currently, these restrictions in the United States limit the amount of irradiation, measured in kilogreys (kGy), that can be used for treating food. The amount of irradiation required to destroy pathogens in meat, fish, or seafood is 1 to 10 kGy; to achieve sterilization, 10 to 50 kGy. Currently, in the United States, raw, packaged poultry can be irradiated at 1.5 to 3.0 kGy.[22]

Chemical preservation, using various "curing" agents, is a universal practice. Most of the chemicals used serve a dual function. In addition to preventing the growth of microbial contaminants, they also serve as flavor enhancers, improve the water-holding ability of the product, or serve as color fixatives. Most of the chemicals, in the quantities used, are nontoxic but some, such as nitrate salts, which can break down to carcinogenic nitrosoamines, are potentially hazardous, and the concentrations are controlled by testing the finished product.

These procedures also can be used to safeguard food for animals. To prevent spread of infection from the dam to newborn calves via colostrum, the calf may be removed from the dam immediately after birth and fed colostrum that has been pasteurized. Adequate cooking of garbage containing pork scraps will prevent transmission of vesicular exanthema virus and *Trichinella spiralis* from this source. The two major limitations to this method are (1) use of equipment that will heat the garbage thoroughly (some means of agitation is usually needed), and (2) adequate supervision (inspection) to ensure that only cooked garbage is fed. Swine also may be exposed to *T. spiralis* by consuming infected rats, common around garbage-feeding operations.[5] Rendering, in addition to providing fats for soap or cooking, also provides an efficient method for using heat to recycle valuable animal proteins not used for human consumption into animal food. Heat treatment of bone meal is an effective method for preventing transmission of *Bacillus anthracis* in animal food supplements.

Disinfection is sometimes confused with sterilization. Disinfection is somewhat akin to pasteurization, i.e., steps have been taken to ensure that pathogenic microorganisms have been removed or destroyed. **Sterilization** means that *all* microorganisms have been destroyed.[12,21,93] In both of these approaches to preventing transmission, prior mechanical cleaning is required to ensure the desired results. It is practically impossible to disinfect or sterilize dirty materials with chemicals because they are neutralized or inactivated by organic materials. When veterinarians scrub their boots with soap and water and then apply a quaternary ammonium compound before proceeding to the next call, they are performing cleaning and disinfection. When surgeons remove organic material from their surgical instruments and then place them into an autoclave and subject them to the proper combination of time, temperature, and pressure, they are cleaning and sterilizing. Disinfection of the hands of hospital personnel by washing with soap followed by a rinse with alcohol or an antimicrobial agent has proven effective in reducing nosocomial infections.[25,46]

Reducing Contact Potential

A basic principle in preventing direct transmission of an infectious agent from an infected individual to a susceptible host is to reduce the opportunity for contact. In disease control, two populations are considered: the known infected and the potentially exposed susceptibles.

Three methods are used: (1) isolation or treatment of cases, (2) quarantine of possibly infected individuals, and (3) population control. Note the different use of terms: isolation of known cases of infection and quarantine of individuals suspected of having been exposed. Simply put, isolation is designed to keep the agent *in*, whereas quarantine is designed to keep the agent *out*. The laminar flow hood, familiar to all who have worked in a microbiology laboratory, is an application of the basic principle of isolation, keeping the agent *in* (the hood), thereby protecting the technician. **Herd immunity**, which will be described under the topic of disease control by increasing host resistance, also is a method for reducing contact potential. When the proportion of immune animals in a given population is sufficiently great, a disease agent transmitted by direct contact cannot enter and spread because the opportunity for contact between infected (shedder) animals and susceptible animals has been reduced.

Isolation of an infected, clinically ill animal has two advantages; it reduces the probability of contact with a susceptible host and facilitates treatment and disinfection. Because this approach depends on early and accurate diagnosis for effective disease control, programs based on isolating and treating cases to prevent the spread of infectious disease agents have serious shortcomings and frequently fail. Furthermore, this approach is generally ineffective if shedding occurs during the incubationary period or if healthy carriers are shedding. An exception is when all animals in a group are isolated as, for example, when individual calving facilities are used in *Brucella* reactor herds.

Quarantine of apparently healthy individuals that may have been exposed to a source of infection had its beginnings during the second plague pandemic. When ships arrived from the Middle East where plague was endemic, the crews were restricted from landing for 40 days after arrival. By experience, the authorities knew that this was how long to wait to see if any human cases occurred. It was also how long it took for infected fleas to die. To be effective, quarantine has to be enforced for the longest incubation period of the disease in question, to see if the suspected infected develop detectable disease. It is not effective with diseases involving chronically infected healthy shedders. The population quarantined may be a single animal, as with a biting dog suspected of being rabid, or may include an entire herd of cows exposed to tuberculosis to see if they become tuberculin positive. Geographic areas that are free of rabies, such as the United Kingdom and Hawaii, utilize a 4- to 6-month quarantine for dogs and cats.[1,10,56]

The **"closed-herd"** concept is actually an application of quarantine. A farmer operating a dairy herd under this principle will raise all replacement stock rather than purchasing replacements and, by so doing, reduce the risk of introducing an agent of disease. This procedure demands an excellent reproduction program but is advantageous because the need for protective immunization is reduced to the bare minimum. Portable pens for raising dairy calves allow some quarantine space between calves to control agents spread by direct contact. Their portability is especially useful in controlling gastrointestinal parasitism, for the pens can be moved regularly to facilitate cleaning the ground to break the cycle of transmission. The placement of animals, whether in laboratory animal colonies, farms, or feedlots, should be done with the principles of isolation and quarantine in mind, establishing flow patterns that minimize contact between healthy, susceptible animals and sources of infection. Animals, animal products, feedstuffs, bedding, vehicles, water sources, and personnel must all be evaluated as potential sources of disease agents.

Health requirements are meant to act as barriers against disease. When applied to animal disease control, they also may act as barriers to trade. Import prohibition usually refers to animals and carcasses known to be affected, as well as to those originating from areas where the absence of such diseases has not been adequately demonstrated. Countries with endemic foot-and-mouth disease (FMD) or rinderpest often are unable to ship beef to profitable foreign markets because of animal health restrictions. To aid developing nations, the Food and Agriculture Organization (FAO) of the United Nations has promoted the creation of **"disease-free zones"** in countries not entirely free of FMD or rinderpest. Some of these countries have certain well-defined zones that are free of these diseases, usually associated with geographic situations favorable for disease control, such as islands, large rivers, or mountain ranges. It is more difficult to create a disease-free zone within the land mass of a country, but it is feasible through the use of a feedlot beef production system in which an abattoir that produces boneless beef (reduces the risk of agent spread) for export is an integral part. A well-organized veterinary program is essential to maintain a disease-free zone, particularly because potential importing countries will require these functions as a condition for accepting imports from the zone. The program should include (1) adequate veterinary staff empowered with legal authority for function, (2) disease surveillance, (3) a laboratory for typing FMD virus and rinderpest differential diagnoses, (4) complete control of domestic livestock movement (including identification), (5) a meat hygiene program under veterinary supervision, and (6) an abattoir that meets the hygiene requirements of importing countries. The zone should be free of FMD for at least 1 year and free of rinderpest for at least 2 years before it is approved.[11,62,64,88,106]

Population control programs are another method of reducing contact. Control may be relatively benign, as is seen with leash laws and with the restriction of movement of sheep through human population centers in towns in the western United States during lambing season (when Q fever occurs from airborne spread). On the other hand, population control may be very drastic, as when population reduction is utilized.

Leash laws have been designed primarily to control rabies and reduce fecal contamination. Dogs, defecating on beaches and parks where there are children's sandboxes, deposit ascarid ova, which if ingested can produce visceral larva migrans (VLM) and hookworm larvae, which can penetrate the skin, resulting in cutaneous larva migrans (CLM). CLM and VLM, as well as toxoplasmosis, are also problems related to cats as a source of soil contamination, but movement of cats is even more difficult to control. Leash laws are theoretically appealing but have never been very effective because of public apathy—if not resistance—and lack of enforcement. This resistance to leash laws was true in 1887, when rabies was made a notifiable disease in

London and is true today.[86] A survey conducted in 1975 discovered that, although 95% of U.S. cities had leash laws, only 52% reported that they were effective in reducing strays.[61] In a crisis situation, however, public awareness and cooperation will increase and may even permit more effective procedures, such as large-scale vaccination programs.

Population reduction may be used to control spread of a zoonosis within a reservoir population. Reduction of the dog population was a key component of the echinococcosis control program in Iceland. In addition, it has been used to control noxious, predaceous, and verminous species. It has been effective in reducing rabies transmission from vampire bats in Latin America and in combatting canine rabies by capturing and euthanizing stray dogs. Sometimes the costs of this method exceed the benefits obtained. Any population reduction program should be carefully planned to assure effectiveness and minimize risk. Poisons, traps, gas, or shooting are all associated with some degree of hazard. Therefore, care must be taken in selecting the most appropriate method for the area. These also may produce an adverse public response based on animal welfare concerns.

As was mentioned earlier, **biological control** of wildlife reservoirs has been effective in a few situations. It is important to realize that the basic concept of this procedure is to restrict population numbers, not achieve eradication. An efficient predator does not eliminate its prey. Predator numbers are dependent on the number of prey. Under natural conditions, a stable relationship develops between the number of each so that neither becomes exceedingly abundant. Sometimes, an accelerated reproductive rate in the remaining members of the population will occur because of less competition for food, thereby reducing the effectiveness of the method. The principle of biological control was applied to vertebrates years ago when snakes were introduced into Puerto Rico to control rodents in cane fields. Then the mongoose was introduced to kill snakes. Today, Puerto Rico still has rats and snakes and, in addition, a mongoose rabies problem.

Increasing Host Resistance

In addition to neutralization of reservoirs or contact reduction, zoonoses may also be controlled by **increasing host resistance** to infection. *Preventing* infection is the ideal, but in many instances, increasing host resistance may only *lessen the severity* of disease, without an equal increase in resistance to infection.

In veterinary medicine, genetic selection for resistance and reducing stress by improved nutrition or better shelter are routine procedures. In Africa, the N'Dama and West African shorthorn cattle breeds, which have been resident there for 5,000-7,000 years, are favored because of their trypano-tolerance.[80] In the southern United States, range beef cattle of European breeds are frequently bred to include a 25% Brahma parentage because of the latter's greater resistance to tick infestation. Maintaining animals at a proper level of nutrition not only increases their ability to resist infection but also increases their ability to respond properly to immunization. In human medicine, genetic selection for resistance may occur naturally, as with sickle cell anemia and resistance to malaria, but is not acceptable as an applied disease control procedure. Reduction of stress, by providing improved shelter and nutrition, is not only an end in itself but is also a means to reduce the ravages of epidemics by increasing the survival ability of the affected populations. This is well recognized, with greater case fatality rates among starving populations during epidemics. These approaches to disease control will not be explored further in this text. There are, however, two procedures for increasing host resistance which are appropriate for presentation: (1) chemoprophylaxis and (2) immunization.

Chemoprophylaxis

Chemoprophylaxis contrasts with mass therapy in that, in the latter, medication is administered on the assumption that the recipient is infected whereas chemoprophylaxis attempts to prevent infection or, at least, reduce the severity of the disease. In contrast to immunization, it is a passive means of increasing host resistance, lasting only as long as the drug lasts. Active response to immunization, however, lasts for months or even a lifetime. Typically, no host response is elicited. Live anthrax vaccine with concurrent penicillin prophylaxis is an example of chemoprophylaxis of the wrong kind, i.e., no infection and no immunity.

Chemoprophylaxis is used in laboratories when personnel are accidentally exposed to an agent (including several zoonotics) known to be susceptible to a drug. This is to *prevent* infection, which differs from mass therapy, which is used to *eliminate* infection. On the other hand, mass therapy may leave some immunity in those who were previously infected. Chemoprophylaxis may involve adverse reactions to the drug. In some instances, the agent may be resistant.

Typically, chemoprophylaxis is applied when no other, more effective means of protecting the host is available. Antimalarial medication for people is an example. The medication does not prevent infection (injection of sporozoites by the mosquito) but reduces the severity of consequences of malaria by suppressing the erythrocytic stage. Malaria drugs are no longer used in those areas of the world where the disease has been eradicated. Chemoprophylaxis is a consideration for any high-risk group when an effective drug is available and suitable immunization or adequate protective clothing is not.

In veterinary medicine, slow- or pulse-released boluses of oxfendazole have been demonstrated to be effective in reducing parasitic gastroenteritis (and pasture contamination) among bovines.[63] Some of the most widely used chemoprophylactic materials for domestic animals are insect repellents to ward off arthropod vectors and anti-heartworm medication for dogs. Both of these procedures are two-edged swords, for they also present risks. Cats are easily made ill by exposure to certain chemical repellents. A prophylactic dose of an anti-heartworm medication given to a dog, already infected with the parasite, can cause death because adult worms are killed and dislodged from their site in the heart, producing emboli.

Immunization

Vaccines are used for two purposes: (1) to protect susceptible individuals from infection or disease and (2) to prevent transmission of infectious agents by creating an immune population. To be most effective in controlling disease, the stimulus of **immunization** should be sufficient to prevent infection as well as disease. In maintenance hosts, no reduction in the reservoir of infection occurs if only disease is prevented. The risk of disease remains for any susceptible individual introduced into the population if carriers persist. The level of immunity needed to prevent disease is not necessarily the same as the level needed to prevent infection. The efficiency of immunization as a method for disease control is measured in terms of the percentage of the population developing the desired level of protection in relation to the resources expended (vaccine, equipment, labor, promotion, etc.). Efficiency increases as the number of doses needed decreases. Assuming a similar percentage of the population reaches a level of protection sufficient for control by either method, vaccine in the drinking water would be far more efficient than administration by injection.

In planning any immunization program, the first step is to identify the population at risk (susceptibles likely to be exposed) and then to decide on the specific disease control goal, e.g., reducing the incidence of disease to just a few sporadic cases vs elimination of the agent. The decision to vaccinate or not to vaccinate is based on relative risk. When choosing which route to take in relation to each disease, ask the questions, Where? When? Who? and Why? The answer to one or more of these questions may be crucial to determine the correct decision.[50,51] For example:

Where? Vaccination is generally recommended for populations in endemic areas. Vaccination against yellow fever is, therefore, not recommended for residents of North America or Europe. Similarly, routine vaccination of livestock against anthrax and many other diseases is not justified in nonendemic areas. If a closed-herd situation exists, such as that described in the Reducing Contact Potential section, the need for many immunizations may be nil.

When? If the disease has a distinct "season," such as seen with vectorborne agents, immunization just before the season will provide the maximum efficiency. Whenever an outbreak of a nonendemic disease occurs (e.g., Venezuelan equine encephalomyelitis in temperate North America), immunizations can be an important means of providing protection.

Who? Individuals about to be subjected to stressful conditions, or those whose occupation puts them at high risk for exposure, are candidates for immunization. Vaccination against leptospirosis to protect workers in rice fields is practiced in several countries. In addition to Japanese encephalitis, Russian spring-summer encephalitis and yellow fever vaccines are used to protect general populations in (or travelers to) endemic areas. Several arboviral vaccines are used in laboratories to protect high-risk personnel. Rabies vaccines are widely used to protect laboratory workers as well as individuals working with wildlife in endemic areas. With some vaccines, pregnancy introduces the risk of producing fetal infection and death. Age differences in susceptibility to disease and ability to produce a response to an immunogen sufficient to provide protection may be critical factors.

Why? For a program of vaccination to be justifiable, the loss caused by the disease must be greater than the cost of immunization. (The definition of "loss" will vary between animals and humans.) Also, immunization should be at least as cost effective as other means of control. When using vaccines, the potential hazards should be considered. Strain 19 brucellosis vaccine, for example, in addition to producing titers high enough to interfere with subsequent testing, can be shed in the milk of vaccinated cows and can produce severe reactions if injected into humans. (In spite of this, the Russians have used strain 19 for immunizing humans.) The risk of adverse effects from the vaccine should be less than that posed by the disease. "Adverse" effects need to be evaluated. For instance, approximately 25% of individuals receiving human diploid cell virus rabies vaccine have mild adverse effects but not sufficient enough to suspend the series of immunizations. For another 6% who have severe side effects, the vaccine should probably be discontinued. A similar situation exists with the newly developed, inactivated Japanese encephalitis virus vaccine, and as a result, it is recommended only for those who will reside in endemic areas, particularly during transmission season.[109]

In addition to being a method for protecting susceptible individuals from infection or disease, immunization of groups frequently has the added benefit of conferring a "herd immunity" on that group. **Herd immunity** was referred to earlier as a method for reducing contact potential. For an agent spread by direct contact only, in which immunization stimulates resistance without development of carriers, such as with rabies virus, immunization of a sufficient percentage of the population will reduce contact potential by the mechanism of herd immunity. Herd immunity is defined as that point at which the proportion of immunes in a given population becomes so great that a disease agent, transmitted by direct contact, cannot enter and spread. A population with 70% of its individuals immune is a commonly accepted proportion to achieve. In the World Health Organization's smallpox eradication program, the herd immunity phenomenon was utilized with the "cluster" immunization technique. After initial wide-scale immunizations had been accomplished, identification of a case would result in vaccination of all individuals within a radius of a half mile and an intensive search for other cases within a 2-mile radius.[36,38,39,41] The effectiveness of herd immunity is influenced by the duration of individual immunity, the duration and amount of agent shedding, infectivity of the agent, population turnover (introduction of new susceptibles), and mobility.

For immunizing large numbers of individuals, a jet injector may be used. The jet injector was introduced in 1947 as a rapid, safe, relatively painless method of mass injection of vaccine under high pressure without a needle. Intracutaneous or subcutaneous injections are produced by forcing the vaccine under high pressure through a very small hole in the instrument into the skin. An orifice diameter of 0.005 inches is optimal for humans, whereas a diameter of 0.009-0.011 inches is best for livestock. Also, a crowned head is preferred for animal use. Measured doses from 0.1 to 1.0 ml may be administered in this way. A two-person team can immunize up to 1,000 per hour by this method, as compared to 100 per hour by conventional syringe methods. When immunizing animals, the speed is dependent upon management practices. Under optimum conditions, 400 horses may be immunized in 1 hour. Other advantages of the jet injector are (1) the possibility of breaking off needles in fractious animals is eliminated, (2) the number of post-injection sterile abscesses is greatly reduced, and (3) it does not transmit bloodborne agents as do contaminated needles (particularly important as regards AIDS). Even though the original monetary investment is greater, a jet injector quickly becomes more economical than syringes and needles. It does, however, require careful maintenance.

Immunization as a method of disease control is generally so effective and commonplace that, all too often, the many variables associated with the procedure are ignored.[7,14,24,32] Immunization failures may occur as the result of failure of the delivery system or failure of the immune response, or they may be iatrogenic in origin.[54,103]

A critical component of the delivery system is proper temperature control. It is naive to assume that a breakdown in the "cold chain" is something that happens only in the less-industrialized portions of the world. Many batches of vaccine have been rendered useless even in highly industrialized nations as a result of overheating during transit, for example, from exposure to summertime temperatures in the trunk of a car. Vaccines have a finite shelf life, even when stored in optimum conditions. Generally, the chemical methods used to inactivate the immunogen are also those used to preserve the vaccine during storage. The critical factor is inactivation of enzymatic activity that will decompose the immunogen. For example, anthrax spore vaccines are prepared by using sufficient heat to inactivate the enzymes in the vegetative cells, yet not kill the inactive spores. The spores will remain inactive, yet viable, as long as they are not exposed to oxygen. The problems of inactivation become more complex as the severity of inactivation decreases (active enzymes remain). Irradiation and disruption may prevent replication, but all enzymatic activity may not be destroyed. Therefore, cold or lyophilization must be used to preserve these products, as well as vaccines containing live (able to replicate) agents. Vaccines in which some enzymatic activity remains when in solution (even under refrigeration) will lose their potency in 2 weeks or less; therefore, after a lyophilized vaccine is reconstituted, it must be used promptly. This is especially important when using vaccines from multiple-dose containers. Also, using a vaccine after the indicated expiration date, for whatever the reason, will almost certainly lead to a less than satisfactory level of protection.

Even though the vaccine is a satisfactory immunizing material, failures may occur because the recipient does not produce a protective level of antibodies. Failure to respond adequately may result from immaturity, the presence of circulating passive antibodies, or a genetic (or innate) or acquired immune response deficiency. This last factor is becoming more common with the use of immunosuppressives following transplant surgery and the increased number of individuals infected with the human immunodeficiency virus (HIV).

It is important for the professional performing the immunization to understand the level of protection conferred. A laboratory worker developed what was considered a protective rabies antibody titer from immunization, but contracted rabies following inhalation (an unusual route of exposure) of a virulent strain. Because the olfactory apparatus has no synapses between the nose and the brain, the virus was able to enter the brain before a protective antibody response could be produced. A similar situation involved a case of pneumonic plague in Vietnam.[20] Sometimes the vaccine will protect against disease, but not infection. This is a problem, for instance, with leptospirosis in which, following immunization, the animal may be spared the clinical disease syndrome but continues to harbor and shed the spirochaete in its urine. It is important to be aware that a vaccine may prevent clinical disease but not infection, resulting in a healthy carrier condition.

Vaccine failure can also stem from using an improper route for injection. The usual routes for vaccine administration are oral and parenteral, which most commonly involves subcutaneous, intramuscular, or intradermal injection. (Ocular and intranasal administration without injection are also parenteral routes.) Hepatitis B vaccine is effective when administered intramuscularly, but produces a much lower rate of seroconversion if deposited in the fatty tissue of the buttocks. Utilization of gluteal tissue as an injection site, rather than depositing the vaccine in the deltoid muscles as per directions, has resulted in death from rabies even though postexposure immunization was performed.

Other reasons for vaccine "failure" include administering a reduced dose of vaccine, failure to complete a full series of doses, and administering a vaccine concomitantly with antibiotics or immunomodulators. Antibiotics may inhibit replication of live bacterial vaccines. For example, concurrent penicillin therapy and use of anthrax spore vaccine is contraindicated.

Finally, a vaccine may fail to provide the desired level of protection because the immunogens present are incorrect. Although it is useful in protecting against *Mycobacterium tuberculosis*, attempts to prevent leprosy in humans by using the vaccine developed by Calmette and Guerin from *Mycobacterium bovis* (BCG) met with equivocal results. Failure also might be the result of genetic drift of the agent, as seen with influenza, or because of host factors, such as is seen in the failure to produce immunity to rabies in skunks or raccoons with a vaccine designed for immunization of foxes by the oral route.[33,34]

Examples: Field Necropsy, Broiler House

Two examples will be used to illustrate the application of reservoir neutralization, reducing contact potential, and increasing host resistance in preventing spread of infection: (1) a field necropsy and (2) a broiler house operation.

Field Necropsy

Field necropsy is required when the whole animal is too large to transport without undue exposure to personnel or contamination of the environment, the distance to the diagnostic laboratory is too great to allow economical shipment of the entire carcass (i.e., only collect and transport selected tissue and fluid specimens), and/or an immediate presumptive or confirmatory diagnosis is critical **and** it can be done based, at least in part, on necropsy observations. Aborted fetuses, always with the placenta, if it can be found, should be placed in a container and transported to a diagnostic laboratory for examination rather than expose the tissues to unnecessary contamination in the field. Dead domestic and wild birds also can be collected easily and placed in a plastic bag for transport to a laboratory where contamination of the diagnostic material is easier to control. Because field necropsies are frequently performed on large domestic and wild animals, they should be carefully planned events to avoid contamination of any tissues needed for microbiological examination, contamination of the environment where the necropsy is performed, or infection of people or animals who may be at risk of exposure. There is a higher potential for transmission of disease agents during and following a field necropsy than exists with a necropsy performed in a laboratory setting, where facilities are available for containing the agent during necropsy. A properly conducted field necropsy has three components: (1) preparation, (2) examination of the carcass and collection of specimens, and (3) cleaning and disinfection.

Preparation to perform a field necropsy requires a history of events leading to the death of the animal and gathering the materials that will be required during and after the necropsy. The first is acquired by interviewing the owner or caretaker of the deceased animal. The second requires careful consideration of all factors related to the actual performance of the necropsy: the species of animal, the location of the carcass, the possible cause(s) of death (based on the history and your prior knowledge of the situation), and specimens that may be required for laboratory analysis. In considering what materials to bring, it is important to keep in mind that the performance of the necropsy, and subsequent cleanup, must be conducted in such a manner that there will be minimal opportunity for transmission of infectious agents to you, to anyone else present or assisting, or to other susceptible animals in the area. During the initial conversation, the owner should be advised not to move the carcass.

Examination of the carcass and **collection** of specimens will vary with the situation. A necropsy of a horse is far removed from the necropsy of a broiler. The precautions taken when performing a necropsy of a cow under a lightning-splintered tree, for insurance purposes, obviously will not require the same precautions as examination of a cow suspected of having succumbed to anthrax. There are, however, some basic rules that apply to all necropsies in relation to preventing the possible transmission of infectious agents. During the necropsy, protective clothing should be worn. The arms as well as the torso and legs should be covered; heavy-duty rubber gloves and boots should be worn; and if there is any suspicion that an infectious agent that can be transmitted as an aerosol is involved, a face mask is essential. Anyone assisting in the necropsy should be similarly protected, and spectators should be kept away from the immediate site and not be allowed to handle any potentially infectious material.

There should be minimal disruption of the carcass during the necropsy to prevent contamination of the area. If feasible, a plastic sheet may be placed beneath the carcass to prevent contaminating the ground. After the necropsy, the carcass can be removed to a site so that it can be cleaned without contaminating the environment and disinfected. If a disease such as anthrax is suspected, the carcass should not be opened because the agent will sporulate on contact with air, forming highly resistant forms that will contaminate the soil. A blood specimen will be sufficient. If an invasive procedure is required, the history should first be considered in relation to possible agents, and only those organ systems requiring inspection and/or tissue collection be exposed. The collection, handling, and shipment of tissue specimens is covered in Chapter 3. Any specimens submitted to a laboratory should include identifying information and, if a zoonotic disease that can be transmitted to laboratory personnel is suspected, adequate warning to that effect must be attached.

Cleaning and **disinfection** following completion of the necropsy are the final procedures, which if properly done, will prevent transmission to other susceptible animals. The protective clothing, including face mask, should be removed and placed in a sealable container. Rubber gloves and boots must first be mechanically cleaned using water and a brush and then disinfected with a suitable chemical. Remember, it is practically impossible to disinfect any surface through a layer of mud, blood, or other dried animal tissue. Instruments used during the necropsy must be placed in a disinfectant solution in a covered container until they can be removed, cleaned, and sterilized.

The final aspect of the cleanup involves the carcass. Once again, the options to be considered depend upon the species (size) and the magnitude of threat to other susceptible animals, including the owner/manager. Normally, burning or burial are the two choices for disposal. Under no circumstances should rendering be considered if a highly infectious agent capable of survival in the environment is suspected. The owner should be advised that transferring the carcass from the farm to the rendering facility can distribute the organism along the entire route, and for this reason, employing a rendering company to dispose of the carcass (or any others that may have died) is not an option. If the carcass is to be burned, the person responsible should be informed that the temperature must be hot enough to completely destroy any infectious organisms and that the carcass should be burned at the site of the necropsy, thereby ensuring destruction of organisms on the ground that may have escaped from the carcass. To ensure complete destruction, the flammable material used must generate a very high temperature as it burns. Soft woods, such as pine, may not accomplish this. Rubber tires, although smokey, generate considerable heat as they burn. In some areas burning may not be an acceptable method because of governmental restrictions. Be sure, before advising. If burial is the choice, the hole must be deep enough to prevent dogs or other carrion eaters from digging up any part of the carcass. As with burning, the burial should be at the site of the necropsy. After the carcass has been deposited in the pit, add a generous coating of lime over the entire surface to hasten decomposition. Finally, any equipment that has come in contact with the carcass should be thoroughly cleaned and disinfected.

The two disease control methods illustrated in this example include environmental manipulation (burning or burial, and disinfection) and reducing contact potential (use of protective clothing and ensuring that the carcass is not moved). On occasion, persons performing the necropsy may be exposed to infectious material, requiring prophylactic therapy.

Broiler House

In a modern broiler production system, day-old chicks are placed in a building consisting of one large common room where they will be maintained until ready for slaughter. This growth period normally is 7-8 weeks. Depending upon its size, there will be 20,000-30,000 chicks per building. Obviously, unless precautions are taken, the potential for a disastrous epidemic is very high. The steps taken to prevent losses from occurring illustrate how the principles of preventive medicine are utilized in an everyday situation. The two areas of concern are (1) the birds and (2) the environment, which includes feed, water, personnel, and the physical facilities (air flow, etc.).

The birds chosen for this type of operation come from strains that are genetically resistant to Marek's disease, which is caused by a lymphotrophic retrovirus. The source flock will have been tested to ensure freedom from *Salmonella pullorum* and *Salmonella enteriditis*. Before the chicks are delivered, they will have been debeaked to prevent cannibalism, and vaccinated against Newcastle disease, infectious bronchitis (usually via an intranasal spray), and Marek's disease. Although acquired immunity against coccidiosis is effective, broilers must be protected from a coccidial infection severe enough to produce clinical disease. This is done with an anticoccidial drug that is used on a continuous basis to increase resistance. (If anticoccidials are used, the proper withdrawal period must be observed to prevent violative levels of drug residues in the slaughtered birds.)

New birds are never added to an existing group. An "all out-all in" policy provides a time barrier between groups, and also provides an opportunity to clean and fumigate the poultry house to prevent possible transmission of environmentally resistant organisms or vectors. Maintaining birds in closed buildings prevents contact with wild birds. An active rodent control program using poisoned baits and traps is essential. Because a large proportion of the feed is often derived from rendered poultry carcasses, the feed must be certified *Salmonella*-free. The water source must be tested to assure it is not contaminated with pathogenic microorganisms or potentially toxic levels of chemicals, and both feed and water must be stored and delivered in a sanitary manner. Floor litter must be kept dry to inhibit sporulation or replication of microorganisms. Great care must be taken to ensure that personnel do not act as sources of infectious disease agents or vectors. Restricted entry is needed to prevent not only transmission from sources external to the farm but cross-contamination between houses. This may include facilities for the disinfection of footwear and/or a complete change of garments.

The disease control methods illustrated in this example include (1) reservoir neutralization by test and slaughter (birds originating from a specific-pathogen-free flock) and by environmental manipulation (cleaning and fumigation between groups; disinfection of clothing and equipment; ensuring a safe source, storage, and delivery of feed and water; and use of a rodent and vector control program); (2) reducing contact potential by segregation of groups with all in-all out production and restricted entry of personnel; and (3) increasing host resistance by breeding genetically resistant birds (against Marek's disease), by chemoprophylaxis (use of coccidiostats), and by immunization (against Newcastle disease, infectious bronchitis, and Marek's disease).

Consumer Protection Strategies

In the modern environment, "consumer protection" can refer to a myriad of concerns, but one of the earliest was related to foodborne disease. Regulations regarding foods of animal origin are found in several major religious texts. As civilizations developed, foodborne disease control became part of the public health activities of governments. In the Western world, antemortem and postmortem inspection of carcasses began in Bavaria in 1615. A system of public abattoirs was established in France in 1807. In the United States, the modern food safety program had its origins around the beginning of the 20th century.[58,86] As an alternative to the prevailing quality of milk, which was often produced under filthy conditions, the American Association of Medical Milk Commissions, a nongovernmental organization, established standards for **Certified Milk**. The program emphasized pure, clean, *raw* milk. Although illness from milkborne pathogens was reduced, pasteurization of raw milk added further protection and, coupled with sanitary requirements for production, eventually became the norm. In meat inspection, the emphasis, until recently, was on inspection during processing, utilizing "organoleptic" testing. Animals were inspected before and after slaughter using the senses of sight, smell, and touch. The pre-slaughter inspection was limited to the premises of the slaughter plant. As the information base relative to foodborne disease accumulated, it became evident that prevention by inspection during processing was not the complete answer. The potential for introduction of agents of foodborne disease existed throughout the food chain: production, processing, transportation, storage, retailing, and preparation.

There is a "Pareto Principle," which holds that a few (the "vital few") contributors to a problem account for most of the problem—perhaps 90%. The remaining many (the "trivial many") account for only a small proportion—perhaps 10%.[16] This concept applies admirably to foodborne disease. Year after year, four agents account for approximately 90% of foodborne disease cases reported by the Centers for Disease Control. Among these four, three are zoonoses having their reservoir in food animals: *Salmonella* species other than *S. typhi*, *Clostridium perfringens*, and *Campylobacter jejuni*. Only *Staphylococcus aureus* among these "vital few" originates primarily from human sources. The prevention and control of zoonotic diseases must, therefore, include strategies for reducing the incidence of foodborne disease.[2]

The traditional quality-assurance approach for meat and poultry has emphasized post-harvest (off-farm) inspection, addressing only one point in the food chain: slaughter and processing. This emphasis on end-point inspection is inefficient because it does not adequately address prevention. To change this emphasis and produce a more-effective foodborne disease control program, a new approach is being adopted. The **Hazard Analysis Critical Control Point (HACCP)** approach to controlling foodborne disease is a procedure developed by the manufacturing industry, whereby the production system is analyzed to determine potential hazards to human health, and the related critical control points are determined.[15,75] It was adapted to food production by the Pillsbury Corporation on behalf of the U.S. government and is being increasingly used by the food industry in the United States and Japan.[102] The "critical" points are selected on the basis of potential hazard to human health. The HACCP procedure, as adapted to disease control, involves four steps:

1. Develop a schematic depicting the life cycle and chain of transmission of the disease agent under consideration.
2. Identify points in the life cycle and chain of transmission that produce the highest potential for animal or human infection. These may reflect spatial or temporal factors that affect the probability of successful transmission. It must be recognized that these factors may change over time as control procedures succeed or fail.

3. Conduct an analysis of disease incidence (= hazard) related to transmission of infection from each of these points. This may be accomplished by retrospective studies, if sufficient reliable data are available, or by instituting appropriate surveillance, which may include population sampling, laboratory testing data, and/or disease reporting.

4. Assess the feasibility of instituting control procedures at each of these points and, after they have been instituted, evaluate their effectiveness in terms of results and cost.

Although inspection during slaughter and processing continues to be a primary activity of the Food Safety and Inspection Service of the USDA, the adoption of the HACCP approach to foodborne disease prevention and control is creating a shift in the emphasis to include on-farm (pre-harvest) inspection. There are two advantages to this approach: (1) the incidence of foodborne disease (and the resultant expense of treatment) as a result of eating meat from infected animals that might be missed during organoleptic end-point inspection is reduced and (2) the financial loss to the producer or processor because of condemnation of tissues or entire carcasses during processing is reduced when the problem is detected and corrected on the farm.

Animal Identification

Accurate animal identification is critical to any effective zoonotic disease risk analysis or control program involving domestic animals. The two areas of concern are (1) individual animal identification and (2) identification of point of origin.

Individual Animal Identification

Individual animal identification is of critical importance. For example, cows determined to be infected with brucellosis or tuberculosis are tagged and branded to ensure that they do not leave the premises except for slaughter. Immunization records of a dog, coupled with accurate individual identification, facilitates determining the potential for transmission of rabies virus to that dog if bitten by a wild animal, or the potential for virus transmission to a human if bitten by that dog. Furthermore, it is reassuring to the parents of a child who has been bitten to know that the animal in confinement is actually the one that did the biting. Serum banks would be almost useless as tools for retrospective studies of infection and disease patterns without accurate species and individual animal identification.[78] Particularly, in this age of rapid transportation, valid health certification without reliable animal identification is impossible.

Ear tagging is the most common procedure for individual identification of ruminants (cattle, goats, sheep). Horses can be tattooed on the mucosa of the lower lip, and dogs can be tattooed on the inside of the pinna of the ear. During antemortem inspection in a slaughter plant pigs found to have some condition that may result in condemnation during postmortem inspection are "slap" tattooed to identify them during the postmortem inspection procedure. A sophisticated improvement in identification of individual food animals is the use of small transmitter chips that emit a signal with a different frequency for each animal on a farm or in a feedlot. The chips are usually inserted in the loose tissue at the base of the ear and removed at slaughter. Smaller chips are available for use in pets and may be linked to a commercial, computer-based program for identification if the animal strays and becomes lost.

Point of Origin

Without an effective identification program, it is impossible to trace an animal back to its point of origin (and, presumably, the source of infection). In the United States, the success of the bovine brucellosis eradication program is dependent upon the "traceback" system in which cows moving through sale barns and slaughter plants are tested, and those designated as reactors are identified by farm of origin. The same concept is utilized in bovine tuberculosis control, but today, animals with visible lesions are usually discovered in slaughter plants. In both instances, the farm of origin becomes the focus of a disease control program that includes individual cow testing and stringent limitations on movement of potentially infected animals from that herd.

Health Maintenance

Zoonotic disease control programs are affected by certain socioeconomic factors. In a typical public health unit, rabies will usually get the lion's share of funds earmarked for zoonoses control programs, whereas others, such as toxoplasmosis, generally are ignored. Sometimes this is as it should be, but often, implementation of control programs is less than optimum because an objective analysis of actual needs is not done. Two factors that need to be considered are (1) the difference between animal health and public (human) health disease control programs and (2) cost-benefit analysis.[23]

Animal Health vs Public Health

As was indicated when describing hazard analysis, effective control programs require reliable disease reporting systems. When public health departments were being formed, certain diseases were considered important enough from a public health viewpoint to be designated as scheduled, or reportable diseases, many of which were quarantinable. This was the beginning of morbidity incidence reporting, which is still the backbone of most public health surveillance programs. In contrast, when agriculturally based veterinary services were created, population statistics for animals (except for specific well-defined populations) were very difficult to obtain. Most food-producing animals experience a very short life span, which ends abruptly at slaughter. The diseases of primary interest were those of economic concern, such as tuberculosis and brucellosis, or those with a potential for major public health impact, such as rabies. As diagnostic techniques improved and tuberculosis skin testing and serologic testing of cows for brucellosis became established (thus detecting infected, as contrasted to diseased animals), the accumulation of information became based on an active surveillance system, rather than passive reporting of clinical disease. Thus, by different processes of evolution, incidence reporting became a basis of public health data and prevalence reporting became a basis of animal health data gathering.[86]

Cost-Benefit Analyses

Cost-benefit analyses, in which the quantitative reduction in monetary losses from disease are compared to expenditures for various disease control stratagems, first appeared in the veterinary literature during the 1970s.[30,31,59] These early attempts to improve economic efficiency encouraged a host of similar studies. Now, some three decades later, this is routinely done in well-managed food animal disease control programs.[44,45]

In human medicine, cost-benefit analyses have not been utilized as much, at least in the developed world, because of the emphasis on curative, rather than preventive medicine. As health costs soar, and prevention, rather than cure, becomes more attractive, cost-benefit analyses are gaining popularity. It is specious to say that one cannot ethically do cost-benefit analyses when dealing with people because human life has no monetary value, such as is true for cows or pigs. For example, a control program that is effective in reducing the incidence of a given disease and costs $10,000 per year to implement is obviously a more cost-effective choice than one that has the same efficiency but costs $50,000 per year. Several studies have attempted to quantify the monetary value of human health as a guide to allocate limited financial resources. At first, these were primarily philosophical in nature,[92,117] but soon, true cost-benefit analyses began appearing.[69,71,72,91] An extension of these analyses has been the concept of using the public's willingness to pay for perceived reduction in health risks. This is widely recognized as the appropriate perspective for evaluating the U.S. Food and Drug Administration's risk management decisions.[74]

Communication

Communication Among Health Professionals

For disease control programs to be effective, a mechanism must be in place that will ensure that information obtained through surveillance systems is made available on a regular basis to the individuals responsible for the success of these programs.[26,42,66,90] To a large extent, these are the same individuals who are involved in the reporting process: private practitioners and workers in laboratories and hospitals. Without an efficient feedback system, few of them will be aware of significant health-related events taking place outside their immediate area. For the health professional in public practice, the receipt of accurate and timely information regarding incidence and prevalence rates, as well as morbidity and mortality data, allows the establishment of priorities to make the most efficient use of time and money for control. For private practitioners, the main value of surveillance reports is that the information keeps them aware of disease patterns in their own area of practice. In addition to being of help in differential diagnoses, the data may also indicate the necessity of instituting preventive measures.

Usually, data gleaned from surveillance systems reflect the endemic situation, i.e., the "normal." This information is important because, just as in any diagnostic procedure, knowledge of what is normal is a prerequisite for identifying the abnormal. Dissemination of these base-line data will depend upon the size and scope of the reporting organization. On an international scale, the World Health Organization issues *Bulletins* and *Technical Reports*. The United Nations Food and Agriculture Organization publishes the annual *Animal Health Yearbook*. In the United States, the *Morbidity and Mortality Weekly Report (MMWR)*, published by the U.S. Public Health Service, Centers for Disease Control, is an excellent example of disease reporting, including information in both narrative and tabular form. On a local level, most state health departments issue monthly reports. U.S. veterinary medicine professionals can glean additional information from the reports issued by the Food Safety and Inspection Service and the brucellosis and tuberculosis eradication programs of the Animal and Plant Health Inspection Service.

A key element in any surveillance system is the inclusion of some method to signal a transition from "normal" to "abnormal," i.e., when an endemic level of disease becomes epidemic. The weekly pneumonia-influenza deaths curve, mentioned in Chapter 2, is an example of one such mechanism. Current incidents are compared to expected values, based on retrospective data that have been plotted on a time line. If the incidence of disease appears to be increasing with monthly reporting, the frequency can be enhanced to weekly monitoring, based on an appropriate fractioning of the monthly threshold value to aid in providing an early warning.[111]

The mechanism for reporting an emergency situation, which often requires an immediate response from health professionals in the field, requires an established system for timely contact. Experience has shown that during emergencies lack of efficient communication often is a weak link in the response effort. Such a system will usually be centered in the state or county public health department or, for diseases of livestock, the state animal health agency. It is essential that the method for prompt communication, including a backup system in case of power failure, is in place *before* an emergency occurs, and that such a system includes some means for communicating with the public as well as with health professionals.[81,94,95,105]

Communication with the Public

The two reasons why a disease control program must include an effective means for communicating with the public are (1) to provide accurate information about a health-related problem and (2) to provide instructions about the response required from the public to solve the problem. A problem exists when a situation has been determined to be significantly different from an accepted standard. Because complete agreement on what constitutes a problem is generally not available, problems identified by professionals are described as "**needs**," and those identified by the public as "**demands**" or "**felt needs**." The greater the overlap of need and demand in any problem, the greater the likelihood of cooperative effort toward its solution. The primary motivating force for disease *control* programs involving animals usually emanates from owners who have suffered economic loss. Diseases in animals that create public health threats provide an additional basis for motivation. When distress is sufficient, the public will demand control programs. Programs to *prevent* disease, on the other hand, generally require additional motivation because an immediate problem is not recognized. For a demand to be generated, the community must be sufficiently knowledgeable concerning its needs. This requires a mechanism for communication between health professionals and the public. Because the general public is not normally privy to the information circulated among health professionals, alternate channels of communication must be utilized. This may be most easily accomplished through newspaper articles or television and radio news stories. If a problem is urgent or requires educational input, special meetings may be conducted or school programs arranged. The local or state public health unit will usually provide the means for channeling this type of communication to the public.

Occasionally, a group of physicians, veterinarians, or other health professionals in the community who are knowledgeable about the problem can serve as a means of communication. The mechanisms used to reach the public will change if a problem expands from a local to a regional or national level. The messages also will change, from specific instructions for local conditions to general guidelines for regional or national problems. If, for example, a mass vaccination program is required to control a local rabies outbreak, there must be a publicity campaign that will ensure that each segment of the population that needs to be reached will not only be contacted, but will also understand the reason for the immunization and the dates, times, and places that public vaccination will be available. If the problem to be addressed is national in scope, i.e., the spread of rabies in a wildlife reservoir such as the raccoon, the emphasis will be on instructing the public to avoid contact with raccoons. The need for immunization of dogs will be explained, but specific details will be left up to local authorities.

Education

Historically, the education of health professionals has emphasized diagnosis and treatment, rather than control and prevention. Education regarding "people skills"—understanding and using felt needs—has been minimal or nonexistent. In veterinary medicine, a series of symposia has resulted in a consensus among U.S. educators that this traditional emphasis ill serves the needs of the profession as it enters the 21st century. Implicit in these deliberations is the concept that education of the public cannot be successful unless health professionals fully understand that education is one of the most effective disease prevention and control tactics.[101]

The success of hydatidosis eradication programs around the world illustrates the value of educating the public to accomplish goals. At the turn of this century, approximately one out of four dogs in Iceland was infected with *Echinococcus granulosis*. The same prevalence of hydatidosis (the larval stage of *E. granulosis*) existed among humans. A key component of the eradication campaign, which included postmortem inspection of sheep carcasses, stray dog control, and dog treatment, was an intensive educational effort. In addition to the distribution of a pamphlet describing the life cycle of the parasite and the means of prevention, a rigorous educational program was instituted in schools. By 1960, the disease had been eradicated from Iceland. Similar campaigns, all relying heavily upon education, have been equally successful in New Zealand, Tasmania, and Cyprus.[8,18,73,85,87] The success of these campaigns was in large part the result of a felt need (demand) by the public that was developed through education.

In today's world, the need for education is no less than it was a century ago. In fact, our highly mobile society coupled with the appearance of "new" disease problems has accentuated the need for more effective education of the public as well as health professionals.

A survey of U.S. pet owners conducted in 1986 revealed a poor understanding of the potential health hazards associated with animal ownership. A third of the respondents were unaware that, with the exception of rabies, diseases could be transmitted from pets. However, 87% of the respondents reported at least one visit to a veterinarian during the past 18 months.[40] Another survey revealed that only a third of veterinarians engaged in private practice routinely discussed the potential hazard of human toxocariasis with their dog-owning clients despite the proven association between dog ownership and the disease.[53] The role of *Toxoplasma gondii* in human chorioretinitis is well understood by health professionals, but the necessity of educating clients *before* pregnancy (most adverse effects occur when infection begins during the first trimester) is not a common practice.

With the advent of the AIDS epidemic, the need for education regarding the potential for transmission of zoonoses has increased dramatically. Toxoplasmosis has been reported in approximately 10% of AIDS patients; cryptosporidiosis in 15%. About 5% of HIV-positive persons develop salmonellosis. The incidence of cat scratch disease, rhodococcosis, campylobacteriosis, microsporidiosis, and *Mycobacterium marinum* infection has also increased.[48] Because individuals afflicted by HIV require emotional support, they are reluctant to give up their pets. It is imperative, therefore, that health professionals working with HIV-positive persons be well informed regarding the reservoirs, life cycles, and methods of transmission of the zoonoses that pose an increased risk to immunosuppressed individuals.[37]

Occupational safety, as related to the zoonoses, is another area demanding improved education. A survey conducted in 1978 among 22 U.S. veterinary schools showed that none of them had a full- or part-time health and safety officer, and only 12 had safety committees.[57] Because one of the functions of these individuals presumably would be education related to occupational safety, it can only be assumed that this responsibility was met on a catch-as-catch-can basis, if at all. Livestock and poultry producers, abattoir workers, veterinary technicians and laboratory workers, animal control officials, wildlife biologists, and pet shop employees are all, by dint of their occupations, at higher risk of infection by zoonotic agents than the average person and need to be educated about the hazards and means of prevention relevant to their situation.[29,65]

Major disasters, whether natural or manufactured, can create a situation in which the potential for a zoonotic disease outbreak is increased.[3,6] A 1989 survey of 26 U.S. veterinary schools revealed that the veterinarian's role in a disaster response was not being taught to most of the students.[70] Without proper education, the average practitioner will be ill prepared to participate in pre-disaster planning, much less to initiate disease control associated with dramatic changes in the status quo following a disaster.[13,28,43]

Foodborne disease has become of increasing concern to health professionals as well as to the general public. In the struggle to control this problem, the need for improved education about the transmission of foodborne disease agents and mechanisms for control becomes obvious. Much of the problem is the result of misinformation, generated by well-intentioned, but misinformed groups and individuals. An example is the current controversy regarding irradiation of foods. Many equate irradiation with carcinogenesis or efforts to hide unhygienic practices and, therefore, are opposed to the incorporation of this procedure in food processing. An apt similarity is the resistance to pasteurization of milk that occurred when this method was proposed as a means of preventing the transmission of *Mycobacterium bovis*. Without a well-planned educational campaign as the initial step in introducing a new procedure, public acceptance of irradiation or any other advancement, may be delayed, and transmission of the identified foodborne disease agents will continue. It is important to learn what the public concerns are and not consider them frivolous.

The question remains, though, how education related to the zoonoses and their control can be delivered. At the professional level, courses in preventive medicine must go beyond the concept of immunization as a panacea for all potential problems. The interrelationships among the agent, host, and environment, and the application of those interrelationships to develop control programs must be taught in the basic curriculum, as well as being offered as special areas of expertise at the graduate level. Continuing education programs provide another mechanism for education of private practitioners. Periodic reinforcement may be needed because each new generation does not always remember why milk is pasteurized.

The responsibility for educating the public belongs to all health professionals, whether engaged in private or public practice. Educational campaigns presented by professional organizations can be effective if focused on a particular problem of current interest. Local medical and veterinary associations can offer programs directed at specific groups such as farmers or wildlife biologists, addressing occupational hazards associated with daily animal contact. Public health nurses and sanitarians can assist in educating the public regarding problems associated with food or the environment.

The major responsibility for educating the public regarding potential zoonotic diseases associated with animal ownership lies with private veterinary practitioners. During their daily contacts, veterinarians have the opportunity to identify potential problems and then educate their clients as to the risks and possible solutions. In a private practice environment, the opportunity for effective, one-on-one counseling is presented many times a day. The catch is that before professionals can be effective teachers they must be convinced that teaching is one of their primary responsibilities.

Summary

Prevention, Control, and Eradication

1. Prevention is defined as inhibiting the introduction of a disease agent into an individual, population, or area.

2. Control consists of steps taken to reduce the frequency or severity of a disease and maintain it at a tolerable level.

3. Eradication is the elimination of a disease-producing agent from a population or geographic area.

4. Total eradication is the complete removal of the agent.

5. Practical eradication is the elimination of the agent from the reservoirs of importance to man or his domestic animals.

Reservoir Neutralization

1. Reservoir neutralization involves preventing spread of infection by removing the infected individuals from the reservoir or by manipulating the environment where the reservoir resides.

2. Infected individuals can be removed by testing and slaughtering, or by mass therapy. Removal of infected animals is most effective with agents spread by direct transmission and in which a limited number of reservoir species are involved.

3. If the agent is vectorborne and the reservoir is a wildlife species, it is usually more economical to control the vector than to try to eliminate the agent in the vertebrate reservoir.

4. Mass therapy is usually restricted to a local situation in which all potentially infected individuals are treated without the use of screening tests.

5. Environmental manipulation can be designed to decrease environmental contamination by acting in relation to the portal of exit from the infected host, or by decreasing exposure of susceptible hosts by acting in relation to the portal of entry.

6. Environmental manipulation is effective only in the immediate area where controls are instituted.

7. The efficiency of environmental manipulation as a method for controlling vectors of disease agents is dependent upon the life cycle of the vector.

8. Vehicle manipulation is used when the source of infection is inanimate. It includes water purification, pasteurization, food preservation, and disinfection/sterilization.

9. Foodborne disease can be controlled by applying heat, cold, dehydration, or irradiation to the food, and by treating the food with preservative chemicals.

10. Pasteurization is designed to kill only pathogens. Sterilization destroys all microorganisms present in the food.

11. To be most effective, disinfection or sterilization must be preceded by cleaning.

Reducing Contact Potential

1. A basic principle in preventing direct transmission of an agent from an infected individual to a susceptible host is to reduce the opportunity for contact between the two.

2. Known cases (sources of infection) are isolated.

3. Susceptible individuals suspected of having been exposed are quarantined.

4. Herd immunity is effective in reducing contact potential because it decreases the proportion of susceptible animals in a population, thereby reducing the likelihood of contact with an infected animal. Herd immunity occurs when the proportion of immunes in a given population becomes so high that a directly transmitted disease agent cannot enter and spread.

5. Population control programs include leash laws, designed primarily to control rabies (prevent animal bites) and reduce fecal contamination, and population reduction to control transmission of an agent spread by direct contact within a reservoir population.

Increasing Host Resistance

1. Increasing host resistance may prevent infection of susceptibles or reduce severity of disease.

2. Host resistance may be increased by genetic selection, stress reduction, chemoprophylaxis, or immunization.

3. Chemoprophylaxis is used to prevent infection or minimize disease, whereas mass therapy is administered on the assumption that the recipients are already infected.

4. To be effective in controlling disease, immunization should prevent infection as well as disease. The level of immunity required to prevent disease is not necessarily the same as that required to prevent infection.

5. The decision to vaccinate or not is based on relative risk. For immunization to be justifiable, the cost of the disease must exceed the cost of immunization.

6. Immunization failures may occur as the result of failure of the delivery system or failure of the immune response, or they may be iatrogenic in origin, i.e., using an improper route of administration, using a reduced dose, failing to complete a series, or administering vaccine concomitantly with antibiotics or immunosuppressives.

Consumer Protection Strategies

1. Among the four microbial agents responsible for most foodborne disease in the United States, three are zoonotic: *Salmonella* species, *Clostridium perfringens,* and *Campylobacter jejuni.*

2. Hazard Analysis Critical Control Point (HACCP) is a procedure that has been applied to foodborne disease control and prevention. The HACCP approach has resulted in an increased emphasis on pre-harvest (on-farm) control rather than depending solely upon end-point inspection during slaughter and processing.

Animal Identification

1. Control and prevention of zoonoses transmitted from domestic animals is dependent upon an effective animal identification method.

2. Animal identification, for purposes of disease control, includes individual animal identification and identification of the origin of the animal(s), e.g., farm or herd.

Health Maintenance

1. Incidence reporting is the basis of public health disease surveillance. Prevalence reporting is the basis of animal health surveillance.

2. Cost-benefit analyses attempt to compare the financial expenditure (cost) for a disease control program with the quantitative reduction (benefit) in monetary loss from that disease.

Communication

1. A system of communication among health professionals must be in place *before* an emergency occurs. It must include a backup system, in case of power outage, and include some mechanism for communication with the public.

2. There are two reasons for maintaining communication between health professionals and the public during an emergency: to keep the public accurately informed about health related conditions and to provide instructions for coping with the emergency.

3. Problems identified by health professionals are called "needs," those identified by the public are called "demands" or "felt needs." The greater the overlap of need and demand in any problem, the greater the likelihood of cooperative effort toward its solution.

Education

1. Education is one of the *most* effective disease prevention and control strategies.
2. Without an initial educational campaign, acceptance of a new control procedure will be delayed.
3. Health professionals in private practice have a major responsibility and maximum opportunity for educating their clients regarding health risks and prevention.

References

1. Acha, P. N., and B. Szyfres: *Zoonosis and Communicable Diseases Common to Man and Animals*, 2nd ed., Sci. Publ. No. 503. Washington, D.C., Pan American Health Organization, 1987.
2. Acuff, G. R., R. A. Albanese, C. A. Batt, et al.: Implications of biotechnology, risk assessment, and communication for the safety of foods of animal origin. *J Am Vet Med Assoc*, 199:1714-1721, 1991.
3. Aghababian, R. V., and J. Teuscher: Infectious diseases following major disasters. *Ann Emerg Med*, 21:362-367, 1992.
4. Andrews, J. M., and A. D. Langmuir: The philosophy of disease eradication. *Am J Pub Hlth*, 53:1-21, 1963.
5. Bailey, T. M., and Schantz, P. M.: Trichinosis surveillance, United States, 1986. *MMWR*, Centers for Disease Control. 37(SS-5):1-8, 1988.
6. Baker, M. S.: Medical aspects of Persian Gulf operations: serious infectious and communicable diseases of the Persian Gulf and Saudi Arabian peninsula. *Milit Med*, 156:385-390, 1991.
7. Bart, K. J., A. R. Hinman, and W. S. Jordan: International symposium on vaccine development and utilization. *Rev Infect Dis*, 11, suppl 3:S491-S667, 1989.
8. Beard, T. C.: The elimination of echinococcosis from Iceland. *Bull WHO*, 48:653-660, 1973.
9. Beck, A. M.: *The Ecology of Stray Dogs*. Baltimore, York Press, 1973.
10. Benenson, A. S. (ed): *Control of Communicable Diseases in Man*. 14th ed. Washington, D.C., American Public Health Association, 1985.
11. Black, R. E.: Prevention in developing countries. *J Gen Intern Med*, Sep-Oct, 5(5 Supp):S132-135, 1990.
12. Block, S. S. (ed): *Disinfection, Sterilization and Preservation*, 3rd Ed. Philadelphia, Lea & Febiger, 1983.
13. Bres, P.: *Public Health Action in Emergencies Caused by Epidemics: a Practical*

Guide. Geneva, World Health Organization, 1986.

14. Brown, F.: Designing future vaccines. *J Hosp Infect*, 18 Suppl:164-169, 1991.

15. Bryan, F. L.: Hazard analysis critical control point approach: Epidemiologic rationale and application to foodservice operations. *J Environ Health.* 44:7-14, 1981.

16. Bryan, F. L.: Risks of practices, procedures and processes that lead to outbreaks of foodborne diseases. *J Food Prot*, 51:663-673, 1988.

17. Bundy, D. A. P.: Control of intestinal nematode infections by chemotherapy: mass treatment versus diagnostic screening. *Trans R Soc Trop Med Hyg*, 84:622-625, 1990.

18. Constantine, C. C., A. J. Lynbery, R. C. A. Thompson, et al.: The origin of a new focus of infection with *Echinococcus granulosis* in Tasmania. *Int J Parasitol*, 21:959-961, 1991.

19. Cockburn, A.: *Infectious Diseases: Their Evolution and Eradication.* Springfield, IL, Charles Thomas, 1967.

20. Cohen, R. J., and J. L. Stockard: Pneumonic plague in an untreated plague-vaccinated individual. *J Am Med Assoc*, 202:365-366, 1967.

21. Collins, C. H., M. C. Allwood, S. F. Bloomfield, et al. (eds): *Disinfectants: Their Use and Evaluation of Effectiveness.* Soc. Appl. Bacteriol. Tech. Ser. No 16. New York, Academic Press, 1981.

22. Conley, S. T.: What do consumers think about irradiated foods? U.S. Department of Agriculture, Food Safety and Inspection Service, *Food Safety Rev*, 2:11-15, 1992.

23. Dargatz, D. A. and M. D. Salman: Decision tree analysis and its value to herd health. *Compend Contin Ed Pract Vet*, 12: 433-441. 1990.

24. Devaney, M. A.: New approaches to animal vaccines utilizing genetic engineering. *Crit Rev Microbiol*, 15: 269-295, 1988.

25. Doebbeling, B. N., G. I.Stanley, C. T. Sheetz, et al.: Comparative efficacy of alternative hand-washing agents in reducing nosocomial infections in intensive care units. *New Engl J Med*, 327:88-93, 1992.

26. Dowdle, W. R.: Surveillance and control of infectious diseases: progress toward the 1990 objectives. *Pub Hlth Rep*, 98:210-218, 1983.

27. Drummond, R. O., J. E. George, and S. E. Kunz,: *Control of Arthropod Pests of Livestock.* Boca Raton, FL, CRC Press, 1988.

28. Dunsmore, D. J.: *Safety Measures for Use in Outbreaks of Communicable Diseases.* Geneva, World Health Organization, 1986.

29. Dutkiewicz, J.: Occupational biohazards: a review. *Am J Ind Med*, 14:605- 623, 1988.

30. Ellis, P. R.: *An economic evaluation of a swine fever eradication program in Great Britain using a cost benefit analysis technique.* Study No. 11. Reading, England, Department of Agriculture, University of Reading, 1972.

31. Ellis, P. R.: *Benefit vs cost of three systems of mastitis control in individual herds.* Study No. 17. Reading, England, Department of Agriculture, University of Reading, 1975.

32. Ellis, R. W.(ed): *Vaccines: New Approaches to Immunological Problems.* Biotech Ser No 20. Boston, Butterworth-Heinemann, 1992.

33. Esposito, J. J., J. C. Knight, J. H. Shaddock, et al.: Successful oral rabies

vaccination of raccoons with raccoon poxvirus recombinants expressing rabies virus glycoprotein. *Virol*, 165:313-316, 1988.

34. Esposito, J. J.: Live poxvirus-vectored vaccines in wildlife immunization programmes: the rabies paradigm. *Res Virol*, 140:480-482, 1989.
35. Feinstein, A. R.: *Clinical Epidemiology: The Architecture of Clinical Research.* Philadelphia, W. B. Saunders, 1985.
36. Fenner, F., D. A. Henderson, I. Arita, et al.: *Smallpox and its Eradication, History of International Public Health*, No. 6. Geneva, World Health Organization, 1988.
37. Filice, G. A., and Pomeroy, C.: Preventing secondary infections among HIV-positive persons. *Publ Health Rep*, 106:503-517, 1991.
38. Foege, W. H., J. D. Miller, and D. A. Henderson: Smallpox eradication in west and central Africa. *Bull WHO*, 52:209-222, 1975.
39. Foege, W. H.: Preventive medicine and public health. *J Am Med Assoc*, 265:3162-3163, 1991.
40. Fontaine, R. E., and P. M. Schantz: Pet ownership and knowledge of zoonotic diseases in Dekalb County, Georgia. *Anthrozoos*, III:45-49, 1988.
41. Foster, S. O.: Smallpox eradication: lessons learned in Bangladesh. *WHO Chron*, 31:245-247, 1977.
42. Fox, D. M.: From TB to AIDS: Value conflicts in reporting disease. *Hastings Center Rep*, 16, Suppl:11-16, 1986.
43. Frace, R. M., and J. A. Jahre: Policy for managing a community infectious disease outbreak. *Infect Control Hosp Epidemiol*, 12:364-367, 1991.
44. Frank G. R., M. D. Salman, and D. W. Macvean: Use of a disease reporting system in a large beef feedlot. *J Am Vet Med Assoc*, 192:1063-1067, 1988.
45. Gardner, I.: Techniques of reporting disease outbreak investigations. *Vet Clin No Amer: Food Anim Pract*, 4:109-125, 1988.
46. Gerber, R. A., R. S. Hopkins, B. A. Lauer, et al.: Increased risk of illness among nursery staff caring for neonates with necrotizing enterocolitis. *Ped Infect Dis*, 4:246-249, 1985.
47. Gibbs, H. C., and R. P. Herd: Nematodiasis in cattle. Important species involved, immunity, and resistance. *Vet Clin No Amer: Food Anim Pract*, 2:211-224, 1986.
48. Gill, D. M., and D. M. Stone: The veterinarian's role in the AIDS crisis. *J Am Vet Med Assoc*, 201:1683-1684, 1992.
49. Gundersen, S. G., H. Birrie, H. P. Torvik, et al.: Control of *Schistosoma mansoni* in the Blue Nile valley of western Ethiopia. *Trans R Soc Trop Med Hyg*, 84:819-825, 1990.
50. Haber, M., I. M. Longini, and M. E. Halloran: Estimation of vaccine efficiency in outbreaks of acute infectious diseases. *Stat-Med*, 10:1573-1584, 1991.
51. Haber, M., I. M. Longini, and M. E. Halloran: Measures of the effects of vaccination in a randomly mixing population. *Int J Epidemiol*, 20:300-310, 1991.
52. Hanson, R. P., and M. G. Hanson: *Animal Disease Control: Regional Programs.* Ames, IA, Iowa State University Press, 1983.
53. Harvey, J. B., J. M. Roberts, and P. M. Schantz: Survey of veterinarians recommendations for treatment and control of intestinal parasites in dogs: Public health implications. *J Am Vet Med Assoc*, 199:702-707, 1991.

54. Hinman, A. R., W. A. Orenstein, and E. A. Mortimer: When, where, and how do immunizations fail? *Ann Epidemiol*, 2:805-812, 1992.
55. Ho, K.-C.: Epidemiologic methodology as used in China. *J Rheumatol Suppl*, 10:82-85, 1983.
56. Hubbert, W. T., W. F. McCulloch, and P. R. Schnurrenberger: *Diseases Transmitted from Animals to Man*, 6th ed. Springfield, IL, Charles C. Thomas, 1975.
57. Hubbert, W. T.: Occupational health and safety programs in schools of veterinary medicine. *Health Lab Sci*, 15:210-214, 1978.
58. Hubbert, W. T., and H. V. Hagstad: *Food Safety and Quality Assurance: Foods of Animal Origin*. Ames, IA, Iowa State University Press, 1991.
59. Hugh-Jones, M. E., P. R. Ellis, and M. R. Felton: *An assessment of the eradication of bovine brucellosis in England and Wales*. Study No. 19. Reading, England, Department of Agriculture, University of Reading, Reading, England, 1975.
60. Hughes, W. I.: A tribute to toilet paper. *Rev Infect Dis*, Jan-Feb 10:218-222, 1988.
61. Hummer, R. L.: *Animal control statistics every city official and taxpayer should know*. Presented at Amer Vet Med Assoc meeting, Cincinnati, Ohio. July 22, 1976.
62. International Office of Epizootics.: *World Animal Health, No.2. Zoo-sanitary Situation and Methods of Control of Animal Diseases*. Paris, France, Office International des Epizooties, 1986.
63. Jacobs, D. E., M. T. Fox, G. Gowling, et al.: Field evaluation of the ox-fendazole pulse release bolus for the chemoprophylaxis of bovine parasitic gastroenteritis: a comparison with three other control strategies. *J Vet Pharmacol Ther*, 10):30-36, 1987.
64. Jamison, D. T. and W. H. Mosley: Disease control priorities in developing countries: health policy responses to epidemiological change. *Am J Publ Health*, 81:15-22, 1991.
65. Kaufmann, A. F., M. D. Fox, J. M. Boyce, et al.: Airborne spread of brucellosis. *Ann NY Acad Sci*, 353:105-114, 1980.
66. Konowitz, P. M.,G. A. Petrossian, and D. N. Rose: The underreporting of disease and physicians' knowledge of reporting requirements. *Publ Hlth Rep*, 99:31-35, 1984.
67. Laird, M. (ed): *Biocontrol of Medical and Veterinary Pests*. New York, Praeger, 1981.
68. Laird. M. (ed): *Commerce and the Spread of Pests and Disease Vectors*. New York, Praeger, 1984.
69. Landefeld, J. S., and E. P. Seskin: The economic value of life: Linking theory to practice. *Am J Publ Health*, 72:555-566, 1982.
70. Linnabary, R. D., J. C. New, and J. Casper: Environmental disasters and veterinarian's response. *J Am Vet Med Assoc*, 202:1091-1093, 1993.
71. Lipscomb, J., J. T. Kolimaga, P. W. Sperduto, et al.: *Cost-benefit and cost-effectiveness analyses of screening for neural tube defects in North Carolina*. Draft report prepared for the state of North Carolina, 1983.
72. Loehman, E. T., S. V. Berg, A. A. Arroyo, et al.: Distributional analysis of

regional benefits and costs of air quality control. *J Environ Econ Manag*, 6:222-243, 1979.

73. McConnell, J. D., and R. J. Green: The control of hydatid disease in Tasmania: Echinococcus granulosis prevalence in dogs and sheep. *Aust Vet J*, 55:140-145, 1979.
74. McDaniel, T. L.: Comparing expressed and revealed preferences for risk reduction: different hazards and question frames. *Risk Anal*, 8:593-604, 1988.
75. Miller, D. G.: Preventive medicine by risk factor analysis. *J Am Med Assoc*, 222:312-316, 1972.
76. Miller, L. H.: Discovery and disease control. *Am J Trop Med Hyg*, 42:191- 195, 1990.
77. Molyneux, D. H.: Selective primary health care: strategies for control of disease in the developing world. VIII. African trypanosomiasis review. *Rev Infect Dis*, 5:945-956, 1983.
78. Moorehouse, P. D. and M. E. Hugh-Jones: Serum banks. *Vet Bull* 51:277- 290, 1981.
79. Murphy, D.: Massive depopulation and disposal by composting. *Proc Ann Mtg U S Animal Health Assoc*, 96:342-347, 1992.
80. Murray, M., J. C. M. Trail, C. E. Davis, et al.: Genetic resistance to African trypanosomiasis. *J Infect Dis*, 149:311-319, 1984.
81. National Research Council: *Improving Risk Communication*. Washington, D.C., National Academy Press, 1989.
82. Nelson, G. .: Microepidemiology, the key to the control of parasitic infections. *Trans R Trop Soc Med Hyg*, 84:3-13, 1990.
83. Nicoletti, P.: Vaccination against Brucella. *Adv Biotechnol Processes*, 13:147-168, 1990.
84. Nutman, T. B., K. D. Miller, M. Mulligan, et al.: Diethylcarbamazine prophylaxis for human loiasis. Results of a double-blind study. *N Engl J Med*, 319:752-756, 1988.
85. Pappaioanou, M., C. W. Schwabe, and K. Polydorou: Epidemiological analysis of the Cyprus anti-echinococcosis campaign. 1. The prevalence of Echinococcus granulosis in Cypriot village dogs, the first dog-test period of the campaign, June-December, 1972. *Prev Vet Med*, 3:159-180, 1984.
86. Pickett, G. E.: *Public Health: Administration and Practice*, 9th ed. St. Louis, Times Mirror/Mosby College Pub, 1990.
87. Polydorou, K.: The control of echinococcosis. Echinococcus granulosis, sheep, dogs in Cyprus. *World Anim Rev*, 33:19-25, 1980.
88. Putt, S. N. H., A. P. M. Shaw, A. J. Woods, et al.: *ILCA Manual No.3: Veterinary epidemiology and economics in Africa*. Addis Ababa, Ethiopia, International Livestock Centre for Africa, 1987.
89. Radostits, O. M., and D. C. Blood: *Herd Health*. Philadelphia, W. B. Saunders, 1985.
90. Raska, K.: Epidemiologic surveillance in the control of infectious disease. *Rev Infect Dis*, 5:1112-1117, 1983.
91. Rice, D. P.: Estimating the costs of illness. *Am J Publ Health*, 57:424-440, 1967.
92. Rosser, R., and P. Kind: A scale of valuations of state of illness: is there a social consensus? *Int J Epidemiol*, 7:347-358, 1978.

93. Rutala, W. A., and D. J. Weber,: Infectious waste-mismatch between science and policy. *New Engl J Med*, 325:578-582, 1991.
94. Ryan, C. P.: Informing health officials of reportable diseases. *J Am Vet Med Assoc*, 197:962-963, 1990.
95. Sacks, J. J.: Utilization of case definitions and laboratory reporting in the surveillance of notifiable communicable diseases in the United States. *Am J Publ Health*, 75:1420-1422, 1985.
96. Sasa, M.: *Human Filariasis: A Global Survey of Epidemiology and Control.* Baltimore, University Park, 1976.
97. Schantz, P. M.: Parasitic zoonoses in perspective. *Int J Parasitol*, 21:161-170. 1991.
98. Schnurrenberger, P. R., and W. T. Hubbert: Problems of animals in urban areas. *Ann Inst Super Sanita*, 14: 185-409, 1978.
99. Schnurrenberger, P. R., and R. S. Sharman: *Principles of Health Maintenance.* New York, Praeger, 1983.
100. Schnurrenberger, P. R., R. S. Sharman, and G. H. Wise: *Attacking Animal Diseases: Concepts and Strategies for Control and Eradication.* Ames, IA, Iowa State University Press, 1987.
101. Schwabe, C. W.: *Veterinary Medicine and Human Health*, 3rd ed. Baltimore, Williams and Wilkins, 1984.
102. Sutherland, J. P., A. H. Varnam, and M. G. Evans: *A Colour Atlas of Food Quality Control.* The Netherlands, Wolfe Publishing Ltd, 1986.
103. Taylor, J. and E. Paoletti: Pox viruses as eukaryotic cloning and expression vectors: future medical and veterinary vaccines. *Prog Vet Microbiol Immunol*, 4:197-217, 1988.
104. Taylor, J. P., and J. N. Perdue: The changing epidemiology of human brucellosis in Texas, 1977-1986. *Am J Epidemiol*, 130:160-165, 1989.
105. Thacker, S. B., S. Redmond, and M. C. White: A controlled trial of disease surveillance strategies. *Am J Prev Med*, 2:343-350, 1986.
106. Trevino, G. S. (chrmn): *Foreign Animal Diseases: Their Prevention, Diagnosis, and Control.* Richmond, VA. United States Animal Health Association, 1992.
107. United States Department of Agriculture, Animal and Plant Health Inspection Service. *Brucellosis Eradication: Uniform Methods and Rules, Effective May 6, 1992.* Washington, D.C., U.S. Government Printing Office, 1992.
108. U.S. Department of Health and Human Services, Centers for Disease Control: Distribution program for Ivermectin seeks to prevent blindness. *CDC/NCID Focus*, 3(1): 1993.
109. U. S. Department of Health and Human Services, Centers for Disease Control. Inactivated Japanese encephalitis virus vaccine. *MMWR*, 42(RR 1): 1993.
110. Warren, K. S. (ed): *Geographic medicine for the practitioner: Algorithms in the diagnosis and management of exotic diseases.* Chicago, Univ of Chicago Press, 1978.
111. Watier, L., and S. Richardson: A time series construction of an alert threshold with application to *S. bovismorbificans* in France. *Stat Med*, 10:1493-1509, 1991.
112. Weinberg, A. N.: Ecology and epidemiology of zoonotic pathogens. *Infect Dis Clin North Amer*, 5:1-6, 1991.
113. Weiser, J.: *Biological Control of Vectors: Manual for Collecting, Field Determina-*

tion and Handling of Biofactors for Control of Vectors. New York, John Wiley and Sons, 1991.

114. Wilesmith, J. W., and D. R. Williams: Observations on the incidence of herds with non-visible lesioned tuberculin reactors in south-west England. *Epidemiol Infect*, 99:173-178, 1987.

115. Young, E. J.: Human brucellosis. *Rev Infect Dis*, 5:821-842, 1983.

116. Young, E. J.: Health issue at the U.S.-Mexican border. *J Am Med Assoc*, 265:2066, 1991.

117. Zeckhauser, R., and G. S. Shephard: Where now for saving lives? *Law & Contemp Prob*, 40:5-45, 1976.

SECTION III

The Future

5

RECOGNITION AND DEVELOPMENT OF "NEW" ZOONOSES

Introduction

Epidemiologists revel in disasters, usually involving others, sometimes themselves. Unfortunately, in the next decade, it is most unlikely that any significant disasters will be discovered to be new zoonoses. In all probability there will be no new zoonoses. The most that can be hoped for are some new genera of arboviruses, but they will certainly be related to already known viruses. And, there are vectors of known *Leishmania* species of humans and animals that have yet to be identified.[53] The discoveries of the last 20 years have amply demonstrated that any novel infectious disease has been around for many years, producing cases that have gone undiagnosed or been overlooked. This will continue to be so. Outbreaks of so-called "new" diseases cause a few but very well publicized cases, garnering attention that is out of proportion compared with their risk, and distracting services from the much more costly but mundane common diseases. It would be a waste of time and resources to intently watch for new diseases, when the old are still with us causing havoc.

The epidemiologic characteristic of the coming decade will be a continuous foreground reprioritizing of diseases because of changes in the frequency and relative importance of various inconstant risk factors and their responses to control. As a certain factor becomes more common, related diseases will occur more frequently. Similarly, changes reducing other factors will in turn result in a lower incidence of other diseases and perhaps a relatively greater dependence on previously minor factors. The importance of viral evolutionary mechanisms and the emergence of new virulence factors encoded by bacteriophages, plasmids, and transposons significantly affecting disease incidence is a matter of heated academic argument.[42,46,57] Meanwhile in the background, and especially in the developing nations, the currently common zoonoses will continue to flourish. In the latter countries, one can travel back in time to see diseases now controlled or absent in developed countries. This has attractions for those wishing to use modern techniques on historical conditions, to prove oneself better than Koch or Pasteur or Gorgas.

Unfortunately, appropriate techniques and chemicals have been misapplied, resulting in the multiplication of resistant organisms and vectors. The stunning emergence of molecular biology and its intellectual excitement has shifted funding and personnel out of the field (and reality) and firmly into the larger, institutional laboratories. In the promise of this new biotechnology, experienced field officers have been "let go," and the dying and retired are not being replaced. Improved diagnosis is confused with cure. The new, cheap, nontoxic chemotherapeutics and insecticides may, if developed, have the potential for more-efficient control and even in a few instances disease eradication. One can only pray that the field expertise will then be available to apply them efficiently and appropriately.

Just as a number of existing systems for disease management will be rightly shown to be no longer appropriate, it is also certain that some old, proven techniques of disease control will be rediscovered and reapplied successfully. Institutional memory seems to last some 20 years or so, presumably reflecting the average scientific career. Thus, we can expect old systems and preexisting knowledge to resurface at similar intervals, sometimes to be hailed as scientific "breakthroughs."

The potential to misapply scientific knowledge for the purpose of offensive biological warfare (BW) has existed for many decades. Nightmares of new biological agents can be readily conjured. So far, they have been no more than that, in spite of the vociferous claims of various groups and conspiracy theorists. But, this is not to deny that the potential does exist, both for agents and toxins. In the past, some signatories of international treaties ignored their obligations and promises, and continued offensive research. Compliance and verification are essentially voluntary. In the rationale of ethnic and tribal warfare, extra-treaty countries may well utilize biological weapons tactically on the battlefield and terrorize civilian populations. In today's world, the latter can be anybody.

Recognition of "New" Zoonoses

Electronic Information Systems

Better health records. The rapid and continuous downsizing of computers and memory systems will continue to introduce more and more powerful computers and related networked systems into the medical and veterinary clinical workplace. In time, physicians' and veterinarians' clinics will catch up with the routine use of computer strength already in such places as supermarkets and franchised fast-food outlets, and change research-oriented special studies into everyday, universal, support services. There is pressure and action to improve the efficient delivery of health care and disease prevention within large health management systems, such as Kaiser Permanente, which by the mid-1990s had 6.6 million clients in six U.S. states, and some European national health services. In New York, for example, there were 11 health maintenance organizations with more than 30,000 enrollees. The utilization of these large medical databases can and should result not just in improved patient care and management, but also in the retrospective recognition of clusters of cases with shared and initially ill-defined characteristics, variable diagnoses, and maybe poor prognoses that constitute possibly "new" diseases and known but missed diagnoses. Institutes such as major teaching hospitals and veterinary schools attract the rare and unusual cases. They start in the normal world, and a fraction are successfully referred and survive to reach these institutes. Artificial intelligence techniques are available to improve the diagnostic capacity of physicians, as well as to sort through the histories, signs, and symptoms of patients, to propose a tactful short list of probable diagnoses. Many mild, rapidly resolving conditions without permanent effects may never be described, without loss to science or academia. Once a condition is defined, however tentatively, epidemiologic investigations become possible, but not before. In its trail will come more understanding and possibly prevention and control.

Electronic mail. We forget how efficient the mail services were a century ago; one should refer to Sherlock Holmes for the frequent and efficient use of telegrams in his albeit fictional investigations. People corresponded by writing frequent letters. Today, with global telephone links, we have a much improved communication capacity. The present explosion in electronic mail (E-mail) communication is phenomenal, probably because systems such as Internet are currently free, but also because the technical wizardry itself is attractive. Anyone using a network knows that a question put to a worldwide group may get a useful answer or two, if one exists, despite the large volume of chatter going on; E-mail bulletin boards improve the efficiency of news dissemination within specialist groups. Internet was used daily by the Cuban Ministry of Health epidemiologists during 1992-93 to mobilize help and worldwide support in their attempts to diagnose and control the island-wide epidemic of a diffuse but crippling neurologic syndrome of unknown etiology.[26]

Global television news and programs, CNN, and satellite dishes. The capacity of "seeing" events as they occur means that outbreaks that were once only of local concern can now be broadcast globally. For example, Lyme disease outbreaks in Massachusetts might stimulate similar reports in Oregon and Ireland. These can find echoes in Rocky Mountain spotted fever cases in suburban Atlanta as well as in Junin fever cases in Argentina, thereby affecting reports of hemorrhagic fevers in eastern Europe and New Mexico. This hypothesis assumes that broadcast journalists competently practice their craft and that facts are reported with reasonable accuracy. It must be kept in mind, however, that the major factor contributing to the recognition and reporting of a condition is probably the personal awareness by medical and veterinary personnel that it exists, and that it possibly exists among their patients and clients. It is interesting that once a single case of a condition currently thought to be absent has been diagnosed, surrounding practices will begin reporting it also.

General Technological Improvements

Diagnostic efficiency will improve as probes and polymerase chain reaction (PCR) techniques, enzyme-linked immunosorbent assay (ELISA), and other novel systems become readily available to hospital and physicians' clinical pathology laboratories and in field kits. Similarly, chemical antigens will increase the diagnostic repertoire of small laboratories, though without improvements in the basic skills of technical staff. Parallel changes will follow in veterinary laboratories. The specific impacts of the new technologies are discussed in Chapter 6.

Similarly, other research technologies will filter outward. Successful disease control and health maintenance programs will remove, or at least significantly reduce, the common conditions to reveal a wide range of "old" diseases of complex and multiple etiology, as well as less-frequent conditions, to which physicians and veterinarians will shift their efforts and concerns. Parkinson's Law applies to clinical medicine and research just as it does to other endeavors. Consequently, laboratories will respond to this increased demand for new diagnostic tests, which before were economically prohibitive. It is interesting to note how a "new" disease is taken up by a research institute with publicity generated in the hope, usually well founded, that it will result in extra funding to replace discontinued funding that supported prior, successful programs.

Publication of Research Results

It is occasionally overlooked and forgotten that medical and scientific research goes on, and graduate students and their professors publish. Sometimes, the answers may be already in the veterinary literature before the medical questions are asked. Publicized events and scientific advances can stimulate further work, occasionally independent of medical or veterinary need. For example, *Yersinia enterocolitica* has been recovered from a wide range of domestic and wild animals worldwide.[35] Many animals are healthy or clinically inapparent shedders. For many years, it was a well-recognized pathogen of some species and an incidental finding in others. Because of the importance of serology in the control of bovine brucellosis, it was known that antibodies to serotype 9 *Yersinia* infections cross-reacted with antibodies against *Brucella*. The serotypes pathogenic for humans can be recovered from pigs, dogs, and cats. Only in the late 1960s was it recognized as an etiologic agent of gastroenteritis and mesenteric lymphadenitis in humans. It causes an acute enteritis, especially in children, and some 10-20% of cases will mimic appendicitis; thus outbreaks can be retrospectively recognized by a sudden increase in appendectomies. Since recognition is laboratory dependent, it is still frequently underreported, if appropriate isolation is not attempted.[19,52,61]

While anthrax has been known for millennia, some major breakthroughs in scientific knowledge have followed dramatic revelations of *Bacillus anthracis* as a BW weapon. A recent example was the 1980 publicity about the human and animal deaths following an accident at a secret Soviet research institute in Sverdlovsk in April 1979. The reactive increase in research funding and effort by the U.S. military resulted in a significantly better understanding of the plasmids' functions and of the pathogenesis of this disease. At that time, the U.S. and British research on anthrax had been inactive for 10 or more years. In 1936, the British government reacted to the perceived threat of German offensive BW by organizing what is now known as the U.K. Public Health Laboratory Service.[34]

A more bizarre version of reactive research occurred in Canada. The Canadian government stockpiled 2,800 pounds of American botulinum toxin in Sheffield, Alberta, in 1946 as a possible weapon in any future confrontation with the Soviets. In due course, this was reported by Philby to Moscow and the Soviets expanded their botulinum toxin program. This in turn was discovered by the Americans, who restarted their botulinum program at Fort Detrick, which is where the Canadian's toxin supply had come from.

Until natural infections with *Mycobacterium leprae* were noted in nine-banded armadillos (*Dasypus novemcinctus*) in Louisiana in 1975[81] as a result of prior attempts to infect wild armadillos,[43] the organism was cultured with great difficulty in the footpads of mice. Other studies could only be done on tissue taken from living or dead human cases, with very limited results. The very large numbers of organisms that can be harvested from artificially infected armadillos underwrote the development of the lepromin skin test and a rapid expansion in research and diagnostic tools. Whether nine-banded armadillos are a reservoir host for this disease in humans is currently unknown. The seven-banded armadillo (*Dasypus hybridus*) is not as susceptible to infection.[7]

A notable difference between humans and animals is the relative difference in known teratogenic and SMEDI (for stillbirth, mummification, embryonic death, and infertility) infections. In humans, the current list is short and essentially limited to four viruses (*Cytomegalovirus, Herpes simplex, Parvovirus* B19, and rubella[44]), three bacteria (*Listeria monocytogenes, Treponema pallidum, Leptospira* spp.), and the protozoan *Toxoplasma gondii; Borrelia burgdorferi* is suspected but, as yet, unproven.[48,71,73] There is very persuasive epidemiologic evidence that A2 influenza infections in pregnant women during the second trimester are associated with the later development of schizophrenia in their offspring.[9,51,58] In pigs, there are significant fetal and perinatal losses from porcine parvovirus, Aujeszky/pseudorabies virus, and the "porcine reproductive respiratory syndrome" agent (probably an arterovirus), as well as from *Leptospira interrogans, T. gondii*, hog cholera/swine fever (*Pestivirus suis*) viruses ("congenital tremor"), Japanese B encephalitis virus, chlamydia, Sendai virus, and porcine cytomegalic inclusion virus.[83] The Flaviruses contain, besides the Japanese B encephalitis virus, Wesselsbron virus, which affects humans and produces congenital hydranencephaly in sheep, and the St. Louis, Murray Valley, Rocio, and West Nile encephalitides. Teratogenic lesions are found in cattle and sheep following infections with Akabane virus (*Bunyavirus*), bluetongue virus (*Orbivirus*), bovine virus diarrhea virus (*Pestivirus*), and the related border disease virus. In the past, many of these teratogenic effects were considered to be genetic diseases.

The relative absence of recognized teratogenic infections in humans relates directly to the haphazard manner in which pregnancy occurs as compared to livestock. Even the best human pathology units rarely autopsy spontaneous abortuses. This is in stark contrast to the high frequency that aborted fetuses and placentae are examined in veterinary diagnostic laboratories. When "outbreaks" of human miscarriages occur, they are usually recognized retrospectively and then the blame is frequently put on presumed toxic exposures from local petrochemical or heavy-metal industries.

Similarly, human milk is rarely examined for infectious agents, whereas it is an everyday event in veterinary laboratories. *Leptospira interrogans* serovar *hardjo* has been transferred from a lactating infected anicteric mother to her infant.[12] *L. monocytogenes* has also been isolated from human milk from an apparently asymptomatic mother. Her 3-week-old infant and a litter of puppies of the same age simultaneously developed listeriosis and from the same serotype, 4b; the mother's surplus milk had been fed to the puppies.[77] Human milk is not pasteurized before consumption.

Following the importation in 1933 from Germany of some sheep that had successfully come through quarantine, there were simultaneous disease outbreaks of unknown etiology on a number of Icelandic farms. The Germans had unknowingly exported *visna-maedi*. This retrovirus infection was facilitated by the prolonged, crowded, winter housing of sheep on the island. The Icelandic sheep also suffered from *rida*, an Icelandic form of scrapie, and *jaagsiekte* from another retrovirus infection. This collection of severe, long-incubation diseases of significant economic import initiated the medico-veterinary research of what was later identified by Bjorn Sigurdsson and his colleagues at Keldur as "slow virus" diseases.[82]

Model situations based on observed events in animal populations, such as the above examples, will act as catalysts to reveal similar but heretofore unrealized situations in the human population. Also, if the normal antenatal TORCH (*Toxoplasma*/Rubella/*Cytomegalovirus*/*Herpes*) serum samples were stored until the pregnancy outcome was known, they could then be used for initial case-control screening material for infectious causes. Complaints about the U.S. government's hiatus on support for human embryo studies are hollow because much can be done without recourse to such experimental material.

Dynamics of Recognition

Why was Lyme disease not recognized until Steere and his colleagues investigated a cluster of pediatric arthritis cases in Lyme, Connecticut, in 1975?[75] "Montauk knee" was already a well-known local condition at the tip of Long Island, a few miles across the sound from Connecticut. The characteristic initial skin rash (erythema migrans) had been described in Europe at the beginning of the century,[1,47] and for 25 years it was known to follow the bite of the European tick, *Ixodes ricinus*,[30] which is closely related to the North American vector, *I. scapularis/I. dammini*. The ecologic conditions necessary for the maintenance of endemic foci of *B. burgdorferi*—appropriate tick species, rodents, abundant white-tailed deer, woodland, and forest—have waned and waxed as the woodland habitat was cleared for agriculture, charcoal, and firewood in the 18th and 19th centuries. Then, as farms were abandoned, it returned from open fields to deciduous forests and the "woodburbs" of suburban residential communities. The latter carry high densities of both deer and humans.[8] At the beginning of the 20th century, the U.S. deer population was estimated to be about 0.5 million; 90 years later it has grown to 15 million.

A similar scenario occurred with infections of *Babesia microti* and is being followed in the recognition of acute pathogenic hantavirus infections—a triggering cluster followed by the reporting of similar cases elsewhere.[15] As there are between 50,000 and 150,000 unexplained human respiratory disease deaths each year in the United States, there are ample opportunities to find more cases.

Where was AIDS/HIV until 1979? The reexamination of stored sera and pathological tissues has shown that this disease existed for decades, albeit sporadically, before it was recognized. The earliest documented and confirmed case was a 25-year-old seaman who died in Manchester, England, in 1959.[17] In 1966, a Norwegian sailor sickened with an HIV-1 infection, which was fatal to him, his wife, and daughter in 1976. In 1968, a 15-year-old African American male who had never gone outside the St. Louis area was hospitalized with what has been retrospectively diagnosed as a fatal HIV-1 infection.[27] HIV antibodies have been identified in a Zairian sample from among 672 plasma specimens collected during 1959 in central Africa (Leopoldville and Stanleyville, and rural tribes in the Belgian Congo, Rwanda, Burundi, and southern Sudan). No evidence of infection was found in 146 samples from Xhosa bushmen (1959), from 118 rural Bantu in Mozambique (1967), or 277 rural Bantu in the Congo (1982).[54]

The paucity of serologic evidence for HIV in archived African serum collections is in stark contrast to the high seroprevalence rates in more current collections. For example, in 1984-85 some 10% of Kinshasa women aged 15-29 years old were HIV positive, and female prostitutes in Nairobi went from 4% seropositive in 1980-81 to 59% in 1985-86. The causes of this explosion in urban Africa in the late 1970s are not fully described but would include the following: opportunities for rapid passage and increased virulence offered by the breakdown of traditional rural living in the post-colonial period; the population shift into larger and larger urban centers; sexual networking and parallel high rates of sexually transmitted diseases aiding heterosexual transmission; the use of unsterilized needles in hospitals and pharmacies; and contaminated blood transfusions.[59,64,66] A genetic comparison of HIV-1 and HIV-2 indicates that the former virus may have evolved from the latter as recently as the late 1940s.[74] Whether it evolved originally from a simian SIV virus or from a nonpathogenic human HIV virus is currently unclear[49] and certainly not without controversy.[24,76]

An undescribed condition can be "discovered" in a laboratory system established for special studies. This specialist laboratory will act as a "trap" for infrequent diseases that are clinically very similar to the designated disease. With their enhanced, specialized experience, the pathologists will notice that some submissions do not match either the new disease or the well-described old diseases. For example, the Lasswade Veterinary Investigation Laboratory in Scotland noted the absence of the characteristic spongiform brain lesions associated with bovine spongiform encephalopathy (BSE, or "mad cow disease"), which is a scrapie-related condition, in two beef cows compulsorily slaughtered with "maniacal" signs. At the time, the United Kingdom had compulsorily slaughtered some 86,500 cows under the BSE Orders. Some 25 animals in Scotland and 2 in England have now been diagnosed with idiopathic brainstem neuronal chromatolysis and hippocampal sclerosis.[36,50] Earlier, a similar situation had occurred with pig diseases and teratogenic infections during and following the eradication of swine fever/hog cholera in the United Kingdom.

The probable components for the recognition of a "new" disease are:

1. A cluster of cases or an "outbreak" that defines itself. The awareness of infrequently occurring conditions is missing until they cannot be ignored.

2. Coincident availability of a competent laboratory and/or specialist, e.g., kuru in Papua New Guinea and Gajdusek, lymphoma and Burkitt in East Africa.

3. Recent development of a new technology, whether or not it has any initial relevance to the problem.

4. Infrequent case numbers but a celebrity patient, or parent, or one who merely pushes doggedly for answers.

5. Deaths—one or more of "our" children, hundreds of "theirs." This did not apply as strongly to the old colonial and tropical medical officers.

6. Legal recourse (a spreading American habit).

7. Parallel epidemiologies—a traditional but productive epidemiologic approach.

8. Negative effects—As diseases and infections become less frequent, they are underdiagnosed and underreported because their possibility is not considered or even remembered by physicians and veterinarians, e.g., rubella and anthrax.

Scenarios That Have or Will Increase the Incidence of "New" Zoonoses

International Travel

Some zoonotic diseases have managed to travel, others have not. This success will depend on the infectivity of the infected, the nature and duration of their shedding and carrier status, incubation periods, the availability and efficiency of potential new vectors, and lethality of the disease, all in relation to the transit time and the nature of the transport.

Chagas' disease occurred in early native Americans when (zymodeme 2 [Z2] *Trypanosoma cruzi*-infected) guinea pigs (*Cavia porcellus*) were domesticated in the high plateaus of Bolivia and, instead of living wild in rock piles with their ectoparasites and triatomine bugs, were raised underfoot in human shelters. The triatomine vectors soon followed. Although *Triatoma infestans* is now highly synanthropic, wild populations have been identified in Cochabamba and Sucre, with their primary habitat among stones.[10] Archeological evidence of the domestic raising of guinea pigs has been found in Peruvian sites dated 2500 B.C. The *T. cruzi* Z2 strain is associated with megacolon and megaesophagus forms of the human disease. Among the first pre-Incaic cultures to abandon the nomadic life for settlement were the Wankarani Indians, who migrated from the Bolivian altiplano to settle in northern Chile. Tombs near their settlements dated around 2500 B.C. contain naturally mummified bodies, and about 30% show signs of cardiac fibrosis or mega-syndromes consistent with chronic Chagas' disease. The relatively benign nature of Chagas' disease in Chile today suggests an ancient association with humans. This chronic infection probably remained a local Andean problem until the emergence of the Inca empire with its considerable organization skills and successful military campaigns. With Pizarro and the Spanish conquest of South America and the subsequent Spanish colonial rule and trade, the Z2-related disease spread slowly throughout southern South America. For example, it only reached northeastern Brazil in the 1970s.[70] The carrier is a chronically infected rural human, a migrant worker in particular, who must be fed upon by a domiciliary triatomine vector for spread to occur to other humans and dogs that can then act as reservoirs. For efficient disease spread, it seems that the human carrier must be accompanied by *T. infestans*, which out-competes and quickly replaces other domestic triatomine species. Where the sylvatic cycle exists, involving the Z1 strain in arboreal marsupials and Z3 in armadillos, human infections are only occasional and of slight public health importance; Z3 is rarely found in humans. In urban areas in Latin America, the major threat is now from contaminated blood transfusions where more than 5% of blood donors can be infected.

It is traditional since time immemorial to hold that plague has been spread by the triad of trade, travelers (commercial, military, and religious), and ships with rats. If so, the rodent reservoir and its fleas, resupplied with susceptible animals by breeding, were important components in maintaining the infection during transit. Others have introduced caveats based on death rates in restricted infected rodent populations, such as in small sailing vessels.[78] However, plagues still broke out in ports. In retrospect, it seems that the Seoul strain of the Hantaan virus has reached almost every port in the world with its unaffected *Rattus norvegicus* host. During and just after World War II, *Angiostrongylus cantonensis*, the principal etiologic agent of human eosinophilic meningitis, spread throughout the Indo-Pacific basin and adjoining lands via infected rats sequestered in shipments of war materials and facilitated by postwar commerce. It has since been identified in tropical and semitropical ports worldwide, affecting humans and even caged primates.[45] The parasite's spread has also been aided by the widely traveled giant African snail, *Achatina fulica*, a popular intermediate host that can harbor between 10,000 and 39,000 infective larvae.[2] The present worldwide distribution of *Triatoma rubrofasciata* indicates that it was transported by 16th- and 17th-century Portuguese and Dutch merchant adventurers from coastal Brazil to the Antilles, Africa, India, and Southeast Asia, where the *rubrofasciata* complex radiated.[70] And ships have transported pathogens, such as *Vibrio cholerae*, and exotic fauna (Zebra mussels) in their bilge water.

With more-rapid transit times, successful travel by infectious agents depended more on shedding by convalescent cases or by a slow spread through a ship's company. Later, cholera and malaria, for example, were successfully disseminated by railroads in India and North America. The introduction of air travel permitted the portage of increasingly ephemeral infections. Travel initially available to a select few is now available to virtually all. Vast numbers travel daily, with hundreds in any one plane, in a churning polydirectional matrix of contact and aerosol opportunities. In 1957, the author of this chapter witnessed the majority of the population in the city of Kaduna in Northern Nigeria afflicted with "Asian flu" (subtype H2N2) within a week of the return of the pilgrims from their Haj to Mecca. The city had welcomed them back with the traditional white horses and accompanied them to their homes. Not only do they share the same air, but airline passengers also eat the same food, which may have been put on the plane with the passengers or at an intermediate stop. Food poisoning has been identified as a leading cause of airline pilot incapacitation.[11] Travel-related stress has immune-suppressing effects. For example, in 1979 72% of passengers on a flight to Kodiak, Alaska, came down with influenza after the plane had been held at the landing gate for 4 hours.

The present global tourist industry has the potential for rapidly transferring exotic infections from one latitude to another. For example, in one study[23] of Swedish tourists who had visited Cyprus in September 1987, 50% had antibodies to sandfly fever after their return to Sweden; in 1985, 11 of 298 United Nations soldiers stationed on Cyprus for 6 months had seroconverted. The emergence of eco-tourism will put increasing numbers of susceptible individuals at risk. Such packages take the tourists rapidly into and out of areas that they would not normally visit, thereby exposing them to new enzootic infections over fairly short periods of 5 to 10 days. This is enough time to develop the clinical disease at home, if not on the flight home while surrounded by other travelers. The use of Cuban soldiers as mercenaries in Africa expanded the range of dengue viruses on that island. The collapse of the largely successful *Aedes aegypti* eradication program organized by the Pan American Health Organization and its member countries has contributed significantly to the increased frequency and size of epidemics of dengue and dengue hemorrhagic fever in the Americas. The arguments[16] for the apparent nonappearance of dengue in North America, in spite of its high incidence in the Caribbean basin countries, might be used to similarly explain the absence of yellow fever.

1. Although *Aedes aegypti* and *Ae. albopictus* are competent vectors, are widely distributed in the southern United States, and occur in the peridomestic environment, their distribution is variable and uneven within the region.

2. Although vector-host contact may be frequent in areas where screens do not inhibit the indoor entry of mosquitoes or in garden areas, the housing types and lifestyles (e.g., screens and air conditioning) of those likely to travel to and from the Caribbean and the Amazon basin preclude human contact with North American vector species.

3. The human population lacks immunity to dengue (and yellow fever) virus; travelers in yellow fever areas (e.g., Darien, the Amazon basin, and Africa) are expected to be vaccinated, but it cannot be presumed. The seasonal occurrence of dengue transmission in endemic areas usually peaks during the winter holiday season in North America, when travel to the tropics is most intense but when U.S. vector populations are at their lowest.

4. Although dengue is endemic in many countries (just as yellow fever is enzootic in forest primates) and the virus may be introduced, the viremia lasts only an average of 4 to 5 days, providing a small window of vector opportunity.

5. The nonrecognition of dengue infections by U.S. physicians may allow local transmission to begin, but the critical vector density necessary for successful secondary transmission in a specific locality may not exist over larger areas. The wild primate hosts for yellow fever are absent outside zoological gardens.

Although dengue may never invade the United States and Canada, this is not to proscribe the arrival and successful dissemination of all other vectorborne infections. Whereas an infection may be naturally absent in an area, the potential native vector population, as yet also unexposed, may be a competent vector when presented with a viremic host. Vectors can also travel. In 1985, *Ae. albopictus* arrived in North America and Brazil from the Philippines and has taken over all but the innermost nuclear areas inhabited by *Ae. aegypti*. There is a possibility that dengue may have a primate reservoir in Southeast Asia. If so, it might utilize new primate hosts as *Ae. albopictus* spreads globally. Although *Ae. albopictus* is recognized for its competence with dengue virus, it is now known to be competent for eastern equine encephalitis virus; other viruses will be identified in due course. In 1930, *Anopheles gambiae*, an African species, was reported in Natal, northeastern Brazil, possibly as a result of early transatlantic flights or via ships. This was followed by a decade of severe malarial outbreaks in that part of Brazil. In July 1977, two cases of *Plasmodium falciparum* malaria were reported in Paris, one in a luggage porter and the other in a person living near the airport. In 1981, there was an outbreak of malaria in the area surrounding the Paris airports. Similarly, in 1983 four cases of *P. falciparum* were found in British residents who had not traveled to malarial countries; two had taken a European flight on a plane recently arrived from Africa and the other two lived near Gatwick Airport, an international airport south of London.[68]

It has been predicted that the global mean temperature will increase by 0.3°C per decade.[79] If correct, temperature increases will be about 1°C by 2025 A.D. The northern latitudes will warm faster than the equatorial, more in winter than in summer, and more at night than in daytime. The ocean level is expected to have risen by about 20 cm by 2030 A.D. The temperature rise in central North America and southern Europe will be greater than the mean and accompanied by a decrease in precipitation. Indirectly, these aggregate events will affect the ecology and thus the interactions between vectors, hosts, old and new reservoirs, and viruses. The viruses will replicate more rapidly and efficiently in their arthropod vectors, which will mature more rapidly and possibly with a shorter life span. In some instances, the latter will prevent the former from being completed. But, in general the disease latitudes will increase as infections and their vectors move toward the poles.

Airplanes carry humans and their waste products. Although sterilizing chemicals are added to the waste tanks containing urine and feces, they may not be fully effective.[41] Cholera cases of uncertain origin in central and southern Europe during 1970-75 underlay flight paths from Calcutta.[67] The ground crews emptying these tanks are at obvious risk. It has been known that members of these crews have arranged to hide delicacies from relatives in their home country in the tail section of international flights. The "contraband" arrives in good order because of the natural refrigeration of high-altitude flight.

Zoonotic diseases, by definition, affect animals. Thus, the agent can be transported when animals are moved. An outbreak of epilepsy among native peoples in Irian Jaya was eventually diagnosed as cerebral cysticercosis caused by *Taenia solium*. Until Indonesia annexed West Irian, this parasite was absent in West Irian and Papua New Guinea. It was traced to a large importation of pigs from Bali, where taeniasis occurs, as a gift from the Indonesian government to community leaders. Pigs occupy a central position in the culture of New Guinea and live in intimate family contact, thereby facilitating the ingestion of *T. solium* eggs. In Hindu Bali, the people bathe frequently, and pigs are managed outside the home. Therefore, the Balinese have taeniasis, not cysticercosis. Because of the severe political and civil problems following the unilateral military annexation, this medical problem in Irian Jaya may have been foreseen.[18] A real risk exists that *Echinococcus granulosus*, and thus human hydatidosis, will be imported into Papua New Guinea via infected sheep. Evidently, the quarantine regulations have not been applied as meticulously as laid down.[4]

During 1989, there were some half million birds imported legally into the United States (Table 5-1). This included 361 species representing 65 avian families, with finches and parrots comprising 97% of the birds imported. Approximately 85% were for commercial sale in pet stores or to commercial aviculturists. Some 14% were dead on arrival or died shortly thereafter in quarantine; this mortality measure is minimal because shipments had been off-loaded in transit and dead birds removed. Even with the available data, 12% of imported shipments had death rates of 30% or higher.

During 1989, 3,507 birds from Honduras and Indonesia were refused entry because of Newcastle disease (ND); 37% were re-exported and the rest died or were euthanized. During the decade 1980-89, more than 2.2% of birds were refused entry because of Newcastle disease; sick and dying birds in quarantine are only routinely examined by the USDA for *Salmonella enteritidis* and hemagglutinating viruses—Newcastle disease (*Paramyxovirus*) and avian influenza infections (*Orthovirus*). Other possible infections are ignored. During the period 1980-84, birds usually imported from the following countries were suffering from Newcastle disease: Africa (Ghana, Tanzania); Latin America (Argentina, Bolivia, El Salvador, Honduras, Mexico, Panama, Paraguay, Peru, Guatemala); Asia (India, Indonesia, Malaysia, Taiwan); and Europe (Belgium). More recently, velogenic viscerotropic ND virus was recovered from five batches of imported birds in 1990, five in 1991, and three in 1992. Considering that ND is an airborne or fecally transmitted infection, depending on the virus type, the extreme stress that these birds suffer through capture, holding, and transportation packed together in less than optimal conditions, the diagnosed incidence of ND may be underestimated as it is based on the birds that survive until landing.

Table 5-1. Regional origins of birds imported into the United States in 1989

| | | % Mortality | | |
Continent	Numbers Imported	DOA[a]	DQ[a]	Total deaths (DOA + DQ)
Africa	206,184	7.0	12.3	19.4
Latin America and Caribbean	117,420	1.2	8.9	10.1
Europe and Middle East	60,957	0.6	6.3	6.8
Asia and Pacific	49,062	1.0	9.2	10.1
Australia	8,370	1.7	3.1	4.9
Unknown origins	19,868	2.8	19.1	22.0
Grand Totals	461,861	3.8	10.4	14.3

Source: Nilsson, G.[56]

[a]DOA = dead on arrival; DQ = died in quarantine or were euthanized.

The experience of the smuggled blue-fronted Amazon parrot (*Amazona aestiva*) is common for many others. It was once extremely common in the Chaco of eastern Brazil, Paraguay, Bolivia, and northern Argentina. But Brazil, Paraguay, and Bolivia prohibit the export of their native birds. The blue-fronted Amazon parrot can only be legally exported from Argentina, and thus large numbers are smuggled into Argentina from the adjoining countries. Despite this influx, there remains heavy pressure to trap those parrots in Argentina. Similarly, birds from Guyana include a significant proportion of birds illegally exported from Venezuela. Similar appearances of non-native birds occur in exports from Singapore. The accompanying documents do not define the true origins. It is estimated that a further 225,000 birds are smuggled into the United States each year, and of these at least 100,000 cross the U.S.-Mexican border. These smuggled birds are not held for 30 days, while any infection resolves itself and the birds stop shedding. These figures give an idea of the potential for smuggling a "new" zoonotic disease into but one country, the United States. Perhaps importing countries are protected by the high death rate of birds in transit.

There is a large international trade in monkeys for research laboratories. This is under increasing national and international control and is already significantly reduced from what it was in the 1960s and 1970s. African hemorrhagic fever, which includes the Ebola and Marburg viruses, has been associated with imported monkeys, initially in research institutes. The true reservoir of either virus has yet to be defined.

Whereas many of the above examples are of diseases traveling from the tropics to wider latitudes, from developing to developed countries, the advanced countries can and do pose serious risks. The United Kingdom imported bulls with enzootic bovine leukosis from Canada and in turn has exported animals affected with bovine spongiform encephalopathy. Whereas the U.K. experience with Canada was more of a nuisance, Albania imported infected bulls from a number of countries with the result that 27 of 28 districts had enzootic leukosis prevalence rates ranging from 14% to 100% infected cattle.[60] Uruguayan sheep carried *Cochliomyia hominivorax* larvae to Libya at a final eradication cost of $82 million.[28] *Haematobia irritans* was introduced from Europe into the United States more than a century ago, and by 1977 its dispersal area was from Canada to Venezuela; it has now reached northern Argentina.[6] A number of importing countries have learned, to their financial dismay, that the certified brucella-free status did not match the condition of the accompanying cattle. The same situation applies to other official "certified-free" states and international bureaucratic constraints on control.[5,33] Less well known infections will make use of similar opportunities.

Regional Travel of Susceptible Populations into High-Risk Areas

When people travel into the surrounding countryside and wildernesses, they can become exposed to novel infections, especially when camping or "roughing it." Giardial dysentery has become sufficiently common that backpacking North Americans are firmly advised to boil or chemically treat all drinking water taken from streams and lakes, even in the most-isolated areas. The protozoan appears to be acquired from naturally infected beavers, moose, and other animals. Higher socioeconomic Mexicans have acquired *Trypanosoma cruzi* infections by having holiday homes in high-risk tropical areas,[80] and people with holiday homes frequently take their dogs and cats with them. Non-voluntary travel by those condemned to internal exile, as in previous decades to Siberia, exacerbated by severe psychological, physical, and nutritional stresses, will have exposed such individuals to, for example, the viral hemorrhagic and rickettsial diseases. During World War II, the German troops suffered extensively from typhus and rickettsial spotted fevers while battling partisans behind their Eastern Front.

A century ago, the majority of the world's population lived in a rural setting with agriculture to match that of small family farms. Now, more than 90% of the global population is urban with many cities with populations in the millions; by the end of the century there will be 425 cities with more than a million inhabitants. This urbanization has not just been a movement toward industrial centers to take advantage of better wages and jobs but also a flight from the countryside as agriculture became more efficient, increasing rural poverty in the face of decreasing facilities and alternative jobs. Thus, a number of cities are now ringed by slums, colonias, and favelas of dense, crowded populations living with minimal shelter, overwhelmed health services, open sewage, polluted drinking water, malnutrition, minimal educational facilities, and a maximum opportunity for crime, both by criminals and the sometimes equally predatory local police. These populations are characterized by a high proportion of juveniles in spite of a high infant mortality rate. With high death rates, come high communal susceptibilities to hyperendemic infections. For those more accustomed to Canberra, Paris, London, or Washington, there is a surprising number of livestock, usually small ruminants and poultry, in these places. All in all, these environments present an ideal opportunity for the maintenance of a multitude of infectious and communicable diseases.[55]

Increasing Proportions and Numbers of Susceptible Human and Companion Animal Populations

A weakening of the immune system within communities can follow from a number of causes. Some can be expected from societal changes, directly related to medical and veterinary responses to changes in the population structure and to the increasing frequency of disease conditions among the elderly. The progressive decline of the immune system in aging individuals is compounded by their economic and psychosocial problems of low consumption of proteins, micronutrients, and vitamins.[25] Reduced communal immunogenicity can follow from a number of causes:

1. Age shift, e.g., aging populations of humans and companion animals.
2. Immunosuppressive treatments, e.g., associated with organ and tissue transplants, anti-autoimmune treatments, chemotherapy for malignancy.
3. Radiation treatment of malignancies.
4. Immuno-suppressive diseases, e.g., HIV, FIV, feline panleukopenia, BVD.
5. Malnutrition.
6. Seasonal weather—extremes of temperature.
7. Refusal of various religious groups to have themselves or their children immunized.

The immune suppressed, rather like a communal polymerase chain-reaction multiplication, promote infections to reveal agents that are otherwise medically invisible either because of normal nonpathogenicity or by being below the diagnostic threshold of recognition. Avian tuberculosis and *Pneumocystis carinii* pneumonia in AIDS patients are examples of this. The question is whether the increased frequency of human and animal passage will result in a change in the pathogenicity, thereby putting the whole population of either or both at increased risk.

Monkeypox is unusual in humans and unlikely to spread beyond the first person. But, in a chain of person-to-person cases involving five young children in two families, two had clinical measles at the same time, suggesting that the other three children may have had subclinical measles infections.[37] Morbilivirus infections suppress the immune response to other coincident infections.

A community failure to acquire immunity is a direct effect of budget cuts and failed vaccination delivery programs. These are exacerbated by reductions in public health programs, especially in relation to pediatric and school health delivery systems. Unfortunately, effective vaccines and public health clinics alone do not ensure that children are vaccinated. And, leaving it to parents to decide whether their children should be vaccinated will significantly reduce the numbers vaccinated. Vaccination programs must involve all levels of the community and a number and variety of delivery systems, and must be proactive if they are to be successful. The same applies to veterinary vaccination programs.

With families worldwide much smaller than they were even a few decades ago, one can speculate as to whether it has made a difference in exposure and randomly acquired immunity. Although smaller families have more time and money to spend on each child, the child contact rate with other children, especially of very different age groups, may be reduced even if the children are in daycare outside the home. This may have the effect of delaying exposure until ages when disease effects can be more severe.

Within small groups and at the local level, the following individual effects will continue to affect immunity: (1) dysmaturity and prematurity of neonates; (2) inherited diseases; (3) malignancy; (4) pregnancy; (5) severe trauma and burns.

Listeriosis is a good example of the above, for local outbreaks affect pregnant women, neonates, and the immune suppressed within the exposed community, which is otherwise unaffected. When patients who are usually severely ill from acute care facilities are mixed with residents in long-term-care hospitals who have decreased immune function because of age or chronic illness, there is a real potential for increased nosocomial infection rates, thus posing a risk to patients, staff, and visitors. The occurrence of such outbreaks can go unnoticed because there are no standardized criteria defining nosocomial infections in long-term facilities.

Water

Water contaminated with animal feces is increasingly being cited as a factor in outbreaks of waterborne disease. Some outbreaks have been spectacular in size, such as the 13,000 persons with gastroenteritis in the U.S. state of Georgia in 1987 after consuming water from a filtered, chlorinated public water supply. *Cryptosporidium* oocysts were recovered from fecal specimens and from samples of treated water; the oocysts are resistant to chlorination. Investigations showed that, although the water met turbidity standards, filters had allowed the passage, for a variety of mechanical and management reasons, of particulate matter likely to have contained oocysts. A blocked major sewer line, allowing a sewage overflow above the water treatment plant inlet of unknown duration, was also noted. In spite of these major defects, cattle were cited as a contributory cause when 3 of 56 (2 were calves) were found to be excreting "low numbers" of oocysts; cryptosporidiosis is a disease of neonatal ruminants.[29] In the latter case, an outbreak of cryptosporidial diarrhea affecting an estimated 370,000 residents in Milwaukee during March and April 1993 was associated with turbid water from a single water treatment plant and employee inexperience, but the blame was laid on the local dairy industry.[21]

The true zoonotic contribution to the epidemiology of this protozoan infection awaits critical studies. A Swiss case-control study of cryptosporidiosis in children found that the highest relative risk was prior contact with a person suffering from diarrhea (20.0) followed by prior travel in a Mediterranean country (5.0); a weak association was noted for contact with cats and dogs failing to thrive (P=0.08, RR=4.0), and consuming raw milk (P=0.10, RR=4.3).[22] An uncontrolled United Kingdom Public Health Laboratory Service study of cryptosporidiosis found that 23% of the U.K.-acquired cases during 1985-87 were associated with exposure to farm animals or raw milk. Subsequent to this study, an outbreak of 84 cases was noted in South Glamorgan, but only 4 had consumed raw milk; 15 of those affected had been on vacation. It was later found that the area had been receiving unfiltered, but chlorinated, drinking water. Again, the blame was put on local livestock without any supporting evidence.[62]

A common epidemiologic error when faced with a lack of positive evidence is to invoke the paradigm. We have all committed this error, and any epidemiologist denying it should be viewed with caution. Paradigms are just *les matrices du jour* (something of the day). Nature and God do not read the literature. This is not to deny that livestock may play an epidemiologic role in human cryptosporidiosis. It merely points out that a defecating cow in an upstream pasture is inadequate proof, just as observing cats in a barn cannot fully explain toxoplasmosis. There are many occasions when other sources are more valid and must be sought and quantified. One must never forget normal infective doses and that the mere presence of an agent is no proof of its vehicle being the cause.

Another aspect confusing the origins and causes of waterborne infections is politics. Recently, a river in southeast Louisiana was found to be highly contaminated with *Escherichia coli*. The contamination was so severe, in fact, that the authorities promptly shut down various leisure activities associated with the river, such as "tubing." The blame was very promptly laid on the less than 300 dairy herds grazing pastures adjoining the river and its tributaries. Very expensive environmental laws were passed to force the dairy farmers to lagoon the bovine feces. What was missing from the public discussion was the fact that 9 of the 11 municipalities on the river had sewage systems out of compliance, and that very many outlying and rural homes had septic tanks that were less than rudimentary with outflows that reached the river. The latter also applied to many weekend homes and hunting camps on the river banks. The political and financial cost of insisting that community and individual systems be upgraded would have been unacceptably high.

An examination of the public health records for this river indicated that the river water may have become a culture medium because there was less variation from north to south than one might expect from only human and animal fecal sources. Chemicals—agricultural, industrial, and domestic—must affect the normal phytoplanktonic population and thus the ability of streams and rivers to absorb these pathogens. Poor water management, excessive sediments, and siltation can only exacerbate the situation. The epidemiology of waterborne infections is very complex and must involve the whole ecosystem, not just feces. For example, environmental reservoirs of toxigenic *Vibrio cholerae* O1 El Tor exist independently of humans in Queensland, the Gulf of Mexico, and other places. Many trematodes live and thrive in a water habitat and have only an incidental, albeit painful, residence in humans. They actually prefer livestock or wildlife hosts.

Regional, Transcontinental, and International Food Industries

With the development of high-quality livestock and poultry (which have very rapid growth rates and uniform carcass standards) and the monitoring that progresses from rearing pen to the local supermarket, the need for the gross inspection of individual animals at slaughter is no longer essential in developed countries. The problem now is microbiologic and chemical contaminants that cannot be seen on inspection. Rapid-screening systems for checking animals and batches on the moving line are needed and will be implemented over the coming decade. Gross inspection will be necessary, though, for the foreseeable future in developing countries. Similarly, it will have to be maintained in developed countries for culled stock, such as dairy cows, which frequently present a number of microbiologic, pathologic, and residual toxicologic problems, including systemic infections and inapparent bacteremias when slaughtered. The multi-state outbreaks of disease associated with *E. coli* O157:H7 highlight this situation.[13,14,38,69] Hamburger meat is derived from the trimmings and less-attractive parts of carcasses. It is then ground and mixed, dispersing the fecal contaminants throughout the whole.

The last two decades have seen the emergence of transcontinental and international food industries, especially poultry and pork products. For efficiency, these industries are vertically integrated from the primary breeder units to the local supermarket. These super-industries have brought to major segments of the population in many countries and regions significant social and economic benefits in the form of better-quality and cheaper food. McDonald's and its imitators have been a force for nutritional good in society.

The food industry in the developed world might be summed up as follows: It is feeding more people (1) simultaneously, (2) in many homes, in few but extensive hotel and restaurant chains, and in institutional catering organizations, and (3) with the same products, which are potentially subject to the same production errors, in fewer but larger plants that have obtained animals and animal products from relatively few but very large farms. Therefore, any errors or accidents will be multiplied exponentially compared to what epidemiologists saw previously when many, smaller farms and local processing were the norm. Along with the vertical integration of these commercial agricultural systems has come less heterogeneity in management systems and a narrowing of the microbiologic environment. While limiting access to many organisms, some of which would have provided cross-immunity and visceral competition, commercial agricultural systems have provided an ecologic opportunity to a few organisms to multiply almost unchecked.

A scenario based on recent experiences with *S. enteritidis* can be proposed. This *Salmonella* emerged out of the geographic cacophony of *Salmonella* serotypes in the late 1970s and the 1980s to be a major human pathogen, and in some areas more common than *S. typhimurium*. In North America, especially in New England and the Mid-Atlantic states, phage type 8 formed 60% of isolates from human *S. enteritidis* outbreaks during 1985-89, with phage type 13A as the runner-up; in Europe, phage type 4 has been most common. A recent abattoir survey of some 117,000 spent layers found that 3% of 23,431 pooled cecal samples were positive for *S. enteritidis*, with one or more positive samples from 27% of 406 layer houses.[20] The epidemiologic factors contributing to this were:

1. *S. enteritidis* can infect poultry at any age, and the common North American phage types were ornithologically innocuous.

2. As laying birds age, their productivity decreases. To counter this, some farmers will stress-moult these birds by such methods as depriving them of food and water and reducing the light. Associated with this is a substantial decrease in cell-mediated immunity and an increase in susceptibility among the molted birds to *S. enteritidis*.

3. It enters the bird through the digestive tract and rapidly invades the blood stream to localize in the liver, spleen, ovary, and oviducts. Within a few weeks, it is found intermittently in the egg albumin, normally at a very low frequency, unless the bird is immune suppressed or stressed.

4. Because *S. enteritidis* can be in the egg, the potential exists for congenital infections and vertical transmission in multiplier flocks.

5. *S. enteritidis* is normally introduced into commercial flocks via contaminated feeds such as fish meal, carcass meal, and poultry and feather meal that have been improperly heated with inadequate quality controls, a problem in small feed mills.[31]

6. Infection can also be introduced by replacement birds that are shedding bacteria. This is possible in multi-age commercial laying operations that constantly replace and deplete stocks. Present-day layer farms can have 1.2 million birds with a wide range of ages of up to 70 weeks. With increased mechanization, buildings are packed together, which facilitates indirect house-to-house spread.

7. Replacement pullets can become infected while being transported in inadequately decontaminated plastic or metal coops or modules; wooden

coops cannot be decontaminated.

8. Rodents can serve as reservoirs able to carry the organism from house to house, and even farm to farm. Some 24% of mice on *S. enteritidis*-contaminated farms may be infected, and this infection can persist in the rodent population for at least 10 months after the poultry houses have been thoroughly cleaned, disinfected, and restocked with clean replacement pullets.[32]

9. In the absence of adequate building decontamination, *S. enteritidis* can persist for more than 6 weeks, resulting in infection of the incoming susceptible flock.

10. Although the number of *S. enteritidis* in an intact contaminated egg is usually no more than 10-100 bacteria, multiplication will occur if the egg is not stored at <7°C. After 20 days, the vitelline membrane enclosing the yolk breaks down, thus releasing iron molecules, which stimulate bacterial proliferation and enhance virulence. The frequency of egg contamination will be increased by fecal contamination by shedder hens of intact and later cracked eggs, poor egg handling and washing, on-farm delays, and prolonged storage.

11. Eggs need to be transported in properly designed containers that consist of inert, clean packing material made to an appropriate egg size. They need to be held refrigerated, whether in wholesale storage or in point-of-sale retail display.

12. Mishandling eggs in institutional and fast-food kitchens serving scrambled eggs and sauces, causing cross-contamination to other cooked foods as well as salads, and inadequate cooking temperatures and refrigeration will exacerbate an already explosive situation. Temperature fluctuations, as occurs with moving eggs between countertops and the refrigerator, also degrade the protection provided by the vitelline membrane. There is a tendency for the bacteria to be more heat-resistant when they proliferate in an aged yolk.

As can be seen, it is the same salmonella epidemiology of old, but with minor but important differences, largely resulting from the nonpathogenic nature of the infection in poultry.

Irradiated foods are available in certain parts of the world, especially Southeast Asia. The legislation is in place both in the European Community and in North America to allow the public sale of irradiated food. Experiments in many countries have shown such food to be safe. For example, with *T. gondii*, a dose of 0.1 kGy of ionizing energy will cause a loss of infectiousness and a dose of >0.6 kGy will kill the parasite; 0.15 kGy will interrupt the intestinal maturation of L1 larvae of *Trichinella spiralis* in pork, thereby preventing muscle invasion and disease; a level of 0.7 kGy has been advised to inactivate any cyst. A dose of 1 kGy will inactivate 99.999% of *Vibrio* spp.

in raw shellfish. The following doses will inactivate 90% of *Aeromonas hydrophila* (0.19 kGy), *Campylobacter jejuni* (0.16 kGy), *L. monocytogenes* (0.77 kGy), *Salmonella* spp. (0.38–0.77 kGy), and *Staphylococcus aureus* (0.36 kGy).[63]

Once one multi-national marketing company has successfully released a product, be it chicken, oysters, or precooked meals, other products will follow, making their way into everyday life. Parallel to this development is the marketing of specific-pathogen-free foods, such as "certified trichina-free pork." This will encourage the consumption of raw and undercooked products, either as appetizers or entrees, and only a small fraction will be certified as pathogen-free. With these will come outbreaks among the trendies and fashionables of toxoplasmosis, taeniasis, cysticercosis, hydatidosis, and anisakiasis.

Emerging Specialist Farms with "Exotic" Species

Safari parks and game ranches are replacing many of the old urban zoological gardens. These have fueled the relocation of the more-attractive species around the globe, especially if they are in danger of extinction, and "breeding" programs, successful or otherwise, add to public support. Parallel to this has been the successful commercial development of farmed deer, antelopes, alligators, crocodiles, turtles, and various ratites. Trout, salmon, and shrimp are commercially farmed in many countries; in Norway, salmon farming went from a handful to more than 1,000 farms in a decade. Fish species, which are at low densities in the wild, are raised in artificially high densities in ponds and estuarine containers. The stresses of overcrowding and feeding provide ideal conditions for *Aeromonas hydrophila,* a common pathogen of fish. This organism and other *Aeromonas* species are being found in immunocompromised persons and those in poor health.

With the exception of turtle farming and salmonellae[3,39,40], these endeavors have been relatively benign, for adequate cooking will kill most organisms. On the other hand, tuberculosis is a global problem in deer, brucellosis in wild ruminants in various national parks, and avian tuberculosis in North American exotic ratite species. Emus and ostriches, which are foreign to North America and its infections, have demonstrated that they are excellent, though expensive, sentinels for eastern equine encephalitis. Large, dense populations of susceptible species have the potential of acting as sources of novel or previously unnoticed infections, especially if the multiplying host is relatively unaffected. Similarly, recent successful efforts to protect marine mammals may be increasing the prevalence and intensity of anisakid infections in marine fish, thus raising the risks for humans eating uncooked fish. On the other hand, the 30-year economic development of the Don delta in southern Russia did not result in the elimination of natural foci for tularemia. The control of the river flow, land drainage, decreased numbers of grazing cattle, and the construction of fish farms changed the rodent and tick ecology that was classically needed for the maintenance of this zoonotic disease. Yet, *Francisella tularensis* has managed to persist[65], possibly because the fish farms in the delta continue to provide a habitat for the water vole, *Arvicola terrestris,* the reservoir host for this pathogen. Economic development and drainage in the forest belt in the Ukraine removed the vole habitat and reduced the vector *Dermacentor pictus,* which was replaced by *Ixodes ricinus,* the vector for *Babesia* spp., *B. burgdorferi,* louping ill, and Russian spring-summer encephalitis—a Faustian exchange.[72]

Social Engineering and Human Behavior

There is no reason to suppose that an existing minor-incident zoonotic disease will not be offered improved transmission facilities, as were given to HIV and *S. enteritidis.* Intuition would suggest that it will involve the increased frequency and density of an existing human habit (e.g., bath houses, IV drugs, gold mining in hazardous environments) and not the emergence of a novel human behavior or circumstance. On the other hand, agriculture is more innovative and dynamic and might well introduce a new ecologic circumstance. And, the inappropriate use of pharmaceuticals and chemicals, a universal problem in agriculture and especially in the United States, will efficiently foster the emergence of new resistant strains.

Diseases and infections that are now uncommon, if not rare, in the developed nations are well and thriving in the developing nations. As these nations are overtaken by civil, ethnic, and intertribal wars and government bankruptcy, the frequency and impact of disease increases, as does the overflow potential through refugees into surrounding countries. It is in this confused milieu that the horrifying potential for biological warfare will be realized. Because soldiers can be and are vaccinated against BW agents, it will be the exposed civilians that will be decimated. Since the end of the Cold War, there has been a proliferation of weapons of mass destruction: nuclear, chemical, and biological. Although much of the technology and expertise involved has been obtained from the West, often covertly and illicitly, a number of countries are quite capable of constructing and utilizing BW weapons without outside help.

The technical ability to control the great majority of diseases already exists, though not always with a desirable efficiency. Unfortunately, it is poverty and politics that are the major obstacles to improved human and animal health.

In the education of veterinarians and physicians, there is a temptation to regard the patient as a cipher with a disease problem and to distance oneself with the excuse of psychological survival. Teaching hospitals, both veterinary and medical, are still located where there is a plethora of clinical material, frequently of the poor and politically disenfranchised. The veterinary profession should not feel superior to its medical colleagues when, collectively, we pay more attention to horses and cattle and largely ignore the problems of the sheep, goats, rabbits, and guinea pigs that feed more people worldwide. The need for statistical significance can further the distancing by epidemiologists. Just as political scientists are absent from the hustings and economists from the market place, some of the superficial attractions of veterinary economic studies are their cleanliness, absence of manure, and apparent detachment. Computers and other technical advances also distance us from reality. By only studying the numbers, we miss the richness of nature as well as new conditions before they become problems. Animals do not have rights, legal or otherwise, but as veterinarians we are primarily responsible for their welfare. As members of the greater medical profession, we must all be aware of the needs of society and animals.

Issues for the Future

1. Even now common diseases and infections (e.g., leptospirosis and congenital *Toxoplasma* infections) are being missed or overlooked.
2. National and industrial health databases will recognize new zoonotic risks and problems.
3. Common diseases will still commonly occur.
4. The "old" conditions must not be forgotten. They can and do return.
5. Infectious diseases, especially zoonotic diseases, are still among the major causes of death but are frequently overlooked and ignored.
6. Novel diseases, while intriguing and sometimes revealing, are not ipso facto a matter of major concern.
7. The fundamental epidemiologic concern is to determine which new diseases will remain trivial and which will present a significant threat.

References

1. Afzelius, A.: Verhandlungen der dermatologischen Gesellschaft zu Stockholm. *Arch Dermatol Syph*, 101:403-406, 1910.
2. Alicata, J. E.: The discovery of *Angiostrongylus cantonensis* as a cause of human eosinophilic meningitis. *Parasitol Today*, 7:151-153, 1991.
3. Altman, R., J. C. Gorman, L. L. Bernhardt, et al.: Turtle-associated salmonellosis: II The relationship of pet turtles to salmonellosis in children in New Jersey. *Am J Epidemiol*, 95:518-520, 1972.
4. Alto, W. A., and L. B. Nettleton: Hydatid disease: The threat within Papua New Guinea. *Papua New Guinea Med J*, 32:139-142, 1989.

5. Anon.: Owner describes consequences of EVA outbreak. *Vet Rec*, 133:488, 1993.

6. Anziani, O. S., A. A. Guglielmine, A. R. Signorini, et al.: *Haematobia irritans* in Argentina. *Vet Rec*, 132:588, 1993.

7. Balina, L. M., R. P. Valdez, M. De-Herrera, et al.: Experimental reproduction of leprosy in seven-banded armadillos (*Dasypus hybridus*). *Int J Lepr*, 53(4):595-599, 1985.

8. Barbour, A. G., and D. Fish: The biological and social phenomenon of Lyme disease. *Science*, 260:1610-1616, 1993.

9. Barr, C. E., S. A. Mednick, and P. Munk-Jorgensen: Exposure to influenza during gestation and adult schizophrenia. A 40-year study. *Arch Gen Psychiatr*, 47:869-874, 1990.

10. Barrett, T. V.: Advances in triatomine bug ecology in relation to Chagas' disease. *Adv Dis Vector Res*, 8:143-176, 1991.

11. Beers, K. N., and S. R. Mohler: Food poisoning as an inflight safety hazard. *Air Space Environ Med*, 56:594-597, 1985.

12. Bolin, C. A., and P. Koellner: Human-to-human transmission of *Leptospira interrogans* by milk. *J Infect Dis*, 158:246-247, 1988.

13. Centers for Disease Control: Surveillance of *Escherchia coli* O157:H7 isolation and confirmation, United States, 1988. *MMWR*, 40(SS-1):1-6, 1991.

14. Centers for Disease Control: Update: Multistate outbreak of *Escherichia coli* O157:H7 infections from hamburgers—western United States, 1992-1993. *MMWR*, 42:258-263, 1993.

15. Centers for Disease Control: Update: Hantavirus Disease - United States, 1993. *MMWR*, 42:612-614, 1993.

16. Clark, G. G.: Dengue and dengue haemorrhagia fever. *J Fla Mosq Contr Assoc*, 63:48-53, 1992.

17. Corbitt, G., A. S. Bailey, and G. Williams: HIV infection in Manchester, 1959. *Lancet* 336:51, 1990.

18. Desowitz, R. S.: *New Guinea Tapeworms and Jewish Grandmothers: tales of parasites and people.* New York, W. W. Norton, pp 39-41, 1981.

19. Doyle, M. P.: Pathogenic *Escherichia coli*, *Yersinia enterocolitica*, and *Vibrio parahaemolyticus*. *Lancet*, 336:111-115, 1990.

20. Ebel, E. D., M. J. David, and J. Mason: Occurrence of *Salmonella enteritidis* in the U.S. commercial egg industry: report on a national spent hen survey. *Avian Dis*, 36:646-654, 1992.

21. Edwards, D. D.: Troubled waters in Milwaukee. *Am Soc Microbiol News*, 59:342-345, 1993.

22. Egger, M., D. Mausezahl, P. Odermatt, et al.: Symptoms and transmission of intestinal cryptosporidiosis. *Arch Dis Child*, 65:445-447, 1990.

23. Eitrem, R., B. Niklasson, and O. Weiland: Sandfly fever among Swedish tourists. *Scand J Infect Dis*, 23:451-457, 1991.

24. Ewald, P. W.: Evolution of HIV in Africa. *Science*, 257:10, 1992.

25. Fattal-German, M.: L'immunocompetance chez les personnes agees. *Ann Pharm F*, 50:13-24, 1992.

26. Gamboa, C.: Pan American Health Organization, personal communication, 7 Oct 1993.

27. Garry, R. F.: Early case of AIDS in the USA. *Nature*, 345:509, 1990.

28. Gillman, H.: *The New World screwworm eradication program: North Africa 1988-1992.* Rome, Food and Agriculture Organization of the United Nations, 1992.
29. Hayes, E. B., T. D. Matte, T. R. O'Brien, et al.: Large community outbreak of cryptosporidiosis due to contamination of a filtered public water supply. *New Engl J Med*, 320:1372-1376, 1989.
30. Hellerstrom, S.: Erythema chronicum migrans Afzelius with meningitis. *South Med J*, 43:330-335, 1950.
31. Henken, A. M., K. Frankena, J. O. Goelema, et al.: Multivariate epidemiological approach to salmonellosis in broiler breeder flocks. *Poultry Sci*, 71:838-843, 1992.
32. Henzler,D. J., and H. M. Opitz: The role of mice in the epizootiology of *Salmonella enteritidis* infection on chicken layer farms. *Avian Dis*, 36:625- 631, 1992.
33. Higgins, A.: Equine viral arteritis. *Vet Rec*, 132:591, 1993.
34. Hugh-Jones, M. E.: Wickham Steed and German biological warfare research. *Intell Natl Secur*, 7:379-402, 1992.
35. Hurvell, B.: Zoonotic *Yersinia enterocolitica* infection: host range, clinical manifestations, and transmission between animals and man. In *Yersinia Enterocolitica*, E. J. Bottone (ed.), pp 145-159, Boca Raton, FL, CRC Press, 1981.
36. Jeffrey, M., and J. Wilesmith: Idiopathic brainstem neuronal chromatolysis and hippocampal sclerosis: a novel encephalopathy in clinically suspect cases of bovine spongiform encephalopathy. *Vet Rec*, 131:359-362, 1992.
37. Jezek, Z., I. Arita, M. Mutombo, et al.: Four generations of probable person-to-person transmission of human monkeypox. *Am J Epidemiol* 123:1004-1012, 1986.
38. Karmali, M. A.: Infection by verotoxin-producing Escherichia coli. *Clin Microbiol Rev*, 2:15-38, 1989.
39. Kaufman, A. F., and Z. L. Morrison: An epidemiologic study of salmonellosis in turtles. *Am J Epidemiol*, 84:364-370, 1966.
40. Kaufman, A. R., M. D. Fox, G. K. Morris, et al.: Turtle-associated salmonellosis: III The effects of environmental salmonellae in commercial turtle breeding ponds. *Am J Epidemiol*, 95:521-528, 1972.
41. Kikuchi, R.: Inefficiency of sanitation measures aboard commercial aircraft: environmental pollution and disease.*Aviat Space Environ Med*,48:654-658,1977.
42. Kilbourne, E. D.: New viruses and new disease: mutation, evolution, and ecology. *Curr Opin Immunol*, 3:518-524, 1991.
43. Kirchheimer, W. F., and E. E. Storrs: Attempts to establish the armadillo (*Dasypus novemcinctus*) as a model for the study of leprosy: Part 1, report of lepromatoid leprosy in an experimentally infected armadillo. *Int J Lepr*, 39:693-702, 1971.
44. Klapper, P. E., and D. J. Morris: Screening for viral and protozoal infections in pregnancy. A review. *Br J Obstet Gynaecol*, 97:974-983, 1990.
45. Kliks, M. M., and N. E. Palumbo: Eosinophilic meningitis beyond the Pacific Basin: the global dispersal of a peridomestic zoonosis caused by *Angiostrongylus cantonensis*, the nematode lungworm of rats. *Soc Sci Med*, 34:199-212, 1992.
46. Lederberg, J., R. E. Shope, and S. C. Oaks: *Emerging Infections: Microbial Threats to Health in the United States.* Washington, D.C., National Academy

Press, 1992.

47. Lipschutz, B.: Uber eine seltene Erythemform (Erythema chronica migrans). *Arch Dermatol Syph*, 118:349-356, 1913.

48. Markowitz, L. E., C. Allen, J. L. Benach, et al.: Lyme disease during pregnancy. *J Am Med Assoc*, 255:3394-3396, 1986.

49. McClure, M. O., and T. F. Schultz: Origin of HIV. *Br Med J*, 298:1267- 1268, 1989.

50. McGill, I. S., and G. A. H. Wells: Neuropathological findings in cattle with clinically suspect but histologically unconfirmed bovine spongiform encephalopathy (BSE). *J Comp Pathol*, 108:241-260, 1993.

51. Mednick, S. A., R. A. Machon, M. O. Huttenen, et al.: Adult schizophrenia following prenatal exposure to an influenza epidemic. *Arch Gen Psychiatr*, 45:189-192, 1988.

52. Metchock, B., D. R. Lonsway, G. P. Cater, et al.: *Yersinia enterocolitica*: a frequent seasonal stool isolate from children at an urban hospital in the southeast United States. *J Clin Microbiol*, 29:2868-2869, 1991.

53. Mutinga, M. J.: Leishmaniasis: what is new in transmission? *East Afr Med J*, 69:1-2, 1992.

54. Nahmias, A. J., J. Weiss, X. Yao, et al.: Evidence for human infection with an HTLV III/LAV-like virus in central Africa, 1959. *Lancet*, I:1279-1280, 1986.

55. Nickey, L. N.: *U.S. - Mexico: Border health and environmental issues*. Document presented to the United States Congressional Border Caucus - Washington, D.C., July 13, 1993.

56. Nilsson, G.: *Importation of Birds into the United States, 1989*. Washington, D.C., Defenders of Wildlife, p. 7, 1992.

57. Nuttall, P. A., L. D. Jones, and C. R. Davies: The role of arthropod vectors in arbovirus evolution. *Adv Dis Vector Res*, 8:15-45, 1991.

58. O'Callaghan, E., P. Sham, N. Takei, et al.: Schizophrenia after prenatal exposure to 1957 A2 influenza epidemic. *Lancet*, 337:1248-1250, 1991. [Subsequent correspondence, ibid 338:116-119,390]

59. Orubuloye, I. O., J. C. Caldwell, and P. Caldwell: Sexual networking in the Ekiti district of Nigeria. *Stud Fam Plan*, 22:61-73, 1991.

60. Ostreni, F.: Enzootishe Rinderleukose in Albanien. *Tierarztl Umsch*, 46:478-480, 1991.

61. Ostroff, S. M., G. Kapperud, J. Lassen, et al.: Clinical features of sporadic *Yersinia enterocolitica* infections in Norway. *J Infect Dis*, 166:812-817, 1992.

62. Palmer, S. R.: Cryptosporidiosis—a zoonotic problem? Proceedings of the Society for Veterinary Epidemiology and Preventive Medicine, University of London, 17-19 April 1991, M. V. Thrusfield (ed.), pp 46-52, 1991.

63. Pan American Health Organization: Final Report: joint FAO/IAEA/PAHO/ WHO technical consultation on irradiation as a public health intervention measure for food-borne diseases in Latin America and the Caribbean (hpv/fos/ 126/92). Washington, D.C., 19-21 October, 1992.

64. Piot, P., F. A. Plummer, F. S. Mhalu, et al.: AIDS: an international perspective. *Science*, 239:573-579, 1988.

65. Protopopyan, M. G., V. G. Naletov, G. M. Medinskii, et al.: (Contemporary structure of the natural focus of tularemia of the Don Delta in relation to

economic influence.) *Zool Zh*, 64:468-471, 1985.
66. Quinn, T. C., J. M. Mann, J. W. Curran, et al.: AIDS in Africa: an epidemiologic paradigm. *Science*, 234:955-963, 1986.
67. Rondle, C. J., B. Ramesh, J. B. Krahn, et al.: Cholera: possible infection from aircraft effluent. *J Hyg (Camb)*, 81:361-371, 1978.
68. Royal, L., and I. McCoubrey: International spread of disease by air travel. *Am Fam Phys*, 40:129-136, 1989.
69. Ryan, C. A., R. V. Tauxe, G. W. Hosek, et al.: *Escherichia coli* O157:H7 diarrhea in a nursing home: clinical, epidemiological, and pathological findings. *J Infect Dis*, 154:631-638, 1986.
70. Schofield, C. J.: Biosystematics of the Triatominae. In *Biosystematics of haematophagus insects*, M. W. Service (ed.), Systematics Assoc Spec Vol 37:284-312, 1988. Oxford, Clarendon Press.
71. Sicuranza, G., and L. Sigal: Lyme disease in pregnancy. In *Lyme Disease*, P. K. Coyle (ed.), pp 184-186, St. Louis, Mosby-Year Book, 1993.
72. Sinyak, K. M., A. M. Kas'yanenko, and T. I. Kas'yanenko: (Prerequisites for ecological prognosis of foci of tularaemia and leptospirosis in relation to economic activity by man.) *Zh Mikrobiol Epidemiol Immunobiol*, 7:62-66, 1983.
73. Smith, L. G., Jr, M. Pearlman, L. G. Smith, et al.: Lyme disease: a review with emphasis on the pregnant woman. *Obstet Gynecol Surv*, 46:125-130, 1991.
74. Smith, T. F., A. Srinivasan, G. Schochetman, et al.: The phylogenetic history of immunodeficiency viruses. *Nature*, 333:573-575, 1988.
75. Steere, A. C., S. E. Malawista, D. R. Syndam, et al.: Lyme arthritis: an epidemic of oligoarticular arthritis in children and adults in three Connecticut communities. *Arthritis Rheumatol*, 20:7-17, 1977.
76. Sternberg, S.: HIV comes in five family groups. *Science*, 256:966, 1992.
77. Svabic-Vlahovic, M., D. Pantic, M. Pavicic, et al.: Transmission of *Listeria monocytogenes* from mother's milk to her baby and to puppies. *Lancet*, ii:1201, Nov. 19, 1988.
78. Twigg, G.: *The Black Death: a biological reappraisal*. New York, Schocken Books, 1985.
79. Report of the Intergovernmental Panel on Climate Change, United Nations World Meteorological Organization & United Nations Environment Programme, Bracknell, UK, 1990.
80. Velasco-Castrejon, O., J. L. Valdespino, R. Tapia-Conyer, et al.: Seroepidemiologia de la enfermedad da Chagas en Mexico. *Salud Publica Mex*, 34:186-196, 1992.
81. Walsh, G. P., E. E. Storrs, H. P. Burchfield, et al.: Leprosy-like disease occurring naturally in armadillos. *J Reticuloendothel Soc*, 18:347-351, 1975.
82. Wilkinson, L.: *Animals and disease: an introduction to the history of comparative medicine*. New York, Cambridge Univ Press, pp 217-218, 1992.
83. Wrathall, A. W.: Reproductive disorders in pigs. Farnham Royal, Engl, Commonwealth Agricultural Bureaux, pp 140-211, 1975.

6

ADVANCES IN THE CONTROL AND PREVENTION OF ZOONOSES

Economic Assessment of Disease

Medical and veterinary epidemiology have advanced along parallel paths, which is to be expected as both are concerned with promoting health in communities, whether of animals or humans. Whereas medical epidemiology has been increasingly concerned with chronic diseases and environmental issues, veterinary epidemiology has maintained its interest in infectious disease epidemiology, especially of parasites, and simultaneously expanded into areas concerned with the optimization of animal production. Because of this, and for historical reasons, veterinary epidemiologists are expected to be knowledgeable about the economics of disease control and agriculture. Unfortunately, a rapid perusal of the literature indicates that this is frequently a superficial acquaintanceship. It has many of the characteristics of the past, when epidemiologists were expected merely to provide gross statistics of reported outbreaks, a situation that still persists in Russia and some eastern European and Third World countries. Just as prevalence is confused with incidence, so is the financial or accountant's assessment with economics (see the *Veterinary Economics* journal). So what is "economics" and what do economists do?

Samuelson[121] defines the discipline as follows: "Economics is the study of how people and society end up choosing, with or without the use of money, to employ scarce productive resources that could have alternative uses, to produce various commodities and distribute them for consumption, now or in the future, among various persons and groups in society. It analyzes the costs and benefits of improving patterns of resource allocation." To which one must append Gilpin's comment,[56] "It is not as a science

152

concerned with the problems of what ought to be, but with the explanation and understanding of what already exists." A further caveat is provided by Keynes, quoted by Gilpin, that the theory of economics does not furnish a body of settled conclusions immediately applicable to policy. It is a method rather than a doctrine, an apparatus of the mind, a technique of thinking that helps its possessor to draw correct conclusions, a formal framework for assembling information to appropriately guide choice. More briefly, economics is the science of choice.

Because of the conflict and chaos in choosing between babies, bicycles, bananas, and comfort, the alternatives are measured in common monetary units. The economist's dollar, for example, is a convenient measure of value that enables the comparison of today's apples with tomorrow's antelopes. It may have a notional or an actual relationship to contemporary currency values. There are occasions when it is more convenient to use other measures, such as gallons of milk or person-years-lost, especially in historical or cross-cultural comparisons. The use of monetary units by economists is difficult for non-economists, as the latter readily confuse them with money in their pockets and compare them to personal income. Thus, they find it distasteful to measure the value of intangibles, such as human lives, convenience, fear, and ease of mind in pieces of silver. It is an index to allow things to be ranked on a scale of bigger/smaller, more/less, better/worse.

Value can be expressed as the "exchange" value or the price possessed by a commodity or service that can be used to acquire other services or goods by exchange. Therefore, if something is treasured but cannot be exchanged, either directly or indirectly, it has no economic value. Value can be determined in a number of ways. A simple but limited measure is the amount of labor expended in producing or acquiring a good or item. Thus, if it takes 3 months to save enough money from one's wages to buy a cow, the cow has the value to you of 3 months labor. A more useful and flexible method is to use the total cost of the various factors employed in the production of a good. This system is frequently used in determining costs and benefits of animal disease control. In many ways, it is merely a restatement of the labor theory of value, expressed in monetary terms from the supply side, ignoring demand. It assumes that the cost determines price on the argument that a free marketplace will enforce the necessary adjustments to the volume of production by contracting or expanding the rate of profit. It does not take into account situations where there are constraints on production, monopolies, or fluctuating demands due to changing taste or fashions. These limitations are absorbed by the marginal theory of value which values any commodity or service by the extent that a customer's satisfaction is increased or decreased if he had one more or less units of that commodity for any particular purpose. The marginal value, therefore, depends on relative scarcity or on demand in relation to supply.

It is independent of the ability to produce and the competitiveness of the market.

The economic approach to solving the multi-dimensional problem of finding the optimum solution among many choices is to find answers to the following four general questions (after Cooper and Culyer[28]):

1. What are the outputs of veterinary services?
2. How does society rank these outputs in priority order?   i.e., benefits
3. What is required in the way of "inputs" to produce any of these outputs?
4. What must society lose, i.e., what will it "cost," by using these inputs for that purpose?   i.e., costs

These can be reworded for the farm, or microeconomic, level as follows:

1. What services can the veterinary surgeon/practitioner provide and how are they affected by external circumstances, such as diagnostic laboratory support, transport limitations, professional education and training, etc?

2. How does the farmer rank these services?

3. What is required as "inputs" from the farmer, the veterinarian, and possibly the community to achieve these results?

4. What must the farmer forego?

A Quick Introduction to the Economics of Disease Control (after McInerney[96])

Very Basic Principles: Economic activity is directed entirely to further the benefit of people, and therefore **value** is derived from what people want and how much they want it. This activity is governed by the resources available. Therefore **cost** is derived from the resources that then have to be diverted from another use. This argument can be restated that all economic activity is made up of two parts: (1) basic resources that are transformed into other goods or services and (2) these goods and services are distributed to be consumed or utilized by people. We can apply this to livestock production as follows:

LIVESTOCK RESOURCES → Production → PRODUCTS → Consumption → PEOPLE

e.g., animals	milk	(value)
grazing	meat	
feed	wool	
housing	pony rides	

In economic terms, disease is a negative influence reducing the amount and/or quality of the product derived from the original resources and thereby diminishing the peoples' benefits. A wide variety of "negative inputs" exist (e.g., extreme weather, industrial pollution, disorganized management, civil unrest), not all of which are claimed to be under possible veterinary control. For the purposes of this exposition, we will limit disease to be some effects associated with zoonotic agents.

It then follows that the significance of a disease in livestock, for example, is because it reduces the welfare of people. Its economic importance is defined solely by the extent to which people are worse off, irrespective of livestock pain. A clinical condition, however nauseating, affecting an animal species of no concern to people is not of economic concern. An economic disease is not defined by its etiology or biological nature. Diseases of farm livestock whose services can be readily measured commercially are not necessarily more important economically than diseases of companion animals that have different social and intangible values and normally no commercial output. It is the income, lifestyle, and cultural levels of a society that determine the economic importance of any animal disease in that society. In prosperous, well-fed countries, the health of the marginal domestic dog or child's pony may be more economically important than the death of the marginal cow; in poor countries the reverse applies. The value of lost livestock is not necessarily related to the importance of the disease. For example, the death of a $10 million stallion may affect the cash flow of its owners but need not affect the economy of the racing industry in the slightest. A cheap cull cow with the wrong disease, e.g., BSE or foot-and-mouth disease, however, can put a national industry at risk.

Disease is an economic process that "uses" scarce resources wastefully and generates an output of negative benefit, especially with zoonotic infections that have the potential of directly reducing human health and well-being. Disease control is also an economic process, for it consumes resources, such as veterinary services, drugs, and management, and provides an output of increased and improved livestock products and services of benefit to the public.

For any structured livestock industry there is a systematic relationship between the quantity of input factors (e.g., feed, labor, transport) and the quantity of output (e.g., milk, liveweight gain, calves, eggs). This is known as a **production function**. In general, it can be shown to be nonlinear, such that the output, though rapid at first, will increase at a diminishing rate as inputs increase; at some point production may even decrease. Production is not deterministic but is the result of an array of inputs, including "disease," and outputs.

This can be demonstrated rudimentarily in Figure 6-1, with two production functions that differ only by the presence or absence of a disease.

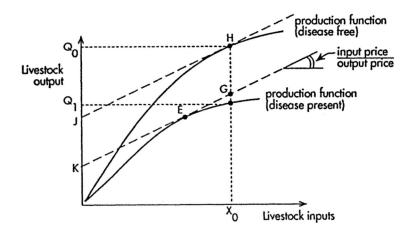

Fig. 6-1. Disease effects on the livestock production function and economic adjustments in response to disease.

The effect of disease is shown by the downward displacement of the "disease" function compared to the production by healthy stock with otherwise the same range of inputs. In reality, there would be a family of such curves resulting from various incidences/prevalences of this disease.

This economic model shows that the loss concept is a relationship and not a number. It will vary depending on the production system. For example, in this demonstration, the output losses are smaller on the left of the x-axis where the system involves low input–low output characteristics than at the more-intensive production level to the right, which involves more inputs and outputs. Economic importance is not uniform across farms, regions, or countries. Similarly, control programs that may be economically justified for intensive systems may not be for extensive systems.

Let us now consider a livestock production system, whether it is an individual farm or representative average, or even a sector aggregate, where there is a continuous output flow from a fixed set of resources. Here the disease effect is to reduce, for example, the growth rate, extend the time to finishing, and affect the final quality. Thus, for a dairy herd the output function could be the average monthly milk production and the input the monthly feed and forage consumed. Alternatively, the quantity and quality of eggs produced by a layer flock would be the output, and the input would be the feed consumed.

Let us assume that the disease-free production system is at optimum efficiency at intensity H such that input X_0 produces the output Q_0. This can be calculated using standard economic analyses for marginal efficiency. It is drawn here (Fig. 6-1) where the tangent to the output curve (indicating the marginal product of the input) is equal to the ratio of the price of input to the price of output. Disease reduces the output so that now only Q_1 results from X_0 inputs. Thus this incidence of disease has a cost in terms of foregone or lost output of $Q_0 - Q_1$. This assumes that the farmer ignores the disease and maintains the input at the original level X_0, even though it is less profitable. On the other hand, we might assume for purposes of discussion that although the farmer will not institute disease control procedures, he will shift his effort to the less-intensive position E on the with-disease production function. He has now saved some input costs, or $X_0 - E$. His new true output loss is now equivalent to JK (= HG), which is less than the original simple reduction in output of $Q_0 - Q_1$.

This loss can rarely be measured or calculated on the basis of simple financial analysis. To achieve it one must have a reliable without-disease baseline, and knowledge of the input-output relationship along which production levels adjust. And unless one is dealing with exotic or unusual diseases, disease is a normal, everyday negative input (or threat of same) on most farms. The response to real or perceived disease or diseases determines the production systems used and the options available to adjust the system accordingly as the prevalence, or incidence, increases or decreases. When this change in output can be attributed to disease, it has only indicated the direct losses.

The approach over the past few decades when assessing the economic aspects of disease control has been to compare the costs incurred with the benefits gained. A worthwhile project has been assumed when the benefits exceed the costs, such that the rate of return is at least comparable with the use of control resources elsewhere. As we are dealing with optimizing choices, the criteria should be whether different control programs, even for another disease, may yield a better rate of return. It is not limited to comparing more or less intensive, alternative control programs but also the possibility, for example, of ignoring the disease problem and using the resources to develop fish farming or tourism.

However, let us consider a livestock disease. It will have a range of prevalences from zero to the normal stable rate in the population without control. To reduce the prevalence will absorb an increasing control intensity and costs. This is shown in Figure 6-2A.

A single control cost curve is shown here. In reality there is a different cost curve for each control procedure that functions at optimal efficiency at different prevalence ranges. For example, general vaccination is generally efficient when an infection is widespread but would be inefficient if the infection is densely localized, or persists in a few residual places. In the latter situation, a highly targeted program would be better. Vaccination itself has large, hidden (i.e., indirect) costs—labor, cold-chain, equipment depreciation, support serologic testing, side effects, litigation costs, and insurance. Also,

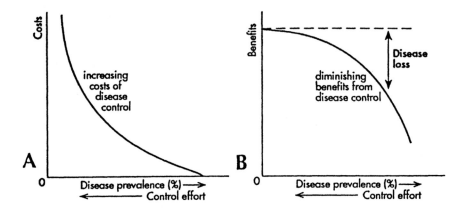

Fig. 6-2. A: Costs of disease control. B: Benefits
associated with disease control.

diseases are dynamic and interact with their control program, with, for
example, the appearance of new or resistant strains that necessitate new
vaccines or drugs and bigger benefits if implemented. In broad terms, control
costs increase as the prevalence decreases.

By definition, the benefits from disease control and a lower prevalence
are the disease losses avoided. Thus, maximum benefits occur when there is
no disease and zero losses. For a number of diseases, the losses increase very
slowly when the disease effects are still small, i.e., losses are minor and
benefit changes are similarly slight. But as the disease rate increases, the
losses can increase rapidly and the benefit curve falls at an alarming rate
(Fig. 6-2B). The higher losses follow from the increasing severity, not from
the direct costs, but from the multiplying secondary effects and wider
indirect costs throughout the production system.

If we merge these two albeit simple curves (Fig. 6-3), it is clear that
there are many disease levels for which the benefits exceed the control costs,
but there is one level at which this difference is greatest. At this disease level
of economic optimality, the gradient of both curves is identical and the
marginal benefits and costs are equal. All else being equal, this is the control
and economic situation to aim for out of all the various alternative programs
available.

The lesson from this is to determine the optimum economic position and
design the control procedures accordingly. Reducing the disease rate further,
just as letting it increase, is not a rational economic move, though there may
be other considerations. It is at this time that (government) accountants can
become extraordinarily dangerous, especially in regard to vector control.
Noting that there is little or no overt disease, they will argue that the control

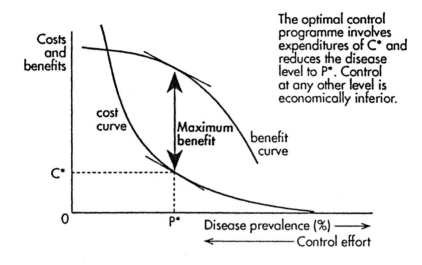

The optimal control programme involves expenditures of C* and reduces the disease level to P*. Control at any other level is economically inferior.

Fig. 6-3. Economically efficient disease control and the optimum level of disease.

program is "too expensive," and the budget is cut back. Depending on the necessary length of the epidemiologic fuse, nothing will happen at first, and then there will be an explosion of new cases exacerbated by the increased susceptibility of the population and, maybe, clinical forgetfulness of the disease by physicians and veterinarians.

Economic and epidemiologic situations are rarely static. What was the optimum yesterday will not be so tomorrow. The efficacy of control programs depends on efficiency more than economics. Control programs involving extensive livestock, for example, are relatively efficiency robust. For example, vaccination will be effective in extensive beef cow-calf operations as long as the vaccinations are to the correct animals and in the proper season, and the vaccine is not thrown out of the ice chest to make room for the soft drinks. But as the system becomes more intense, timing and efficiency must tighten up (for example, the preconditioning, dosing, and handling of calves before and on arrival at feedlots); the most efficiency-sensitive are probably large commercial poultry units.

The risk of disease spread is seldom a simple function of prevalence. For example, babesia incidence can be very unstable below a 30% prevalence with high mortality rates, but the epidemiological situation rapidly improves around 5% prevalence. Similarly, if one is meant to be free of a disease, such as yellow fever in the Trinidad human population, one case can be as expensive as 10 because the indirect costs are binomially determined at this low incidence(for example, cruise liners do not stop and carnival tourists stay away equally whether it is 1 case or 10). The point is that in reality the curves are not necessarily simple but may be more in the way of S-shaped curves or even snakes and ladders. The economic model must be holistic to include all the ways that a disease impinges on economic values from the affected herd, for example, outward to the livestock sector and the community, and through time; that is, from the microeconomic and financial levels upward to the national macroeconomic level (see Table 6-1).

In most if not all national livestock disease control programs, society benefits at the cost of the farming community. The first herds or flocks encouraged to join, frequently with minimal or no disease, profit. The last, compulsorily and sometimes with significant problems, join to minimize losses. For example, both the U.K. and the U.S. national brucellosis campaigns involved significant costs to the individual herd owners. Therefore, society should be sensitive to the communal responsibility shown by herd owners and mitigate these costs as much as possible.

Mathematical Comparison of Costs and Benefits

Any decision involves choosing between alternative proposals or situations. Various techniques are available for comparing the values of the costs and benefits. Partial budgets are appropriate for control programs of chronic disease within a farm or limited series of enterprises. It concerns itself with the components of benefit and cost influence by the control procedure and is best suited to simple problems with relatively prompt responses that do not affect the total management of the farm or enterprise. It allows comparisons between different strategies but does not necessarily produce optimal solutions. Margin analysis is better used with complex endemic conditions, especially integrated health programs, where there may be a number of variable inputs, which will vary with the gross output. It has a limited ability to handle time and subsequent industry expansion in the succeeding absence of the problem. Payoff tables and other forms of decision making under circumstances of risk and uncertainty are used when the disease is inconstant or sporadic. When the probabilities of events are known, they are an extremely valuable decision-making tool.

Benefit-cost analysis has time as an integral part of the analysis and is used widely as a result. The decision criteria are net present value, benefit-cost ratio, and the internal rate of return, which measure different aspects, and any decision will have attempted to balance all three. The usefulness of the analytical techniques is to improve the decision-making process. They are not substitutes for judgment and common sense.

Table 6-1. Losses due to animal disease at various economic levels

Economic Level	A: Disease generally present, but varying in degree per farm	B: Incidental outbreaks of contagious diseases on a national/regional scale	
		B1: With foreign trade restrictions	B2: No restrictions to foreign trade

From Microeconomic

Economic Level	A	B1	B2
1. Farm/individual producer	Direct relationship between loss and incidence/prevalence and morbidity on farm; most severe effects on pig and poultry incomes	Large incidental loss even if the farm is not affected by the disease; possible compensation for destroyed animals	Great loss on affected farms; possible compensation for destroyed stock; advantage for farms not affected
2. Sector/joint stock farmers	Loss insofar as the price does not adapt itself; insufficiently large market (e.g., EU) hardly any relation between level of disease and income of stock farmers, due to price adaptations	Significant loss, particularly with export products, resulting from dropping prices due to failing demand	Moderate loss, depending on possible compensation and on degree of price adaptations
3. Supply and processing industries; service and trade	Price changes are presumed to be passed to the consumer fast and completely but this depends entirely on the elasticities of demand and supply in the system.		
4. Consumer	Loss due to higher prices	Incidental advantage	Slight loss
5. National economy	Loss due to inefficient use of resources	Disadvantage very much less than loss to sector (2B1) famers	Disadvantage may be more than to sector farmers (2B2) but is less than 5B1

To Macroeconomic

Source: After Dijkhuisen, Huirne, and Renkema[38]

Benefit-cost analysis. Something happening today is valued more highly than the same event tomorrow; having a dollar today is better than $1.50 tomorrow. Discounting is the technique by which future cost and benefit streams are reduced to their present worth. If a borrower promises to pay us $1,200 at the end of 5 years, what is that promise worth to us today at an annual interest of 8%? It is $1,200 ÷ $(1.08)^5$ or $817—put another way, if we invest $817 today at 8% compound interest, we will have $1,200 in 5 years. This same calculation can be applied to an income stream. Thus, if one was to receive $6,438 every year for 9 years, it would total $57,942; with each year discounted at 15%, its present worth is $30,722. The discount rate is the opportunity cost of capital. In 1994 this was 12% for the World Bank and similar agencies. One can use the borrowing rate that the government must pay to fund the project, but this will impact on the choice and range of possible projects. For financial and microeconomic (farm) analyses, the discount rate is the marginal cost of money, i.e., the interest rate at the local bank.

Net present value [NPV]. The present worth of the incremental net benefit stream of a project is the present worth of the benefits minus the present worth of the costs; present worth is the value at present of an amount to be paid or received at some time in the future and is determined by multiplying the future value by the discount factor. A project is viable if the NPV is positive, but it provides no ranking for the order of implementation. It can sometimes ignore large costs, which are better appreciated by benefit-cost ratios. When analyzing mutually exclusive alternative programs or projects, one looks for the alternative with the greatest NPV.

$$\text{NPV} = \frac{B_0 - C_0}{(1+r)^0} + \frac{B_1 - C_1}{(1+r)^1} + \ldots + \frac{B_n - C_n}{(1+r)^n}$$

$$= \sum_{t=0}^{n} \frac{B_t - C_t}{(1+r)^t}$$

where:

C_t = measure of costs incurred in time t
B_t = measure of benefits gained in time t
r = discount rate or opportunity cost of capital
n = life of project

Benefit-cost ratio [B/C]. The present worth of the benefit stream divided by the present cost of the cost stream is the benefit-cost ratio. A project is viable if the B/C ratio is equal to or greater than 1; high values (e.g., >15:1) should be viewed with caution. It is very responsive to which discount rates are used and therefore a sensitivity analysis must be included. It may give an incorrect ranking for independent projects and cannot be used for choosing among mutually exclusive alternatives. The selection criterion is to accept all projects with a B/C ratio of 1 or greater, for high ratios are not better than low ratios. It is not presently used with human health projects.

$$B/C = \sum_{t=0}^{n} \{B_t/(1+r)^t\}/\{C_t/(1+r)^t\}$$

$$= \sum_{t=0}^{n} \frac{B_t}{C_t}$$

Internal rate of return [IRR]. The internal rate of return is the maximum interest that a project can pay for the resources used if that project is to recover its investment and operating expenses and break even. Specifically, it is the discount rate that just makes the net present worth of the net benefit stream equal to zero.[57] If the IRR is greater than the actual interest rate, the project is economically worthwhile. It favors short-term advantage over the more distant. It is the calculation preferred by WHO and similar funding agencies, for it is technically the most-correct and dependable tool in guiding decisions. It is calculated by solving r such that:

$$NPV = \sum_{t=0}^{n} \frac{B_t - C_t}{(1+r)^t} = 0$$

Social cost-benefit analysis. This analysis adds in the frequently intangible social benefits and costs of a project beyond the merely pragmatic. Such intangible benefits as well-being, better schools, and agricultural flexibility, and costs such as disruption of traditional values, cultures, and scenic values are real and reflect true values but are difficult, if not impossible, to evaluate. For example, what is the value of your children to you, on a good day? Of your life?—but that is another intangible. They should be carefully identified and, when possible, quantified. When possible, they should be translated into monetary terms; this is usually easier with costs than benefits. The tangible and intangible social factors of a project are considered in the final decision making largely through a subjective evaluation, for intangible costs can be significant and the benefits can make a significant contribution beyond the immediate project.

A major benefit of successful disease control, or eradication, is the **public good** benefit (e.g., something of general benefit—health, welfare, happiness), which accrues to all members of society. Depending on the disease, the attributes may include increased migration and settlement in previously endemic areas, reduced public and private expenditures on disease control activities (e.g., vector control), reduced prophylactic consumption, increased recreational use of previously denied resources (e.g., rivers and lakes), and a generally improved attitude of the public concerning health and confidence in the future.[41] These have the potential for increased savings and investment in both physical and human capital. With a parallel increase in female education, a decrease in child mortality can fuel a switch from investing in child quantity to quality and thus in time to a reduced rate of population growth.

Cost-effectiveness analyses. These analyses are used either where the benefits are hard or impossible to quantify or where the decision has already been made and it is merely necessary to decide between alternative technologies. The cost stream is discounted as in a cost-benefit analysis to determine its present worth. The major forms of analysis involved are based either on (a) constant effects or (b) constant costs. The former uses least-cost analysis to determine the least-cost alternative of reaching a prestated level of benefits, e.g., a defined and hoped for lower prevalence. The constant-costs method calculates the cost per unit of benefit or cost-effectiveness ratio, e.g., the cost of permanently reducing the mortality by one. Because the desired effects are unitized, they can be manipulated in a number of ways without giving them any monetary values. For example, they can be weighted such that early events such as deaths prevented are weighted more heavily than those occurring, or prevented, in the future; or one can have a mix of events of equal weighting; or of unequal individual weighting such that alternative programs are ranked on their effect "score."

Cost-of-illness analyses. Cost-of-illness analyses are in the nature of financial analyses but frequently employed and quoted. The costs are calculated for the various parts involved on the basis of **direct** and **indirect** costs. The former are the immediate costs of treatment and care, and in agriculture, from the reduction in livestock inventories and output. Intangible costs are ignored because they do not directly affect output. Similarly, it ignores quality-adjusted life years gained. The indirect costs are those associated with loss of income from illness, disability, or death; and associated societal effects; and in agriculture, those costs manifested outside the production enterprises. It is the indirect losses which usually have the greatest economic impact. It is a ledger book approach, facilitated by bank accounts and farm receipts, and the results are easily misused and abused, sometimes with absurd implications.[106] Common errors are to ignore multiple disease problems in affected individuals, assuming that all deaths occur on January 1, and the variable quality of morbidity data. But it is useful in getting a first approximation and identifying the major components at the local (familial or farm) and national levels, especially when a more-complete economic analysis is not possible. Conceptually, it is like finding a clock in pieces. It does not explain how it works, but one gets an idea of what is involved—how well depends on how many unknown pieces are missing.

Some of the costs and benefits associated with foodborne outbreaks of disease have been identified as follows:[117]

Costs:
Individual costs:
"Trousseau" (being suitably dressed to visit physician/hospital)
Consultation
Prescriptions
Hospitalization
Loss of income/productivity
Pain and suffering
Leisure time lost, including foregone holidays and related expenses
Child care and home care costs
Risk aversion costs
Averting behavior costs
Travel costs (to/from medical care for patient, family, and hospital visitors)
Industry costs:
Product recall
Plant closing and/or cleanup
Product liability costs
Reduced product demand
Public sector costs:
Disease surveillance costs
Outbreak investigation costs
Public share of medical, hospital, and ambulance costs
Cleanup costs
Lost taxes
Staff opportunity costs
Reduced tourism
Benefits (medium and long-term):
Racheting up of control awareness, less complacency, more exacting standards, refocus of objectives
Improvement in one area improves others (e.g., *Mycobacterium bovis* control/eradication and improved shelf-life of milk)
Improved industry quality
Price preference to good quality with reduced price/margins for lesser quality
Improved quality of animal feed if food is recycled

But it should be noted that if the opportunity is missed and not utilized, e.g., information suppressed, all potential benefits become negative. The more rapid the management response, the less the immediate costs and the greater the medium and long-term benefits. It is similar to a restaurant kitchen inspection by a competent health officer when immediate negative criticism has the positive aspect of getting improvements from the owner and senior management that may have been long demanded by kitchen staff and previously ignored.

Another example: **Congenital toxoplasmosis** has been costed as follows (Table 6-2).[154]

Table 6-2. Lifetime costs for special services, based on 3,300 affected infants born each year.

Service	Cost ($U.S.)
Yearly ophthalmologic follow-up care	4 million
Special schooling for visually handicapped	68 million
Special schooling for moderately retarded	23 million
Institutional or state-supported foster care for severely retarded	301 million
Aid to totally retarded	33 million
Total: in 1985	430 million

Plus: Pain and suffering of affected babies; suffering of parents, as 15% affected babies die; reduced earning capacity caused by toxoplasmosis; and lost income through parents caring for infants.

Human Life Value

In the attempt to quantify the benefits of medical care, one of the common measures used is the years of life not lost. These are calculated from the appropriate life tables in relation to age, sex, and ethnicity at the time of treatment. An alternative is the increase in life expectancy beyond the normal demographic forecast. The argument is that more years are better than fewer. When used with bimodal conditions where cure is excellent or death occurs, or the condition is prevented, the interpretation is straightforward and initially relatively simple. If the murder or rabies rate, for example, is reduced, the exposed group will live longer and, it is hoped, generate more income (i.e., an increased economic output for society). The general improvement in human health in many countries during the past half-century makes this a valid economic measure.

But the situation is more complex when cure may not be complete and there are long-term sequelae or when the intervention is in the premature/dysmature neonate or in old age. For these there are two scenarios: the optimistic and the pessimistic. The optimistic scenario is based on an equal delay of both death and the prevalence of disease and morbidity in, say, the hale "wrinklies." In the pessimistic scenario, only death is delayed, bringing more morbidity in the interim to the decrepit "crumblies." The development and severity of that morbidity considerably influences the social and economic consequences of life extension, such as the demands on health care services, and the socioeconomic and sociocultural position of the elderly or family when the affected are younger. For example, 6-month survival rates for infants with birth weights under 600 g or 25 weeks gestational age are poor and expensively achieved, with various degrees of intracranial abnormality. For those born at less than 25 weeks gestation and surviving for 4 years, 80% may have moderate-to-severe functional handicaps.[61]

Clearly, in economic terms, prevention is cheaper and better than cure.

In the optimistic scenario, the pressure on the care services is about the same as it would be in a normal demographic forecast. For the elderly, the increase in life expectancy will result in higher public social security/welfare costs but extended incomes for those on private pension schemes. Both scenarios are affected by the percentage of people incapable of work, the age of retirement, the position and status of the elderly employee in the labor force, and the norms and values of old age in society.[83] Good nutrition, exercise, and medical advances are already keeping people healthier longer, and it is part of a long-term trend. However, while the number of frail old people may not increase as fast as the overall number of the elderly, that overall number will be climbing to new heights. Thus, the number of disabled old people could still rise in absolute numbers, with parallel costs.

If the intervention prevents debility and premature death, one has two time components (i.e., years) to consider, which are not necessarily weighted equally. For example, it can be argued that complete disability, e.g., blindness, is economically worse than death because of the complete nonproductivity of the affected individual and the demands imposed on society to support that individual, and the reduction, therefore, in overall production. As this argument raises complex questions, 1 year of complete disability is at least equal to 1 year of premature death. While the prevention of child mortality might appear to be more valuable than preventing adult mortality, if only because children live longer, the initial years saved are nonproductive. Thus, it is usual to assign a positive weight to years saved during the active ages between 15 and 60 years. And as it is more important to add the initial years than the more distant, one can discount years added by, say, 10%. Such considerations can reorder the cost-effectiveness of competing programs.[110]

Overall, governments must be able to put monetary values on life and limb so that the cost of diseases and disease prevention and control can be weighed against the benefits. The value of human life varies considerably from country to country (Table 6-3), with the cost of nonfatal injuries usually

Table 6.3. Cost of a road accident death

Country	$U.S. ('000)
United States[a]	2,600
Sweden[a]	1,236
New Zealand[a]	1,150
Britain[a]	1,100
Germany[b]	928
Belgium[b]	400
France[b]	350
Holland[b]	130
Portugal[b]	20

[a]Willingness-to-pay basis.
[b]Human-capital basis.

calculated as a fraction of the cost of a fatal condition.

Some costs are easy to calculate, such as hospital costs and lost wages, but these are only a fraction of the total. For example, in Britain the medical expenses comprise only 5% of the costs of a serious accident and less than 0.1% of a fatal accident—death does abruptly terminate medical care. The rest of the costs comprise lost output, pain, and grief. Easily read, harder calculated.

One approach, **human-capital,** calculates the lost earnings potential of the victim.[33] This method has problems with housewives, whose output is not subject to the marketplace and whose value has to be indirectly estimated (i.e., guessed). If one were to discount the future earnings of small children against their immediate costs of care and education, infants might have a negative value. People are worth more than what they produce, economically and philosophically.

The human-capital method can be modified to correct for this defect. Arbitrary amounts can be added for "pain, grief, and suffering." Germany crudely boosts its value by not discounting the future value of lives saved. Because of the innate flaws, many countries have abandoned this method.

Most people are willing to pay more than their future earnings to avoid death or injury. **Willingness-to-pay** studies assess what people would pay for tiny changes in risk and then calculate a value for one "statistical life."[76,94] These studies place a higher value on life than human-capital. The estimates are found by either asking people directly what they would be willing to pay to avoid a hazard, or they are calculated indirectly by examining prices in markets where risk-pricing plays a part. For example, workers in dangerous occupations should be paid a premium in compensation for the greater chance of death and injury. Neither is foolproof. There are many influences on wages, all of which have to be disentangled before a safety premium can be agreed upon. It is hard for people to put values on tiny changes of already small probabilities. Those who are without experience of serious injuries are ignorant of how much they want to avoid it. It is because of this ignorance that people are willing to pay much more to cure disease when they are afflicted than they are to prevent it. All of which produces differing estimates.

The value of life is not necessarily independent of the cause of death or disease. People who think they have more control of their fate will take more risks than those who do not. Similarly, the more seemingly random and inexplicable an event, the more people will avoid that risk if it can bring harm and, similarly, take it, if beneficial (e.g., buying lottery tickets). For example, physicians and veterinarians will routinely handle and treat infections that concern the occupationally exposed and severely frighten the general public, who are rarely at risk. Likewise, in the face of a few bloody and well-publicized lethal terrorist attacks on international flights and airports that were part of the Arab-Israeli conflict during the early 1980s, there was a precipitate and massive fall in international tourist air travel. The risk of falling victim to such a terrorist attack was minuscule, less than the chance of buying a winning national lottery ticket or of having an accident while driving to the airport. But the public judges the speed and everyday convenience of car travel to be worth the very much greater risk of driving the family car. Similarly, there was significant public alarm in relation to the perceived risk of chemical contaminants (e.g., pesticides, drug residues, growth hormones, and food additives) but much less over microbial contaminants (e.g., bacteria, parasites, viruses, and fungi), which are opposite to reality; latterly this has changed with the reports of salmonellae in poultry.[118]

In general the inflationary/deflationary perception of risks, and thus the willingness to pay or make someone else pay to be safe, is affected by the following:[58]

1. Risks that are imposed loom larger than those that are voluntary.
2. Risks that seem unfairly shared are more hazardous.
3. Risks that people can control are more acceptable than those beyond their control, though those steps may not in fact be taken.
4. Natural risks are less threatening than man-made ones.
5. Risks associated with catastrophes are especially frightening.
6. Risks from exotic technologies (e.g., DNA engineering) are feared more than those involving the familiar (e.g., automobiles and trains).
7. "Bad" news is given more weight than "good"; this can be exaggerated by the imprimatur of the news media.
8. All the above are affected by "outrage factors" that make people feel that even small risks are unacceptable.

Some lives are economically worth more than others. Richer countries and individuals will pay more and have more capacity to reduce risk. For example, the above differences in valuations between New Zealand and the United States can be explained largely by the differences in per capita gross domestic product. Also, as the probability of a person's survival approaches zero, the willingness-to-pay can increase exponentially, but this can be inversely related to education. Because of misperceptions, as the number of lives saved increases, the willingness-to-pay does not increase proportionally. Consequently, the value per person saved is lower for hazards affecting large numbers with large potential lifesaving benefits. For example, the value for saving 100 lives may be only 5 times that for saving one, while saving 10,000 persons may be only 12 to 13 times the value of saving one. Peoples' values are complex.

A hybrid approach has been proposed to bridge the gap between the two methodologies.[84] All in all, the various calculations provide a range of estimates, which are only of value when the various diseases are compared using similar methodologies and arguments. Otherwise the comparisons degenerate into juvenile but sophisticated assertions that "My costs are bigger than your costs!"

Value of Livestock to Small and Landless Third World Farmers: A Caribbean Example

How and why livestock are kept by small, marginal, and landless farmers in developing countries is best documented for the sub-Sahelian zone but little recorded in the Caribbean. Livestock censuses published by the various Caribbean Ministries of Agriculture reveal little beyond the stark data. Horowitz's classic study[65] of village life in Martinique makes only passing reference to livestock and then in a purely sociologic context. In the Caribbean, if one asks, one is frequently told that these marginal livestock owners keep their animals as a bank to be drawn on in an emergency. But no one seems to know how this "bank" is structured and how stock are valued. An unpublished study by Herman McKenzie and the author on Jamaican peasants' livestock, indicated that one of the attractions of livestock as savings is that there are delays that reduce the risk of dissipating savings. Formal livestock marketing systems are rare in the Caribbean; informal arrangements between individual farmers and buyers is the mode.

Where land is either scarce or costly, livestock may be regarded as an intermediate form of investment to the purchase of land;[21] this is part of the rationale behind landless farming and the use of "long-pasture" or roadside verges as grazing. On Nevis, returning migrants have invested in livestock since the late 19th century because land was unavailable for sale.[115] Whereas land on the islands can be owned through purchase or inheritance or by the family as a whole, animals are always owned by an individual and are not in common ownership, as, for example, are fruit trees.[25] Berleant-Schiller[13] has described how men on Barbuda accumulate cash but more importantly prestige by cattle keeping and without emigrating. In the Caribbean, livestock have different economic and social values to the owner, to the community in which they live, and to the state. A superficial examination reveals that this marginal stock is not as productive as even modest commercial units and that minor losses can be catastrophic because of the small herd/flock size. But livestock will be kept in spite of their lower economic productivity compared with horticultural crops.[42] Their management is conservative and traditional. Therefore, an island veterinary service to these livestock may appear to produce only small economic benefits to the community at great unit cost, compared with the greater return from the care of the few large herds and flocks. Thus, any veterinary attention given to this marginal livestock has, in the absence of epidemic disease risk, a potential **opportunity cost** on the limited island veterinary time available, measured through the reduced productivity of those larger herds on which the urban populations may depend for fresh meat and milk. An opportunity cost is the benefit foregone by using a scarce resource for one purpose instead of for its next best alternative use. But the productivity of small and landless farmers in relation to the feed and grazing resources available may be better than is initially apparent.

A small study of some 34 small (no more than 5 acres of owned or rented grazing) and landless long-pasture farmers in St. Lucia provided some insight into the structuring of these superficially marginal herds and flocks. The conclusions suggested the hypothesis that these small and marginal farmers were converting and storing their one available commodity (time) into something (e.g., male small ruminants) that later can be harvested to feed their families or that can be exchanged (e.g., by the sale of cattle) for goods and services. These farmers differ from commercial farmers who use their capital by investing in buildings, land, and improved stock, and their available credit in purchased feed or specially grown forage, hired labor, and other services. This valuation of time would seem to be more important than their reported reasons (e.g., liking animals).

This hypothesis can be taken one step further: the St. Lucian cattle owner has a "stock train" and its length is fixed by the owner's major constraints (time, access to grazing, and whether the owner wished to also keep sheep and goats). For example, the maximum number of stock kept by landless farmers was five adult cattle and five adult small ruminants. The stock gets on this train at "1 year old" (the St. Lucian appreciation of livestock ages appears to be not truly chronological and this age of 1 year is probably declared when a calf is weaned and needs individual care). The bulls alight when they are sold at 24-36 months old (at this time they are becoming difficult to handle and are at risk of being stolen) and cows by 6 years old (having produced two calves). When a calf gets on this train, it pushes a cow or bull off the other end, though maybe not immediately. Although these herds are small, expansion is very difficult because of time and land limitations, such as the need for extra forage in the dry season. There are limited opportunities to reinvest this sale money in extra young stock. The product, therefore, might be interpreted in a number of economic ways, one of which is as the dividend on a fixed investment (the stock train); by maintaining this moving train, the owner has savings "on the hoof" for emergencies or against planned future expenditures (e.g., house repairs, Christmas, school expenses, children's clothes). This value might be regarded, therefore, as the net profit after subtracting the opportunity labor costs, for the widespread use of common and other "free" grazing results in small or even zero land costs; or as the windfall cash value received from the butcher; or as a social value, which might be estimated from the butcher's retail value of the beast; or even as a welfare value because it provides a safety net to those at financial risk. This livestock system has an internal, dynamic imperative in that the animals cannot be ignored and must be handled daily. Thus, to regard it as passive savings, such as with money in a bank, is not only overly simplistic but also false. While this system is efficient for subsistence, it does not allow for expansion or increased productivity.

There is also an important societal or personal value placed on livestock ownership in St. Lucia, for owning livestock was ranked first by both cattle and sheep owners. To quote an old woman at Gros Islet, speaking about her bull recovering from dermatophilosis, "If I sell the bull, what do I have? Money. But if I do not sell, I have cattle."

While it was abundantly clear from these study data that sheep and goats were important for family nutrition in St. Lucia, it was too small a study to determine how many ewes and does are needed to feed the average rural family. How many are needed to provide additional animals for social activities and to foster relationships? What proportion of urban and rural families keep small ruminants, and how might these figures compare with the other Caribbean islands, and why do they differ? These are not idle speculations. Thanks to enzootic cowdriosis, Guadeloupe has a fraction of the small ruminant population seen on other islands in the Lesser Antilles. Widespread predial larceny in Jamaica is so severe that the island has to import goat meat and carcasses from Central America. Small and landless farming form an important component of Caribbean life as it is lived and are integral parts of the social fabric. The provision of adequate and appropriate veterinary services on islands such as St. Lucia is complex, largely un-described, and must be responsive to these social dimensions as well as the usual economic, commercial, and ethical considerations.

Veterinary Economics

A continuing problem in veterinary economics is the depth of knowledge and information needed for the various models and calculations. If a general criticism is to be made, it is that too often the "economist," whether professional or amateur, has displayed a lack of knowledge of the epidemiology of the condition, allied with a blind trust in the quality of data used. It is traditional in economics to use secondary or tertiary data and rare to find an economist who has generated his or her own data; when done, it is commonly at the microeconomic level of a clutch sample of herds or flocks. The variable range of data sources used provide a wide range of results and negate the comparability of notionally similar studies.[124] Sometimes, the social impacts of disease are too subtle or complex for ready evaluation, and are thus unavailable or too variable in the literature. Many have tried to overcome these deficiencies with sophisticated analyses, preferably on a powerful computer and certainly well distanced from the farmyard and reality. A simple answer is that the economist has to be a member of a team so that there is access to sufficient information and advice on production, statistics, and epidemiology to construct a valid and sufficient argument. For example, in many situations losses may be treated in a modular fashion; an abortion is an abortion whatever the cause; a gallon of milk lost through mastitis is a gallon of milk lost; a dead cow is its average live market value plus the present value loss of projected income from calves and milk adjusted for age. But when there are long-term impacts with suboptimal production and management constraints, they must be included in the analysis, such as the within-herd impact of FMD in Latin America, which can take 2 years to work out in an affected herd, or with coccidiosis in spring lambs on the Welsh border in the United Kingdom with excess pneumonia and poor-doing among the survivors during the subsequent autumn, or the possible concatenation of many events such as in a brucella-related abortion storm. However, not all epidemiological components of a disease or health program will significantly affect the precision or accuracy of an economic assessment. Some will merely add an air of verisimilitude. Search long, but the results should be short, simple, and truthful. Or in the words of Francis Crick, one should "make sense of the information...[and] express it in a compact and well-organized manner."

A historical criticism can be made of veterinary economics, that of bias. There are still very few academically trained economists in animal health. This has produced a very "vet centered" perspective of what is important in the economics of animal health and disease, probably exaggerated by the veterinary profession's awareness of its value to society and the pressure to continually reappraise it. They have been happy to live with the kind of economics that provides a favorable B/C ratio. It must look up to wider horizons. One sometimes gets the uncomfortable impression that veterinary economics has concerned itself more with the fly on the axle than the chariot; more with mastitis, for example, than the management of the whole dairy enterprise inside a national industry. Vic Beynon of Exeter University once commented in the early 1970s that if one added up all the animal disease costs in circulation in the United Kingdom, it would be in excess of the GNP. This might have been a modest hyperbole but it accurately reflects a common problem. Conservative estimates of costs, benefits, and risks are not always welcomed, however accurate, because of the advantages of extended and prolonged projects. A minor adjustment in the discount rate has sometimes turned an unprofitable proposed project into a "winner." It is equally strange how often the utility values of a project are only wheeled into action when B/C ratios are near parity, which reinforces the impression of how often the discipline is abused, for economics is not just about measurement—it is about understanding how the whole system works.

To sum up, effect has precedence over cause, before effect comes impact, and before impact there is cost.

Some Economic Studies of Zoonotic Diseases (Table 6-4)

Table 6-4. Some good and bad economic studies of zoonotic diseases

Specific Zoonotic Disease	Animal	Study—Place
Brucellosis	Cattle	Cost-benefit analysis—England and Wales[66, 86]
		Cost-benefit analysis—New Zealand[131]
		Cost-benefit analysis—United States[4, 37]
		Costs and benefits—Louisiana[155]
		Costs and benefits—Chad and Cameroon[39]
		Costs—Ivory Coast[7]
		Social restraints on control—Argentina[31]
		Control benefits—Kirgizia[157]
		Model projections—Ivory Coast[23] (+ trypanosomiasis)
	Human	Socioeconomic costs—Spain[27]
	Review	Americas (34 countries)[53]
		Nigeria[2]
Chagas disease	Vector	Cost-effect analysis of vector control[104]
		Cost-benefit analysis of vector control[126]
	Human	Social costs[20, 132]
Foodborne diseases	Man	Human diseases—Review—United States[92, 116]
		Human diseases—Review—Canada and United States[142]
		Hydatidosis—Cost-effect analysis—Sardinia[9, 18]
		Hydatidosis—Cost-effect discussion—Australia[54]
		Salmonellosis, total case estimates—United States[24]
		Salmonellosis, private and public costs—United Kingdom[135]

Table 6-4. (continued)

Specific Zoonotic Disease	Animal	Study—Place
Foodborne diseases	Livestock	Hydatidosis—Review/Annotated bibliography[140]
	Pigs	Echinococcosis—Costs—Hungary[32]
		Trichinelliasis—France[136]
	Sheep	*Taenia* and *Echinococcus*—New Zealand[85]
		Echinococcus—Spain[114]
Leptospirosis	Cattle	Impact—New Zealand[29]
		Decision analysis—New Zealand[128]
	Pigs	Impact—Argentina[122]
	Various	Impact—Belgium[35]
Listeriosis	Sheep	Flock vaccination assessment—Norway[144]
Liver flukes/	Man	Public and private costs—Thailand[89]
fascioliasis	Cattle	Control trials—Belgium[55]
		Disease costs—Jamaica[22]
Plague	Human	Cost-benefit analysis—United States[80]
Rabies	Dog	Review of cost-effect studies[17]
		Cost-benefit analysis—Philippines[51]
	Foxes	Cost-benefit analysis—France[150]
	Raccoons	Cost-benefit analysis—United States[143]
Tuberculosis	Badgers	Cost-benefit analysis—United Kingdom[95, 109]
	Cattle	Costs—Belarus[156]
		Costs—Nigeria[3]
		Costs—Ukraine[103]
		Eradication costs—TB and Brucellosis—Australia[6, 64, 138]
		Eradication Costs—Irish Republic[102]
		Possum control—New Zealand[88]
		Production losses—Argentina[99]
	Deer	Costs—New Zealand[127]
		Reviews[26, 113]
	Human	Benefits of bovine TB control—United States[119]
Trypanosomiasis	Human	Cost-benefit analysis[130]
	Cattle	Costs and benefits of tsetse control[71, 72, 129, 153]
		Costs—Kenya[152]
		Costs—Zambia[112]
		Data requirements[77]
		Linear programming model[60]
	Goats	Breed effects on costs[79]
Vector control		Cost-effect analyses[19, 108]
		Willingness-to-pay[47, 73]

Note: Basic texts:

Dijkhuizen A. A., R. B. M. Huirne, and J. A. Renkema. *Modelling Animal Health Economics*. Department of Farm Management, Wageningen Agricultural University, 1991.

Gittinger, J. P. *Economic Analysis of Agricultural Projects*, 2nd edition. Baltimore, Johns Hopkins University Press, 1982.

Little, T. W. A, and J. A. Mirlees. *Project Appraisal and Planning for Developing Countries*. New York, Basic Books, 1974.

Samuelson, P. A. *Economics*, 11th edition. New York, McGraw-Hill, 1980.

Control Programs and the Prevention of Zoonoses

With the increasing global suburbanization and abandonment of rural living, the intimate association with livestock, so characteristic of the early decades of this century, is becoming a matter of the dim memory. Along with the widespread loss of this reality has risen the demand for risk-free living, in part a most-valid rejection of the foul adulterations and unhygienic conditions of that golden age. It sometimes includes a nonnegotiable demand for an unrealistic reengineering of the animal industries that somehow will be able to maintain production to feed an ever-larger population at everyday prices. The more "natural" husbandry systems of 100 to 200 years ago fed an essentially rural population and therefore collection, storage, and transport was a local problem. Then, farmers' wives and their strawyard flocks were the producers of eggs; today such a system is impossible if everyone is to be able to buy eggs at a reasonable price. The universal health of any nation depends on good nutrition at an affordable price. This, at an equal pace, locks in the intensification of the various livestock industries and their increasing efficiency. None of these industries is disease free, though the rates may be relatively trivial compared to the past. In production medicine, it is a fine balance of economics and epidemiology, and to improve beyond that can involve exponentially higher costs for negligible gain. And in the absence of antigenic stimulation, we may be facing higher risks of disease than before.

Similarly, for zoonotic diseases with wildlife reservoirs, the cost of preventing all outbreaks can be in excess of the benefits. Bluntly, for some diseases communities will just have to live with a certain annual incidence, be it sylvatic plague, Rocky Mountain spotted fever, Lyme disease, leptospirosis, or aseptic meningitis. And even if control were possible, the opportunity cost of transferring staff and facilities from other programs may be too high.

But given that a zoonotic infection or disease can be controlled and the incidence reduced, and that it is feasible and economically worthwhile, who should be responsible? The animal owner or the government? The simple answer is that it depends on who benefits. For example, because of the direct losses from livestock helminths, the farmer should be responsible for their control, just as it is more efficient to have the processing plant responsible for hazard analysis critical control point (HACCP), because the marketplace should reward success and punish failure. Similarly, for brucellosis eradication, it is more of a community problem because of the complexity of any program, and the community is the major beneficiary. The real world is more complicated, but this is not a bad starting position.

Total responsibility cannot be left to government, however paternal it might be and passive the population, because bureaucracies have an unfortunate tendency to be self-serving. Similarly, all parts of society must assume responsibility for disease prevention; just because food is carefully processed and inspected does not obviate the personal responsibility to handle it properly in the kitchen. Pragmatically, hybrid systems work more efficiently. Involving local cattlemen's associations in brucellosis eradication may not of itself guarantee rapid success, but it significantly reduces the probability of failure. The more short term and local the gains, the more the public will want to be involved and willing to directly contribute to the costs. Likewise, the more areas involved, the greater the need for coordination and agreement on common standards. The more intense an industry, the more it will undertake by itself; the more diffuse, the more likely that coordination and supervision will be external to that industry. Similarly, the more long term the program, the more government will have to be involved. The longer the term, the more the program responsibility will shift from local agencies to state or provincial or even federal levels. Government programs have the capacity to transfer benefits from one part of society to the other, which is one of the reasons for having government and not anarchy. For example, research is a transfer benefit to the community; the hog cholera/swine fever research costs at the U.K. M.A.F.F. Central Veterinary Laboratory were less than 1/20th of the total British government costs of the eradication program. But without it, it is doubtful whether the program could have succeeded profitably.[43] A property of government programs is that their innate generic actions can have multiple benefits.

Unforeseen Effects

These effects tend to be binomially distributed as zero or catastrophically successful.

An excellent example of the former situation was the provision of a live Newcastle feed–baited vaccine for smallholder poultry flocks in five Southeast Asian countries. This competent vaccine provided no production advantage to protected flocks. In that harsh poultry world, the village environment harbored such a complex of hazards for the birds that the entire biological capacity of the flock was taken up with maintaining numbers with little or no surplus available for production. However, subsequent modeling showed that if modest husbandry improvements, e.g., hens less likely to go broody and strategic supplemental feeding, were introduced along with vaccination, the poultry could be twice as productive at little extra cost. Because of the gross inefficiencies of the existing system, a single technical innovation had a trivial impact.[75]

The introduction of the successful Marek's disease vaccine in the early 1970s to the efficient layer industry was catastrophic. At that time this disease was a major constraint on egg production; layer flocks in the United

States overstocked by 10%-15% to allow for losses and by up to 20% in Germany and the Netherlands. The vaccine's introduction resulted in an immediate overproduction of eggs in an industry with already minuscule profit margins; the price of eggs fell, and many producers and breeders were in severe financial trouble. The breeders took up to 2 years to recover, and the industry longer to settle down. The U.K. situation was different because there was a coincident Newcastle disease epidemic throughout the country, with massive mortalities in affected flocks. This buffered the temporary negative economic effects of the successful Marek's vaccine by maintaining profit margins in unaffected flocks. The economic impact was described dryly as follows: "After the short-run economic adjustment problems were overcome, the poultry industry as a whole, however, gained some long-run benefits in terms of its competitive position in relation to that of other foods. Also the nation has benefitted because fewer resources are necessary to produce the same number of broilers and eggs that were produced before."[111] Eradication and control usually aids the already efficient and produces too much competition for the small or less-efficient producer, with their removal from the industry.

Somalia had a successful contagious caprine pleuropneumonia (CCPP) vaccination program in the late 1970s to early 1980s in the central range-lands. This was part of the national "Great Illiteracy Campaign" started in 1974 using representatives from various ministries (e.g., public health, livestock, agriculture, and veterinary extension) and specially selected and trained village Voluntary Self-Help Volunteers, who, apart from other duties, vaccinated millions of animals with the PG3 vaccine. This effective vaccine contributed to a glut of small ruminants, extensive and severe overgrazing, and parallel disease problems. Although Somalia has a nomadic livestock-rearing tradition, it was an efficient system within the severe environmental limits.

Must Ontogeny Follow Phylogeny? Or, Do Developing Countries Have to Follow the Same Path as Developed Countries?

In theory, developing countries with significant disease control problems ought to be able to utilize existing knowledge and technology to leapfrog over history into an improved future. The bad news is that they are usually in this situation because of a past history of poorly trained and directed, ill-rewarded veterinarians, and inadequate infrastructure and financing. These are not corrected overnight. Secondly, when they turn to international agencies, they can and frequently do become victims of "experts" with little or no knowledge of the country and sometimes even of the disease in question—consultants with solutions looking for profitable problems. Each disease has acquired traditional tried-and-true methods of control, which work, more or less, in the countries where they evolved. But, assuming no significant strain differences in the agent, each national disease situation differs because of its cultural and agricultural practices. For efficient control, consideration of these factors is more important than the agent itself. Thus, importing a methodology seldom works of itself. The good news is that problems define their solutions. All possible contributing factors, veterinary, societal, cultural, economic, and agricultural, should be examined before a solution is proposed. Secondly, a flexible, step-by-step Darwinian approach will encourage the optimum national campaign to evolve relatively quickly. Thirdly, because of prior experiences elsewhere and advances in technology, there are shortcuts if one has the creativity to find them and the courage to use them.

Homework *before* Campaign

Over a 10-year period, the Inter-American Development Bank (IDB) in Washington, D.C., disbursed some $100 million for the control of FMD and brucellosis in Latin America. In 1985-86, it did an in-house, retroactive assessment of its programs in Brazil, Colombia, Ecuador, Peru, and Central America. Each team reported that there would have been significant (20% to 30%) savings in money and time with parallel improvements in effectiveness if a proper baseline of epidemiological data had been acquired *before* planning and initiating each project. In retrospect they realized how expensive it was to collect that information after the start of the formal programs. In each case, a delay of 2 years to collect the necessary epidemiological data would have made it more likely that the projected IDB investment benefits might have been achieved. Skimping on the planning budget is expensive.

Risk Analysis

Risk analysis is eclectic and draws on information from a wide spectrum of sources to estimate the probable frequency of an unwanted future event, e.g., importation of a chronically infected carrier and how to manage and inform about that possibility. It supports decisions made in uncertainty, in the absence of hard data. It is made up of three intercommunicating parts: **risk assessment, risk management,** and **risk communication.**

Risk assessment. Risk assessment is the use of the existing available factual base to define the health effects of exposure of individuals or populations to hazardous materials or situations.[101] It is driven by the need to make informed and timely management decisions, sometimes despite very limited data and information.[81] It "is a complex formal process organizing and interpreting scientific information. It includes the identification and documentation of uncertainties; the estimation of risk for specific (predefined) scenarios; and the presentation of findings in concise, organized formats to facilitate informed decision making. This formal scientific process provides a sound foundation for management decisions."[82] It constructs a common structure for those involved in making and implementing regulatory decisions and, thus, for effective communication between them. If it has been rigorously designed, there is the potential to rerun the process as more and better data and information are acquired and, thus, to regularly review a program. It is used in drawing up regulations concerned with importations and food safety, including chemical and biological hazards, exposure to chemicals in the environment, and occupational chemical exposure.

It involves the sequential qualitative description of what can go wrong, followed by the quantitative measure of the likelihood and impact of that event if it should happen. Or, it involves "the characterization of potential adverse effects of exposures to hazards; including estimates of risk and of uncertainties in measurements, analytical techniques, and interpretive models. Quantitative risk assessment characterizes the risk in numerical representations."[100] Risk assessment is composed of four parts:

1. *Hazard* or *risk identification* involves a comprehensive review of all the possible events associated with a situation or potential scenario. If a particular hazard has not been identified, the probabilities of it occurring cannot be calculated, nor can management formulate steps to reduce that risk. For example, to evaluate a proposal to import an animal species, one must list all the pathogens that could be associated with that species in the country of origin and then to identify the possible routes by which those potential pathogens might spread to susceptible animals within the importing country.

2. *Dose-response assessment* or *hazard characterization* is the determination of the quantitative relationship between the magnitude of exposure and the probability of health effects. In certain very infrequent circumstances, a binomial/threshold situation might exist, e.g., the condition is seen/not-seen.

3. *Exposure assessment* is the determination of the extent, frequency, and duration of human or animal exposures before and after the application of regulatory controls.

4. *Risk characterization* brings together the previous three parts to predict the nature, magnitude, and likelihood of the various outcomes in the exposed populations, including uncertainty. It will review the assumptions, the representativeness, reliability, and applicability of the data used to indicate probable level and range of risk. Because of the absence of hard data, confidence intervals cannot be calculated, for it is not a statistical estimate.

Risk management. Risk management is "the evaluation of alternative risk control actions—one choice being no action—and their implementation. The responsible individual or office (i.e., risk manager) sometimes oversees preparation of risk assessments, risk control assessments, and risk messages." The government office can, for example, decide either to refuse importation altogether or to require mitigating measures if a particular level of risk, following importation, is accepted. Such mitigating actions might be the treatment of an animal product to reduce an unacceptably high risk to a more tolerable level, or the use of a highly sensitive diagnostic test to exclude possibly infected animals. While risk assessments are sometimes not without controversy, management processes are usually more available to objective quantification. It is obvious that there must be a dynamic conversation between assessor and manager, for the activities of one will modify the arguments of the other. The objective of risk management is to identify, document, and implement measures that will reduce the risk to a tolerable level.

Risk communication. Risk communication involves the joint discussion of the risk hazard by all concerned parties. The definition is not quite as clear: "An interactive process of exchange of information and opinion among individuals, groups, and institutions; often involves multiple messages about the nature of risk or expressing concerns, opinions, or reactions to risk messages or to legal and institutional arrangements for risk management." (The committee responsible for this definition had obviously never read Gowers.[59]) Those making the risk assessment must be able to explain the process so that the decision-makers, the stakeholders (e.g., the affected livestock industry), and the public (who can also be stakeholders) understand. Similarly, the concerns of the stakeholders must be heard and adequately addressed.

Risk is used in the context of the probability or frequency of occurrence of a predefined hazardous event. While the magnitude of an event is assumed to be significant, the interpretation of the risk probability should be agreed by all. For example, a **negligible risk** that all parties accept under most circumstances is usually 10^{-6} in most human health and environmental risk studies; a tidy number, if not necessarily meaningful. On the other hand, some veterinary proponents of risk analysis have introduced the concept of **acceptable risk**. This is a subjective management decision about the safety of a regulatory decision or permissibility of a hazard—it may involve substantial disagreement and can be fraught with problems of public perception, however sensible the decision might be. The acceptability of a risk will vary in its interpretation, particularly when the benefited group is different from those put at risk. Thus, potential benefits and effects must be identified, described, and if possible, quantified. The generally accepted RA term is therefore **tolerable risk,** which indicates the compromises involved and the temporary nature of the decision. The potential for misunderstandings, both among the experts and with outside groups, is omnipresent, especially when there is fundamental disagreement; these misunderstandings can be reduced largely by agreeing on terms and their definitions. An effective, open communication system and structure is, therefore, vital.

Risk analysis must be "transparent," that is, information used must be properly organized, carefully documented, and available to all. And, the risk assessment should be dynamic, flexible, and capable of absorbing and utilizing new information, as on the health status of the exporting country and new diagnostic techniques. The assessment should be performed independently from the regulatory decision making to maintain high standards of integrity, scientific and bureaucratic. The evaluation standards used for one must be the same consistent procedures used for all. This may appear to be a utopian position, but pragmatically, it is one that produces many, many fewer problems than partiality and bias.

An example of risk assessment. This is a very simple and incompletely documented assessment, based on a published set of calculations.[63] It estimates the risk to New Zealand, which is anthrax-free, of acquiring *Bacillus anthracis* spores and anthrax as a result of importing green hides from Australia, which does have livestock anthrax.

The annual probability (T) of introducing anthrax through unprocessed hides was defined as a function of the probability (p) that a hide contains spores and the number of times (n) that animals would be in contact with those spores, assuming that spore contact has a binomial distribution (i.e., yes or no).

$$T = 1 - (1 - p)^n$$

When T is very small, e.g., 0.001, this may be simplified to:

$$T = pn$$

The probability that an Australian hide imported into New Zealand contains anthrax spores might be assumed to be:

$$p = is$$

where **i** is the probability that an Australian sheep or cow had anthrax when skinned. Between 1970 and 1981, the annual incidence of reported livestock anthrax was 19 per year and ranged from 9 to 42 cases; the maximum risk may then use 40 cases, ignoring the declining trend of this disease. During

1989-1990, some 40.23 million sheep and cattle were slaughtered in Australia; during the 1980s it was in the range of 37.2 to 42.3 millions; therefore **i** was estimated to be 40/40.23 million, or 9.94×10^{-7}. **s** is the proportion of spores surviving until arrival in New Zealand (anthrax spores are traditionally very robust, so **s** was given the value of 0.9). Therefore **p** may be estimated to be:

$$0.000000994 \times .9 = 0.00000089 \text{ or } 8.9 \times 10^{-7}$$

The number (**n**) of occasions or days that susceptible New Zealand livestock will be exposed to viable anthrax spores may be estimated to be:

$$n = gtvfd$$

where **g** is the number of Ministry of Agriculture and Fisheries–approved tanneries, or 23; **t** is the proportion of such tanneries with the opportunity of contaminating pastures with wastewater during seasonal flooding (there was no information so it was approximated at 20% and 100%); **v** is the average number of days each year on which this flooding occurs (the estimated range was 20-30 days, or an "average" of 25 days); **f** is the probability of processing contaminated hides during periods of flooding (or 25/235 average annual working days, or 0.11); and **d** is the duration in days that an infective dose of spores would be available in the grazing (historically this can be almost any number one cares to consider, but let us use 1 and 100, assuming that ultraviolet light will sterilize surface spores and rain will wash others away). Therefore,

$$n = 23 \times 0.2 \times 25 \times 0.11 \times 1 = 12.65 \text{ days}$$

Thus, a first estimate of the probability of introducing *B. anthracis* onto New Zealand pastures downstream of approved tanneries, or **t**, is 0.00000089×12.65 or 1.13×10^{-5}.

If we are more conservative, or health protective, and assume that all tanneries can contaminate pastures for at least 1 day after flooding, the probability becomes 5.63×10^{-5}; if we then include the maximum number of days (30) on which flooding occurs historically, the probability is 6.76×10^{-5}; and then presume prolonged survival in the grazing (100 days), the probability is now near 0.007.

The "real" risk is somewhere in a range of probabilities. By using a range of values for each variable in a stochastic or Monte Carlo model over a large number of iterations, e.g., 1000, one can derive a final risk estimate as a probability distribution. The sensitivity analysis of this albeit simplistic model would be achieved by replacing each variable with a single most likely value and then increasing each in turn by a factor of 10 to identify the most critical variables. Attention can then be focused on parameters, where a small or moderate change makes big differences; better information is then sought and used in designing and implementing better and more efficient risk- reduction measures.

When one then considers the chances of a grazing animal acquiring an infective dose of still-viable spores and the normal procedures in Australian abattoirs, the probability is certainly less than the maximum probability shown here. On the other hand, in advanced countries, anthrax-infected hides rarely come through abattoirs but from hides salvaged from animals found dead or dying; in contrast, anthrax is common in animals slaughtered at village "slaughter slabs" in West Africa. Anthrax occurs in well-delineated areas in Australia and is not widespread. This would suggest that if spore-contaminated Australian hides were imported, it might be in a hide or hides from a single "knacker" as a special shipment to one tannery. Historical experience of this disease near tanneries in Canada, England, Germany, and presently Italy indicate that anthrax is not a risk to be taken lightly.

Risk analysis provides a philosophical structure for risk control in uncertainty. First, in the progressive reduction of international trade barriers, trade agreements such as the General Agreement on Tariffs and Trade (GATT), the North American Free Trade Agreement (NAFTA), and the European Union (EU), borders are no longer used to delineate trade and to control the movement of animals and animal products. Second, there is no biological situation with zero risk. The manipulation of any biological system involves risks. Third, extremely restrictive policies or any beyond those required for biological safety invite smuggling and the gross evasion of responsibilities, which can initiate a train of uncontrolled events. Too often, extreme restrictions can be imposed that only serve to protect bureaucratic anatomy. A reasonable position invites compliance and encourages everyone to support standards because all benefit. Fourth and last, no infection can read an atlas. Put another way, infections know no boundaries but diseases do. Agents of disease are never homogeneously distributed, but are functions of climate, geography, host range, and livestock husbandry, all of which ignore national boundaries. The benefits, other than trade, come from the requirements to improve and maintain animal health and the surveillance systems to demonstrate that status.

A present shortcoming in risk analysis is verification. The mere fact that the feared event has not occurred, following implementation, does not confirm that the right management procedures were designed **and** used. The system may have been overcautious with additional indirect costs or it may have been irrelevant to reality, rather like the Surrey gentleman who tore up telephone directories and threw the pieces out the train window to stop elephants from invading the English countryside, however scientifically structured. Post hoc investigations are needed to discover whether the event ever occurred or is above the projected frequency and, even in its apparent absence, to discover what is actually being done or did happen.

One of the problems in risk analysis and in disease eradication is how do we know when a disease, or infection, is **not** present. The statistically minded would state correctly that one can never know. However big the sample, there is always the possibility that there are still 100 or 10 affected individuals out there. This is the epidemiologic version of Zeno's arrow, or that military jock Achilles' futile efforts to catch a tortoise. But arrows hit targets and diseases do get eradicated and others are truly absent from parts and regions of the world where they might otherwise be expected. With zoonotic diseases there has to be a chain of infection, and "miasmas" ceased to play a meaningful part in disease causation long ago. Beyond a certain very small prevalence or risk, one must abjure statistics and use epidemiological common sense. At this point, one employs disease "traps." When one is poaching rabbits, one does not spread snares all over the countryside but only in those few places where the most rabbits are most likely to be running. Similarly, when one has a disease surveillance system that has actively watched these sites and found nothing over a reasonable period of time, the disease does not exist. The opposing argument is to question whether all possible and improbable sites and modes of spread have been considered. One does not know everything, but minor epidemiological modes of spread, known or yet-to-be-discovered, will seldom be sufficient to maintain an infectious disease at very low incidence rates except possibly in a few nidi. These extreme possibilities can be ignored when proper (post-eradication) surveillance is maintained.

Hazard Analysis Critical Control Point (HACCP)

In the 1930s, S. C. Prescott and K. K. Mayer in the United States and Sir Graham Wilson in the United Kingdom introduced the principle of taking preventive remedial measures rather than examining the final product. This proactive concept of control was ignored and thus the disease rates and economic impacts of foodborne diseases from microbial agents continued to rise and new agents were identified. The breakthrough came with Dr. W. E. Deming's theories of quality management and the development of Total Quality Management systems in the 1950s. The HACCP (Hazard Analysis Critical Control Point) concept was pioneered by the Pillsbury Company, the U.S. Army, and NASA in a collaborative development of safe foods for the Mercury flights. NASA wanted "zero defects" to guarantee safety for the foods consumed by astronauts in space. With Gemini, the problems were magnified because of more-complex foods and longer flights. By the time Apollo landed on the moon, HACCP was developed. Within 2 years of the moon landing, HACCP was in commercial use in the manufacture of consumer foods at Pillsbury. They had concluded that the only way they could succeed in having safe food was to have control over the raw materials, the process, the environment, and people, beginning as early in the system as possible. The principles embodied in HACCP are used now by Australia, Canada, the United States, and the European Union, with coordination deliberations through the United Nations Food and Agriculture Organization, the World Health Organization, and the pertinent Codex Alimentarius committees. The strategy was first initiated within the USDA in 1970; this program is still developing even now. The U.S. National Academy of Sciences recommended in 1985 that the HACCP approach be adopted in food processing establishments to ensure food safety.

HACCP relies on (1) the meticulous identification of hazardous practices and locations, i.e., "critical control points"; (2) the elimination of such hazards by developing processing techniques, or general management practices[48] (GMP), that will control food contamination and colonization; (3) validation of GMPs through risk assessment; and (4) introduction and ongoing evaluation through monitoring representative samples.

The Canadian Food Safety Enhancement Program (FSEP) utilizes the HACCP principles but limits them to the harvesting and commercial processing of food. Within a food processing system, this involves steps based upon HACCP principles that are mutually developed with the commodity industries:[1]

1. Identification of hazards that may be present from harvest through ultimate consumption and the preventive measures for controlling them.

2. Determination of critical control points (CCP) required to control identified hazards. A CCP is a point, step, or procedure (e.g., cooking or rapid chilling) at which control can be applied and a food safety hazard prevented, eliminated, or reduced to acceptable levels.

3. Establishment of critical limits, a value that separates acceptability from unacceptability, that must be met at each CCP.

4. Appropriate CCP monitoring procedures; these are planned sequences of recorded observations or measurements of critical limits designed to assess whether a CCP is under control.

5. Establishing predetermined and documented corrective actions implemented when a deviation occurs at a CCP.

6. Developing and implementing verification procedures for a HACCP plan, i.e., confirm that it is working.

7. Documenting all procedures and records concerned with steps 1 through 6.

An Example of HACCP; Fish and Fisheries Products, FDA[49]

Hazard: Parasites in fish species disposed to them.

Hazard statement: Parasites in wild caught fish and shellfish are an unavoidable defect. Control by fishing only selected areas may be possible, but the data necessary to choose reduced-parasite fishing grounds are not available in most regions. Some species, due to their feeding habits or natural resistance, are less likely to have parasites than other species. The best available control measure is visual examination and physical removal of the parasites. This method, termed candling, can reduce, but does not eliminate, the parasite burden in white, translucent-fleshed fish.

Engineers have not yet developed a nondestructive method to detect and remove parasites from pigmented-fleshed fish or opaque, white-fleshed fish. Parasites in these species cannot be controlled through in-process controls. However, trimming to remove the belly flaps may be effective in reducing the parasite burden in certain species.

In translucent, white-fleshed fish, parasites are considered filth, and the significance of their presence is evaluated by the FDA on a case-by-case basis when they are detected. Translucent, white-fleshed fish are responsible for more than 95% of the parasite-related consumer complaints received by the FDA. The FDA samples finished products and will seize or deny entry to product lots that contain an excessive number of parasites.

Parasites consumed in uncooked or undercooked unfrozen seafood can present a human health hazard. Some products that have been implicated in human infections are ceviche (cibichi), lomi lomi salmon, salmon roe, sushi, sushimi, green herring, drunken crabs, cold smoked fish, and undercooked grilled fish. The FDA discourages the consumption of raw seafood products. Freezing ($-20°C$ [$-4°F$] for 7 days or $-35°C$ [$-31°F$] for 15 hours) of fish intended for raw consumption eliminates the possibility of human infection. This is recommended in the retail food protection manual and in the Food Code. However, all species that are intended for raw or marinated consumption and that have a known parasite danger should be treated as suggested in Option 4 (below).

Critical control point: Receiving, storage, or processing. There are four separate options available:

Option 1: When the processor receives fish without knowledge of its parasite burden (based on past experience with the species and harvest area).
Option 2: When the processor receives product from an area with a known

high parasite burden (i.e., above 1 parasite per kg flesh based on past experience with the species and harvest area).

Option 3: Where the firm receives fish from an area with a known low parasite burden (less than 1 parasite per kg flesh based on past experience with the species and harvest area).

Option 4: Where the firm markets fish to firms that produce cold smoked or marinated products or markets fish to sushi or sushimi restaurants.

To understand what is involved when an option is chosen, assume Option 2 is the option of choice.

Control measure:
1. Candle the entire lot. The production line candling operation should be designed to remove all visible parasites.
2. Monitor the effectiveness of the candling operation by having a representative of management or quality control candle a representative portion of each lot before packing.

Frequency: For candling, each lot. For monitoring, each lot.

Critical limits: The action levels are as follows:

Tullibies, ciscoes, inconnus, chubs, and whitefish—50 cysts/45.45 kg (100 lbs) flesh.

Blue fin and other freshwater herring averaging 1 pound or less— 60 cysts/100 fish, if 20% of the fish examined are infested.

Blue fin and other freshwater herring averaging over 1 pound— 60 cysts/45.45 kg (100 lbs) flesh, if 20% of the fish examined are infested.

Rose fish (red fish and ocean perch)—3% of fillets examined contain one or more copepods accompanied by pus pockets.

Other fish, crustaceans, and mollusks should have visible parasites removed.

Records: The records should describe the results of the candling examinations for each lot.

Corrective action: Destroy or reprocess any lots that exceed the critical limits after production candling to eliminate the defect, keeping full records of the reprocessing. Any critical limit deviation should cause a timely reassessment by management to discover whether the process or HACCP plan needs to be changed to reduce the risk of recurrence of the deviation, and to take appropriate follow-up action.

By implementing *pre*harvest quality control, not only should livestock and poultry be in a more-optimum condition at slaughter, but there are major savings through minimal need for condemnation and lower processing inspection costs.[93] These have been implemented in the poultry industry for a decade, with farm managers getting, sometimes hourly, reports from the processing plants. Similar programs have been in place for pigs in the Netherlands for a number of years. This is relatively easy, though technically complex, for large, vertically integrated systems (e.g., poultry, pigs, and a few beef and dairy groups) with computerized communications and accurate farm batch identification. Fish farms will join this system as hazards are identified. Western Australia instituted a system in 1991 for monitoring the prevalence of 13 chronic conditions in sheep and 22 in cattle seen at slaughter. These data form the basis of "Health Reports" to the individual farmers along with extension advice. Quite apart from helping improve farm productivity, the cumulative database is a valuable epidemiologic resource.[105] The long-lasting problem will be animals harvested from small farms, both because they are small and therefore collectively expensive to supervise, and because such farms tend to collect culled stock from larger units. The solution will lie in developing predictive farm profiles for specific problems, be it *E. coli* O157:H7, *Listeria*, or drug residues, and proactively visiting, inspecting, and advising high-risk establishments.

Two Brief Control Case-Studies

Rabies: an example of international research and government action. This century has seen the sudden emergence of two vulpine rabies pandemics, whose origins are obscure. The first began around 1935 on the Polish-Soviet border where the principal vectors were the red fox (*Vulpes vulpes*) and badgers (*Meles meles*), and moved centrifugally, but especially southwest, aided by the upheavals of World War II. In the western USSR, it was also in wolves (*Canis lupus*) and raccoon dogs (*Nyctereutes procyonoides*). By 1988, rabid red foxes had reached central France and northern Yugoslavia. The other pandemic started in the Arctic and was first noted in the interior of Alaska in 1945-47 in red foxes. It was widely distributed in arctic foxes (*Alopex lagopus*) north of the Alaska Range, from the Bering Sea to the Arctic Sea and adjoining Canada in Aklavic and on Banks, Somerset, and Baffin Islands. By 1952, it was clear that the disease was enzootic throughout the Canadian North West Territories and affected a range of secondary species, including sled dogs, wolves, and ermines (*Mustela arctica*). It was reported in Greenland in 1957.

Epizootics of arctic rabies appear to be related to periodic high densities of foxes, and these are associated with 3- to 4-year population cycles in lemmings (*Dicrostonyx torquatus*) and ptarmigan (*Lagopus lagopus*), and 8- to 11-year cycles in snowshoe hares (*Lepus americanus*).[30] During the winter of 1950-51 rabies appeared in northern Alberta, Manitoba, and Quebec, and spread south. In Alberta it moved rapidly as it utilized coyotes (*Canis latrans*), but eventually burned out. It reached southern Ontario in 1956, and spread to New York (1961), Maine (1962), and Vermont and New Hampshire (1963). It soon became established in southern Ontario in striped skunks (*Mephitis mephitis*), which became the second most important wildlife vector.[139] At the time, only one virus strain was responsible for terrestrial rabies in northeastern United States and Canada, Ontario, Quebec, North West Territories, and Alaska.[133] These isolates are distinctly different from recent European epizootic strains.

The European red fox is the premier host for rabies.[15] It has the highest susceptibility to rabies virus ($10^{-0.5}$ MICLD$_{50}$, or mouse intracerebral 50% lethal doses compared to $10^{3.5}$ in the cow and 10^6 in the dog), but is less susceptible to non-vulpine virus biotypes. The European and North American red foxes are equally susceptible. More infected foxes excrete virus ($\geq 90\%$) than any other species. Broadly, the lower the infecting dose, the more likely the animals are to have virus in their saliva and at above average titers. Few individuals excrete high titers. That is, the virus titer in saliva is likely to be at the optimum low level for infecting other foxes and is insufficient to kill skunks. Post-infection immunity to the fox virus biotype is essentially absent.[14]

Although the virus thus has the advantage of not building up an immune barrier, in a sufficiently dense population it must infect a new host about every 4 weeks to maintain spread, for there can be no break in the chain of infection. The virus survives self-destruction because low infecting doses can result in prolonged incubation periods (up to 266 days and possibly longer) and in virus reactivation, which may occur much later, possibly triggered by stress. This delay will hopefully bring it with its unwitting carrier into a new, dense, opportunity-filled, population of foxes. The red fox facilitates this role by its circumpolar palearctic distribution; its ecological flexibility, from woodlands to urban suburbs; its intelligence, allowing it to avoid problems and pass barriers; its fertility and longevity; and its behavior as a sociable, familial, and territorial animal in contact with other foxes. Late spring and summer are peaceful for foxes, but autumn and winter are seasons of agonistic encounters. Dispersal is in the fall, with young males traveling further and more frequently than females. Some adults will take up new home ranges. Sexual activity is maximal in January and February; rabies incidence starts increasing in the fall and sharply peaks in March, largely in adult foxes.

It had been noted in Europe that there was a relationship between fox rabies incidence and population density. Simply put, fox rabies disappeared where rabies and control efforts had reduced the population density to a low level—empirically when the regular hunting had annual fox kills five- to tenfold below the usual level; that is, to less than 0.35 foxes/km²/year killed by hunters. Rabies did not enter areas with traditional small game hunting (e.g., hare and pheasants) where foxes are systematically controlled. Nor is it seen in areas with low carrying capacities (e.g., marshes and high altitudes; see later section on Ontario). And in fox rabies areas when fox rabies disappears, it also disappears in other terrestrial species. But, campaigns to reduce fox populations were expensively unsuccessful, except for local areas, and then only in the short term. Populations rebound quickly through their innate fertility, improved cub and juvenile survival, and immigration. An area with an 80% reduction can return to normal in 4–5 years.[16]

Gassing dens was used in the 1950s and 1960s in Europe. But foxes are not bound to certain dens; they visit and utilize a range of shelters, badger earths, caves, empty barns and buildings. Only earth dens can be efficiently gassed. Though this will kill litters in springtime, adult foxes do not rest with them and are therefore missed. Once a den has been gassed, the foxes will avoid it during the following breeding season and shift to sites that cannot be gassed. For example, after a gassing season (1969) in canton Basel-Land, only 63% of litters were in burrows and after the second year (1970), probably much less than the 49% observed.[147] Because of public pressure, cost, and the later emergence of successful oral vaccination, gassing was abandoned. Hunting and trapping have had variable success and in brief there is scant relationship between hunter effort and percentage of the fox population killed. Hunters and hunting clubs vary in efficiency and keenness; they are also affected by weather. Hunters tend to kill juveniles, which are poor survivors anyway. Anyone with experience in dealing with foxes knows that they are not fools.

The Canadian experience with hunting and poisoning has been equally unrewarding.[90] The hunting exception that proves the rule was the successful gassing and bounty hunting in South Jutland, Denmark, a peninsular area uniquely favoring this technique.[98] A sophisticated version using immunocontraception is under development by CSIRO Division of Wildlife & Ecology to reduce the European red fox in Australia.

Following a preliminary success in the early 1960s and the research of others,[11] Baer and colleagues successfully orally vaccinated foxes with SAD-ERA strain 10 years later.[10,34] All these foxes developed antibodies to $10^{4.5}$ $TCID_{50}$ Street-Alabama-Dufferin (SAD) virus when the vaccine was put in their mouths, and 10^6 $TCID_{50}$ when put in bait; higher levels are used now. The high virus titers needed are readily produced in tissue culture, making the vaccine inexpensive. The *breakthrough* provided by the CDC workers was picked up by researchers at the National Center for Studies on Rabies in Malzeville, France; State Veterinary Research Institute, Frankfurt, Federal Republic of Germany; Swiss Rabies Center and the Institutes of Microbiology & Zoology, University of Berne, Switzerland; Wildlife Research Division of the Ministry of Natural Resources, Maple, Canada; New York State Health Department Laboratory, Albany; and USPHS Centers for Disease Control, Atlanta, Georgia. Coordination was by the World Health Organization. SAD virus is stable and easily stored. Over the years new vaccine virus substrains (ERA/BHK, SAD-Berne, B-19, P5/88-Dessau), mutants (SAG$_2$), and virus recombinants (vaccinia rabies glycoprotein [VRG] recombinants), and human adenovirus 5 ([HAV5-RG] rabies glycoprotein recombinants) have been developed. VRG works well in foxes, dogs, and raccoons but poorly in skunks, but HAV5-RG functions well in all these species.

The requirements for a live attenuated rabies oral vaccine to be used for free-living wild animals are:[148, 149]

1. It should orally immunize target animals.
2. It should not be pathogenic for humans, the target species, or other species eating bait.
3. It should not be excreted.
4. It should not be oncogenic.
5. It should not easily revert to higher pathogenicity, either by acquiring virulence during replication in the vaccine or by recombining with naturally occurring viruses and result in viable pathogenic progeny.
6. It should be free from pathogenic contamination.
7. It should be storable.
8. It should be stable at ambient temperatures for several days, but not for prolonged periods.
9. It should be easy and inexpensive to produce.
10. It should bear at least one genetic marker.

Early studies showed that the vaccine virus must infect the oral and pharyngeal tissues to provide immunity because the virus is destroyed in the stomach. Therefore, the vaccine should be in a liquid form to contact the buccal and pharyngeal mucous membranes. However, lyophilized and enteric coated virus may safely pass through the stomach and induce an immune response in the intestine. Apart from the obvious risks to those involved in producing these vaccines, safety tests are needed because baits will be taken up by other species, such as wild boar, dogs, and cats, which can then expose hunters and the public. This presents an additional risk to immunocompromised humans and animals (e.g., possibly cats with FeLV, FIP, FIV infections, but the evidence for this is mixed[45,46]). Some strains are pathogenic for rodents, but fortunately, this has proven epidemiologically irrelevant. While HAV5-RG's are very stable, the vaccine virus is excreted by target and nontarget species.

The requirements for baits to be used as vehicles for a live attenuated rabies vaccine are:

1. They should be attractive (e.g., smell, texture, shape) to target species, triggering an eating desire.

2. They should be eaten without being cached.
3. They should be rejected by other species, including humans.
4. They should reach a large proportion of the target population.
5. They should not inactivate the vaccine.
6. They should deliver the vaccine into the oral cavity.
7. They should be able to incorporate a biological marker, such as tetracycline.
8. They should be easily available and inexpensive.

Hamburger was tried, but it is attractive to humans, while chicken heads are not. Though chicken heads are cheap and foxes like them, processing them is time consuming. For example, it takes a dozen workers a week to prepare 30,000 chicken heads to bait 2,000 km². The development and successful field testing of the Tubingen machine–made bait (fat and fish meal), which is cheaper and more easily produced (2.6 million Tubingen baits were produced in 1987), allowed the expansion of the Federal German program in 1985 and the initiation of the programs in Italy, Austria, Luxembourg, Belgium, and France. While the field acceptance rates were the same, 75% vs 73%, more were immunized using the Tubingen bait, whether grossly (74% vs 58%), and with higher antibody titers (73% vs 57% at ≥ 1:180).[125] But these differences should be interpreted with caution, for the German workers merely pushed the blister packs into the mouth of the chicken heads instead of using the Swiss technique of stapling them under the scalp.

For maximal efficiency, the greatest proportion of baits possible should be picked up by foxes and not by other nontarget species and eaten before the vaccine has lost its potency. It also helps if animals will eat additional baits, thereby boosting their titers. The Swiss found that there was no significant difference in take-up rates between baits placed within forests, along forest edges, and in fields and meadows. Because foxes live in permanent family territories, it is better to disperse baits uniformly and extensively so that every fox has access to a few baits; this would not be the case if bait stations were used. This can be done by hand or from airplanes. The normal density is 12-15 baits/km², with dense populations 25 baits/km². When there are other target species such as skunks and raccoons that have smaller home ranges than foxes, the baiting density should be 48/km² to 120/km², to get adequate acceptance by these species. In the Bavarian model, the tactical planning of the campaign is done by the county veterinarian and hunting authorities, with private hunters voluntarily distributing the individual baits. The latter's participation makes it "their" campaign; this has additional advantages later during surveillance. Because of logistics and the nature of the countryside, the Canadians[74] have always preferred aerial distribution, which is cheap at $1.45 (in 1988 Canadian dollars)/km² at 1.25

flight lines/km; the French have found that aerial coverage was 18% faster for mountainous areas but no more expensive than ground distribution.[150] Aerial dispersal by helicopters and airplanes is now common in Europe.

Rabies should disappear from a vaccinated area within two to six baiting campaigns. Surveillance must be intense if this is to be achieved.[146] The three major components of this surveillance are as follows:

Epidemiologic: Rabid foxes should be sought and collected and their geographic positions logged. Viruses from rabid animals should be characterized by monoclonal antibodies (MAbs) or other suitable techniques to check against the usual field strains, the vaccine virus, and possible virus mutants. Nontarget animals should also be examined for the vaccine virus. Unexpected epidemiologic events can only be noted when one is already actively watching for the normal and expected in relation to epidemiologic pattern, host biology, and environmental conditions.

Herd immunity: If possible, healthy foxes should be trapped or shot and bled at a minimum rate of 1 fox/10 km^2, over 1,000 km^2. Successful baiting programs have had $\geq 50\%$ of the foxes demonstrating serum neutralization titers of over 1:20, despite Anderson's simplistic prediction[5] to the contrary. Present target population immunity levels are $\geq 70\%$. The testing is not internationally standardized, but a number of laboratories now use a competitive ELISA test. Bounty-paid trappers can be successfully trained to take blood samples.

Bait uptake: While a number of biomarkers have been tried, the most economical are tetracyclines. A fox ingesting a dose of some 30 mg/kg will incorporate a sufficient amount in bone tissue for it to be visible by fluorescent microscopy. Because tissue turnover does not occur in teeth, dentine marking is preferred for juvenile and subadult foxes. Because dentine is laid down in a daily rhythm, by examining teeth it is possible to determine not only how often but when baits were taken, which can then be related to specific bait attractiveness and caching. In foxes over 1 year old, the dentine deposition is so insignificant that tetracycline may be undetectable and von Ebner lines cannot be seen. Bones are more reliable with such foxes.

In 1978, the Rhone valley in the Swiss Alps was threatened by an advancing wave of fox rabies along the shore of Lake Geneva and toward the mouth of the valley. During October of that year, 4,050 blister-packaged SAD-baited chicken heads were distributed over an area of 335 km^2 in and around Martigny, Canton Valais. The disease failed to cross this barrier where the fox population had a 60% herd immunity. The barrier program was repeated in the following spring and autumn. Similar strategic immune-barrier trials were done elsewhere and in no instance did the disease cross, thereby eventually freeing the entire Swiss Alps. In 1982, the clearance of the Swiss Midlands was started. This time the country was divided not into valleys but into epidemiologic compartments, utilizing natural (lakes and rivers) and artificial (canals and fenced highways) barriers. The foxes were immunized in each compartment in turn. Barring a few foci, the country was free of fox rabies in 1986.

In 1982 Germany started planning for field trials, which were initiated the following year. Following the successful development of the machine-made Tubingen bait, its use was expanded; in 1985 the bait was introduced into other European countries. By 1989, Austria, Belgium, Czechoslovakia, Germany (DDR and FDR), Finland, France, Italy, Luxembourg, The Netherlands, Switzerland, and Yugoslavia were successfully participating in cooperative projects; Hungary followed later.

Following two decades of Canadian bait and vaccine experiments, the first oral vaccination field trial was conducted in southern Ontario in 1985, using sponge baits soaked with SAD and dropped from aircraft; trials were repeated in 1986 and 1987. Later, this bait was replaced by a blister pack vaccine container and field tested in a major Ontario trial in the fall of 1989, when 290,000 baits were airdropped over 15,000 km^2. This "walled off" the central area of eastern Ontario, which was in the midst of a rabies outbreak. In the autumn of 1990, the 30,000 km^2 of the 12 easternmost counties of Ontario were vaccinated with 573,416 SAD-ERA/BHK-laced baits at a density of 20 baits/km^2. This was repeated annually in 1991, 1992, and 1993. The response was impressive—against a 20-year annual average of 385 rabid animals, the counts were (1989) 397 with 206 foxes, (1990) 291 with 146 foxes, (1991) 116 with 30 foxes, (1992) 34 with 8 foxes, and (1993) 16 with 4 foxes. The 1993 total included seven bats and one fox with the same bat strain; four foxes appeared to have come from Quebec.[8]

It is notable that the rabid rates fell for all animals including skunks, confirming what had been believed for some time: that skunk rabies, in this area, was fox-rabies dependent. This is important because SAD-ERA does not immunize skunks. The simultaneous fox-baiting and skunk-trap-vaccinate-release program in Toronto has been equally successful. The program by the provincial Ministry of Natural Resources in eastern Ontario is now one of defense not offense.

A characteristic of the Ontario program has been the intimate and successful integration of mathematical modeling into the strategic and tactical planning. A number of rabies models exist.[134] The Ontario program used the spatial and stochastic simulation model[91, 141, 145] of Voigt, Tinline, and Broekhoven, which has a strong ecological base and has undergone extensive testing and continual validation and verification.

In Ontario, the mean size of fox litters is 6-8 cubs, compared to 4.7 cubs in Europe, with the Canadian foxes living at very sparse densities with larger territories. The population is responding to a high-mortality pressure with a maximum reproductive capacity. Thus, a simple transfer of the European vaccination model was fraught with danger. An optimum fox rabies habitat is "patchy." The "good" patches have a mix of forest and fields, good natural drainage (usually associated with hilly terrain with sandy or clay loam soils), pasture rather than cash crops, smaller fields with a large number of environmental "edges," and soils or geological structures favoring denning. The "poor" patches are flat and have poor drainage, e.g., marshes, and large fields with limited edges and few denning sites.

For sustained rabies there must be a heterogeneity of good and bad patches and a diversity of vegetation. A homogeneous habitat made up only of good patches will ignite too quickly and soon burn out, and a similar but poor area with a thin fox population will not sustain rabies. There must be a balance of good and poor patches sufficient to maintain spread at a modest rate so that the fox population can rebound; remember that these vixens are already at their maximum reproductive capacity. Ontario contains some 10 to 12 clusters of counties with similar rabies patterns, one of which is eastern Ontario, which is isolated from the rest by the fox-sparse Canadian Shield to the west and north, and by the Ottawa and St. Lawrence rivers to the northeast and south. There, rabies was concentrated in a five-county core area surrounded by periphery counties with weak cycles, irregular periodicity, and few cases. Also, this core area comprises some 5,000 km^2, which is larger than the persistence threshold of 4,000 km^2.

The Canadian model is particularly sensitive to four parameters: rate of contact between foxes; rabies incubation period; density of the fox population; and a density-dependent feedback that reduces recruitment when the number of foxes becomes high. The latter adjusts non-rabies mortality. Early runs of the model suggested that if 70% of the foxes were immunized, the disease would promptly die out. But if only 60% were vaccinated, the effectivity was assured only if it were applied just after a rabies outbreak when both fox density and rabies prevalence were minimal. The same level of vaccination applied 1 year before the outbreak would be ineffective. This model was used to time the initiation of the eastern campaign, i.e., after the 1989 outbreak, and then tactically for bait dispersal and to predict and interpret the response.

In summary, the design, planning, and running of a successful wildlife oral vaccination program is complex and follows from decisions in consideration of:

1. Nature and size of area to be covered and whether for eradication or boundary protection.
2. Number of baiting campaigns.

3. Baiting season(s), in relation to vaccine and bait stability, and host population dynamics.

4. Intervals between campaigns, with respect to host population dynamics.

5. Bait and type of vaccine, noting host preferences, competitors, and safety.

6. Bait distribution techniques, for available manpower, technical resources, administrative structure, safety, terrains.

7. Surveillance organization.

Tsetse flies: an example of government research and local action.[40,70] Livestock trypanosomiasis is widely regarded as the single, most-important livestock disease of Africa. It affects an area comparable in size to the continental United States.[151] The various fly species of *Glossina*, or tsetse flies, are vectors of the various human and livestock trypanosome infections. Tsetse control is not without controversy, for the fly is perceived as a guarantor against overstocking and land degradation in Africa, not an invalid argument when the inappropriate use of fly-freed land has merely expanded the demand for more land and put regions with a fragile ecosystem and limited agricultural potential at risk.[12] And insecticides are polluting Africa, and wildlife can be a better choice than cattle.[78] It is a complex situation without simple holistic solutions.

There is a long history of trypanosomiasis and tsetse fly control and attempted eradication in Africa. Following the importation of rinderpest-infected cattle into Somalia and the ensuing pandemic of 1895, it was noted that the tsetse fly disappeared along with the game in the Limpopo and Zambezi basins, except for a few, small, widely scattered foci.[52] This demonstrated that the fly and the disease could be removed by eliminating the wild hosts. In Tanganyika this technique was followed in the 1920s by clearing bush. Both systems were used enthusiastically but destroyed valuable resources, and bush clearing encouraged erosion.

Prophylactic and therapeutic drugs can be used to control nagana when there is a low challenge, but resistant strains of the parasite soon appear with a medium to high challenge. Trypanotolerant cattle, such as the N'Dama, can be used where there is a low challenge, but they do not do well in the harsh rangelands common in many parts of Africa; they do best in the moist southern areas of West Africa.

Tsetse flies are very sensitive to insecticides, and in the 1950s DDT and dieldrin were introduced. These residual insecticides were sprayed on tree trunks and low branches where tsetse flies were likely to rest during the hottest and brightest hours of the day. These chemicals were replaced by the ultra-low-volume aerial spraying of endosulphan, an organochlorine compound with low residual effects. The optimum tactic is to kill all the adult flies with the first spray and then repeat four or five times at 10-day intervals to catch the flies emerging from puparia. Where a high level of expertise and discipline is available, this can be effective against open country species like *Glossina morsitans* but is unlikely to be as effective against forest and riverine species; it is better to spray the latter habitat using helicopters rather than fixed-wing aircraft, but the costs are 10 times higher. While there have been successes with this technique, they have been in areas that are at the edge of the flies' ecological range, e.g., South Africa, Zimbabwe, Nigeria. Attempts at exporting this technique have failed for a variety of reasons, but mainly because of reinvasion from surrounding areas. Also it necessitates high expertise and running costs. Aerial spraying has a place with isolated fly populations and in checking parasite transmission during human epidemics to gain time for the insertion of long-term measures.

Trapping flies was first used successfully on the island of Principe in the Gulf of Guinea in 1914 by catching *G. palpalis* using boards covered with a sticky material and carried on the backs of plantation workers. This concept fell into disrepute following its failure to control *G. pallidipes* in Zululand in 1920-40. Interest was revived in the 1970s with the development of biconal black and blue cloth traps and the discovery that flies of the *morsitans* group and *G. tachinoides* of the *palpalis* group were attracted to host odors (e.g., acetone), phenols in cow urine, and 1-octen-3-ol, by which trap efficiency can be increased up to 30 times. The success of trapping reflects the K-strategies[137] of tsetse flies: medium to large flies, low fecundity, and a long generation time. The low reproductive rate is complemented by a high survival rate, for the larva is protected inside the adult uterus. Thus a female tsetse fly will produce only a few larvae in her 2- to 3-month life, while other insect species lay hundreds or a thousand eggs. With a pupal and pre-adult period of some 6 weeks, there is a maximum possible population growth rate of 2% per day.[120] Thus, daily trapping of 4% of an isolated population will reduce it by 99% in 6 months; at 3% it may be eradicated within a year. While traps require more maintenance than targets, the people see the dead flies, reinforcing the trap's local importance and lessening the risk of damage and theft; targets work on the same attractant principles but use insecticide-impregnated cloth. Traps can be constructed by villagers and dispersed at a density of 2/km^2; density depends on the fly—*morsitans* species disperse rapidly and are very efficient at finding hosts and responding to host odors and visual clues, while the forest-dwelling *fusca* disperse slowly and need a higher density of traps. The cost of building and maintaining traps is about 25% less costly than using chemotherapy, and it is more efficient. Increases in local livestock productivity provide additional direct benefits, reinforced by indirect social and marketing benefits.

Low-cost tsetse control, organized and run by local communities with much-reduced chemotherapy, is a realistic approach to the problems of animal trypanosomiasis in much of Africa. Since control is ongoing, invasions of flies from neighboring areas can be absorbed. In marginal areas near the limit of a species' distribution, fly mortality rates are high and population increase is slow. Toward the center where fly mortality rates are lower, reinvasion is more rapid. Local control works well at the 100-km^2 level when the community is actively involved. In comparison, many national eradication programs have been costly failures or, at best, insubstantial successes.

The tradition in Africa, as in many other Third World regions, has been for high-technology approaches (e.g., aerial spraying), an addictive dependency on foreign aid (fostered by donor agencies and "expert" consultants—the "Lords of Poverty"[62]), and a reliance on central government to provide solutions (this follows the colonial precedent and the political patronage of independence). Thus, government staff, whose necessary resources are at best unevenly available, have been trained to carry out control procedures, with a high opportunity cost of national expertise and of financial and technical support. The development of pastoral ecosystems should build on and facilitate pastoralist strategies rather than constrain them. The tradition in semiarid areas is to build up herds in the good years in the hope that enough stock will survive the bad years of drought and disease to allow herds and flocks to be rebuilt. This minimizes the risk of disaster. But there is evidence[44] that when the risk of disease (and disaster) is reduced, African communities respond by adopting new management strategies to increase the benefits from their livestock.

Remote Sensing (RS) and Geographical Information Systems (GIS)

GIS involves the analysis and display of co-registered, geo-referenced, digital data. RS data collected from satellites and airplanes are specialist datasets but within the wider GIS context. Because the data are co-registered, one can mathematically explore what qualities and quantities are found together, their distance from others, and thus how they vary from other places or regions. It is not primarily the manipulation of maps, although the production of maps is a mundane function of GIS and RS; the latter is still important for areas either without current maps or where national security agencies restrict their safe use and availability. GIS is a tool to bring together features not commonly found together in the same map. It can adjust the scale and projection for special, one-off purposes cheaply. It is excellent for preserving and efficiently using old maps, which are often too frail and faded for everyday use. Overlaid with later maps, one can both see and measure changes with time. All in all, constructive serendipity.

RS data is of the emitted and reflected energy from the earth's surface. As the energy enters the satellite or airborne sensor, it is split into wavelengths and passed over an array of electronic sensors. It is the structure of these sensors and mirrors, together with the platform's altitude, that determines the resolution of the individual datum. With airplanes, the resolution is from <1 m to 9 m depending on altitude and device; with satellite spotting and tracking (SPOT), it is 10 m or 20 m, depending on the system being used; with Landsat-TM, the resolution is 30 m for bands 1-5 and 7 and 120 m for the thermal band 6; and with advanced very high resolution radiometer (AVHRR) it is 1.1 km. These are nadir resolutions and they get larger toward the edges because of the curvature of the earth. The minimum of co-registered data in the image is known as a picture element, or *pixel*. They are set in regular rows and columns with a digital number for the intensity of the electromagnetic energy measured for the area of ground represented by that pixel. In a 185-km by 170-km Landsat-TM scene, there are 5,667 scan lines, each with 6,167 pixels for each band, or 34.9×10^6 pixels per band. With all seven bands, there is a total of 244.3×10^6 pixels per scene. The low resolution thermal data are replicated providing a comparably structured dataset to the other bands.

The bands measured depend on the satellite; SPOT has a panchromatic mode (510-730 nm) and a multi-spectral mode (green, 500-590 nm; red, 600-680 nm, and near infrared, 790-890 nm); Landsat-TM measures blue, green, and red in the visible spectrum, three infrared frequency bands, and one thermal; AVHRR has a red, near infrared, and three thermal bands. The most commonly used single band is the near-IR, for this frequency responds most strongly to vegetation and clearly differentiates land from water. Each of the bands has different characteristics and uses.[68] The images can be enhanced to define edges and linear features. In the context of disease control, they can be used to measure and display ground/water temperature, water sediment levels, soil moisture, and biomass (vegetation indices) and vegetation classes. The latter can be used, with suitable ground truething and principle component analysis, to map habitats.[67]

Side-looking airborne radar (SLAR) can "see" places obscured by clouds. It can provide equally accurate habitat identification but at a higher resolution and cost for limited areas. It utilizes signal polarity and frequencies between 0.8 and 100 cm. The longer frequencies have the advantage of measuring ground characteristics under a forest canopy, such as flooding and therefore mosquito egg-laying sites in mangroves and forests. Passive microwave has very poor resolution but can measure water salinity.

GIS data is defined by two formats: raster (spatially similar to a satellite pixel) and vector. The vector can be used to define a line (e.g., a road or coastline, or a change in parameter value), or a point or site, or it can enclose an area to form a polygon. Parameter values in a separate database can be given to each of these, so that for each polygon, for example, the number of registered voters within each electoral ward or livestock within a farm boundary from a census are recorded; or at a site, the depth of the water table or the position of a tagged fox on a certain day. These data can be manipulated using Structured Query Language (SQL), such as in a Boolean search to identify sites or areas by their characteristics; classifications using Bayesian or neural network analyses; statistical analyses using spatial correlation and association, autocorrelation, and trend analysis; modeling; and a series of techniques that are emerging for time analysis.

The limits of GIS for epidemiology and disease control have yet to be fixed, for it is presently in a stage of almost exponential growth and exploration. The existing software demands technical expertise, and the statistical tools are still few. Also data quality can be very variable in availability and reliability, especially in regard to human and animal health and disease. The emerging uses are in:

1. Health care delivery and optimization, e.g., hospital and clinic siting.
2. Logistic and transport networks, e.g., real-time routing of ambulances and livestock.
3. Environmental and epidemiological studies, e.g., disease ecology and urban clusters.
4. Emergency response, e.g., EPIMAN-type systems for livestock diseases.[97]
5. Improving tactical and operational efficiency in disease surveillance and control programs.
6. Real-time environment surveillance, e.g., water quality in oyster beds, off-shore red tides.
7. Regional strategic policy making, e.g., identification of areas at high/low risk.[107]

Animal-Farm Permanent/Temporary Identification

A vital component in the control and eradication of disease is the ability to trace animals' movements, either retrospectively to find where infected animals came from, or to ensure that only identified and documented animals may enter or be in controlled areas or herds or flocks. The development of small, subcutaneous microchip devices for animal identification has had mixed success. Although originally designed for dairy cattle and technically very accurate, they have only found a significant animal market with race horses, parrots and ratites, and zoo animals. In some areas, they have been used successfully with domestic dogs, but overall the owner response has been poor. Instead, dairy farmers are presently using recoverable external electronic ID collars and only for on-farm monitoring. Microchips have been approved by the USDA for use on sheep in the Voluntary Scrapie Flock Certification Program; they are implanted in the ear, and ears must be discarded at slaughter. National programs in which every bovine is uniquely identified will find microchips invaluable; thus they were a key factor in the successful eradication of brucellosis in Malta. Currently, all resident Louisiana horses must have microchip identification as part of the compulsory annual equine infectious anemia surveillance.

Tattooing of companion animals, including horses, and branding of livestock are still the generally preferred methods, if only because they are markedly cheaper than the microchip devices and ancillary readers. Microchips currently cost around $4.50-$7.50, which is cheap for high-value animals but excessive when the animals are of marginal value in a large feedlot or extensive beef operation. Notching ears (e.g., for camels, llamas, alpacas, pigs) functions adequately at the intra-herd and village level, but no further. Numbered ear tags have been used for many years for stock participating in national disease control/eradication programs. Unfortunately, ear tags on cattle have a limited life, largely dependent on environmental factors. If individual animal identification is vital for some time (e.g., a 3-year research project), multiple ear tags should be used. A farm identification system that has worked well for almost two decades is the Australian tail tag. Each station has a unique tail-tag number and every animal leaving the property has to carry such a tag on its tailroot or ear; these cheap plastic tags are designed to stay on the animal for a month, essentially while the animal is in transit. Adding a check digit to this number has significantly reduced the number of transposition and reading errors that resulted in "ownerless" tags. Presently, each state has its own numbering system and an Australia-wide property identification system awaits implementation. Similar farm identification exists in the European Union for sheep and pigs, but again, each member country has its own standards; under EU regulations each bovine must be uniquely identified.

Whereas most humans will know their name and may provide it when asked, their names provide poor record linkages, except in relatively small databases, because of their lack of uniqueness. Some societies will have high repeat rates because an individual is known as *someone* (son or daughter, or niece or nephew) of *someone else* and thus have limited identification; i.e., less than names squared for binomial naming because some names will be more common than others and usage is therefore nonrandom. The situation can be markedly improved by using identification numbers, such as a social security number or a national ID card number if the individual has one; infants may be difficult to enumerate. Whatever system is used, great care must be taken, for all are open to abuse. Confidentiality must be commensurate with the risk and the desires of the individuals; it is always wise to err on the side of caution.

Future Technologies

Technology is not science. It is engineering. The objective is to have something better, faster, and cheaper, but the difficulties of improving the components are seldom easily overcome. Innovative technology, when successful, can become the paradigm with the frequent unfortunate result that associated research becomes technology driven, not problem orientated. With that caveat, if technology is to be innovative, it must be used in real situations, challenged, and refined; then it will progress and develop. Any new technology needs a critical mass of users, sustained interaction, and more than a few attempts and failures to get it right and accepted. Modern technology can and will produce more-precise results than traditional techniques. An associated problem is that the federal or international regulating agencies may not respond and inflexibly insist on using the old methods.

Vaccines

There are several reasons for developing new vaccines, even when adequate vaccines already exist:

1. Because otherwise adequately attenuated vaccines can still occasionally produce clinical cases.
2. Because inactivated vaccines may sometimes contain live organisms. As vaccine strains are selected based on various criteria, including the ability to multiply in culture and produce antibodies when inactivated, the live strain can sometimes produce clinical cases of a bizarre nature; the author once witnessed an abortion "storm," following the use of an inadequately inactivated commercial FMD vaccine with live, non-vesiculating FMDV O1.
3. To reduce or remove the side effects from lipids, pyrogenic polysaccharides, and other substances involved in culturing and processing.
4. To obviate the logistical and financial constraints of having to maintain and transport the vaccine via a cold chain.
5. To reduce the production costs.
6. To extend the shelf life.
7. To reduce the exposure risks to production staff processing large volumes of bacteria and viruses; it is not just the pathogenicity of these agents, but the risk of hyperallergenic reactions from aerosols generated by defective centrifuges or imploding freeze-drying vials.
8. Because some viruses do not presently produce large enough titers in culture for commercial production, or cannot yet be attenuated sufficiently to be used safely.
9. To increase the level and duration of protection; the Stern anthrax vaccine has been outstandingly successful but protection lasts for only 12

months—a longer duration is needed.

10. To reduce delivery costs; injections are the most expensive system, and oral systems are generally cheaper.

11. To provide protection but without interfering with serological screening for natural infections and carrier/reactor animals.

Assuming efficacy, the primary consideration for human vaccines is safety and for veterinary vaccines the benefit:cost ratio. While the former may be relatively expensive, the latter must be both cheap and have demonstrable, competitive advantages over existing animal vaccines. Four genetic engineering approaches have been utilized:[36]

1. The simplest is to chemically synthesize a peptide with the amino acid sequence corresponding to that of a continuous epitope on the antigen capable of producing the appropriate antibody. But in some instances, even when the correct proteins have been isolated, the new 3-D conformation may be different—the protein may not fold in the appropriate manner with the antigenic site being hidden, shy, and non-stimulating. This problem is surmounted by mimotope peptides whereby amino acid residues within synthetic peptides are repeatedly replaced until a sequence is obtained that mimics the natural epitope.

2. Having identified the genes coded for individual proteins, they can be isolated and cloned into suitable prokaryotic and eukaryotic cells where they have the potential of providing a wealthy source of immunizing proteins, free of the rest of the pathogen. The purified antigens can be used directly or manipulated to improve their stability or antigen presentation (i.e., immunosomes, virosomes, or iscoms). The expressing cells themselves, such as *Escherichia coli*, can be used locally (e.g., in feed) to stimulate the mucosal immune systems of the gut, and with other appropriate delivery systems, of the respiratory or urogenital tracts. There is also the potential for more-sensitive diagnostic and screening kits.

3. Mixed or recombinant viruses result from using one virus as a vector to express the antigens of another virus. These may be either replication-defective vector viruses or replication-competent viruses. The former produce infectious progeny only via complementation by specially transformed cells or by helper-virus superinfection. A variety of such viruses have been so used—simliki for small epitopes, adenovirus for single genes, vaccinia and other pox viruses for multiple genes especially for veterinary purposes, and herpes viruses for neuronal deliveries. Canary pox, for example, if injected into humans, will reproduce, but the virus progeny are incomplete and cannot. Enough antigens are produced but without provoking illness. The large vector viruses have the capacity for additional vaccination "markers," so that vaccinated stock can be differentiated from reactors.

These are not without problems, for they all have complex in vivo replication needs, some virulence characteristics, and sometimes undesirable host range traits. Of course the latter can also be a benefit, for the vector will preferentially deliver to one species (e.g., dogs) but ignore another (e.g., owners). Herpesviruses typically have specific host ranges but not necessarily the convenient habit of life-long persistent infection. While theoretically valuable, this would be disadvantageous if one vaccination precluded the effectiveness of subsequent vaccinations. Recombinant DNA viruses are genetically stable, as compared to attenuated live virus vaccine strains that always have to be proven safe, lot by lot. This simplifies safety and quality-assurance testing.

4. Virulence genes can be deleted from live vaccines, leaving those for antigenicity. Similarly, regions can be removed, thereby decreasing the possibility of reversion.

In general, the problem with vaccines is not that they are ineffective, it is that they do not survive the problems of administration and delivery. Even with the very best vaccines, failures will be nonrandomly distributed. This can obviate the benefits of herd immunity thresholds.[50] Each vaccine has a different schedule from the others, and then there is the need for a reliable cold chain between storage and eventual injection. If it were possible to combine antigenic parts of different organisms into a single vaccine, it could confuse the antibody response. And if multiple injections are needed, the optimum interval varies from vaccine to vaccine. The need for repeated doses might be solved by encasing the vaccines in different biodegradable surfaces that will dissolve and liberate their contents at different time intervals. The dream vaccine is one that combines multiple antigens in a single dose, induces lifelong immunity, is swallowed not injected, is effective any time after birth, is stable in tropical heat, and is affordable and accessible to all.

Advanced Diagnostic Techniques

> So with a hundred "modern improvements"; there is an illusion about them; there is not always a positive advance. The devil goes on exacting compound interest to the last for his early share and numerous succeeding investments in them. Our inventions are wont to be pretty toys, which distract our attention from serious things. They are improved means to an unimproved end.
>
> HENRY DAVID THOREAU, *WALDEN*

When deciding on appropriate techniques for the screening or diagnosis of zoonotic infections, they should fulfill **all** the following criteria: (1) what is needed; (2) what is good enough; (3) what are the time constraints; and

(4) what is affordable. Frequently, John Pierpoint Morgan's demand applies—"I don't want it perfect. I want it Thursday!" Keep in mind that screening tests are used on large numbers of individuals, both sick and healthy, shedders and non-shedders, usually in large batches, and are subject to economic decisions; diagnostic tests are used on individuals already believed to be affected and are chosen financially.

One must remember that the diagnostic facilities aboard Star Trek's starship, the *USS Enterprise* NCC 1701-D, are in the 23rd century and may not be available even then. The modern equivalent, similar to the automobile computer chip, is limited to some toxicology laboratories and then only for drug screening. In the meantime we must use what is currently available. Do not overlook the old-fashioned, classical glassware technology, which has a long and productive, cost-effective history. For many circumstances these flexible techniques are reliable and perfectly adequate, like the DC-3 and low-tech airfields still in common use throughout the world. Like the 50-year-old Dakota aircraft, they have certain limitations: they are capable of a moderate throughput, therefore one must not cram more aboard than they are designed to carry safely; they tend to be labor intensive and relatively slow—they cannot fly themselves nor as fast; you may have to train your staff yourself, for technical support may not be available; materials may have to be made from scratch, which is traditional with such technology. Spare parts are hard to find; you may have to be strict about equipment maintenance and quality control because when things go wrong, there are fewer and fewer deeply experienced laboratory technicians to bail you out—the guy who sold you the DC-3 is dead or has slithered away. One of the great strengths of the traditional techniques is that they do not presuppose a specific pathogen. But, narrowing down takes time.

In the realities of this world and disease control, the laboratory technology should be of a type that can be used and understood by medium- or even low-grade technical staff, perhaps with only a secondary education. It is better if the system can be maintained by such staff. The higher the educational demands of the technology, the greater must be the daily throughput and sensitivity and specificity of the results. Continuing education and training for laboratory staff is never wasted, but is too frequently completely forgotten. If they are to maintain high standards, they must understand the scientific principles as well as the applications.

This is not the place to review the rapidly advancing new technologies; refer to any appropriate text for them: polyclonal and monoclonal (MAb) antibody preparations, polymerase chain-reaction (PCR) techniques, enzyme-linked immunosorbent assays (ELISA), radioimmunoassay (RIA), immuno-fluorescence, and such. These are all immensely valuable, especially with infrequent conditions or circumstances where rapid results are needed, either in elapsed time from taking the samples or to having a diagnosis in advance of the disease and/or shedding; to identify latent and chronic infections so that current or potential shedders can be removed or isolated, especially when the agent cannot be seen or isolated using standard techniques or because it is present in very small numbers; to define the agent more exactly, either through ELISA MAb pattern response or immunoblot patterns with both polyclonal and monoclonal antibodies, through RNA and DNA fingerprinting, by adhesion and virulence factors, or through antibiotic resistance patterns and gene loci; to identify and count a few specific chemoluminescent organisms in a large volume of carrier material; or to identify host immune functions—a rich cornucopia of epidemiologic tools.

The use of ELISA techniques in serum surveys has increased present sample sizes by two to three orders of magnitude at a fraction of the previous unit cost. The results from these tests and chemical analyses are adjunctive and should not be interpreted in isolation. In many instances, the results should be confirmed further by using the appropriate classical microbiological and pathological techniques. The demands of producing adequate volumes of specific MAbs and polyclonal antibodies, primers, and probes is such that a laboratory will soon be dedicated to one or a very limited group of organisms.

Advanced field diagnostic kits have been proposed for use in developing countries,[87] because of (1) insufficient and poorly motivated laboratory technicians, (2) scarcity of well-equipped diagnostic laboratories with well-trained staff, (3) extensive livestock systems with poor communications and transport facilities, and (4) nonexistent or poorly maintained and inadequate cold chains.

A result of these multiple defects is that what disease information does exist can be unrepresentative of the country as a whole and is sometimes based only on clinical reports without laboratory confirmation. This impacts on international trade and the ability to mount appropriate disease control programs. These problems are structural and are not going to be solved just by issuing kits, but they might be part of a larger solution that includes staff training, infrastructure strengthening, and using the kits only for herd diagnoses, especially in severe outbreaks, of suspected conditions inadequately served by classical microbiological and pathological techniques. Their ability to identify latent and chronic carriers is very valuable, if you know what they are likely to be carrying or the program focus is only on a few agents.

Mobile field laboratories have been successfully used in many projects in a number of countries. If that is not possible, one can set up a local "hub-and-spoke" system to rapidly and efficiently transport samples, under wet ice if necessary, to a forward (permanent or temporary) laboratory with refrigeration, clean and distilled water, water baths, etc. Couriers on motorcycles are cheaper and more efficient than using four-wheel drive vehicles, which are expensive and always ill-maintained in developing countries. Such a laboratory could undertake such advanced testing away from the central laboratory.

At this time specialized veterinary diagnostic kits are limited in scope and robustness. As a result, the country must put them together itself or depend on uncertain international aid. In any case, kits must be thoroughly tested for their sensitivity and specificity under local conditions.

Molecular methods require that one knows what the problem is from the start. When running a PCR-based test, for example, one will be 100% right or wrong. But if one already knows what the disease is, why run the test? So, such exquisite tests should be kept for specific surveys, for diagnosing agents difficult to culture or isolate, or when identifying one or a very few organisms. One must also reverse the question. What does it mean if an animal or person is PCR positive? With HIV or rabies the person will die. For virtually everything else, one is ignorant of whether one has found a dead agent or 10^{12} live organisms and therefore of the significance of the result. It can only be interpreted in relation to clinical history and other test results. Quantitative PCR analyses are still in their infancy.

The gene "jocks" have identified an ever-increasing number of single-gene-related disorders (currently some 4,000 have been identified, from the rare (severe, combined immunodeficiency) to the relatively common (cystic fibrosis). It is reminiscent of the flowering of medical microbiology during the latter decades of the 19th century and the excited reporting of "the cause" of related diseases; some will, in time, be found to be statistical quirks. However, this has led to the genetic screening of the yet unborn as well as for diseases appearing later in life. The opportunity for a wide variety of medical and ethical abuses is large, as well as for benefits through gene therapy and more mundane appropriate preventative actions. Until the genetic potential can be mitigated or at least better understood, one should remember Sophocles' remark, "It is but sorrow to be wise when wisdom profits not." Most genetic tests do no more than rule harmful genes in or out. They do not yet predict how severely or when the owners of unwanted genes will be affected, if at all. For most, these genes are evidence of a risk, not of an unavoidable destiny. In time there will be a reacceptance of the multifactorial theory of disease and a realistic medical reappreciation of the importance of environmental and other factors in the development of human diseases.

Because of the breeding management of livestock, poultry, and horses, and to a degree even of companion animals such as dogs and cats, the veterinary problem of high-risk genes is usually relatively trivial. Once identified, such stock can be culled from breeding groups; sometimes it is not as efficient as one might wish, but it is achieved eventually. But, just as the careless use of helminthicides and antibiotics can encourage the agent population to become resistant, the protection of stock from agent pressures can allow an increasing proportion of now genetically susceptible animals that are dependent on protective measures. The veterinary pressure will be for the identification of resistance genes in stock, be they fish or fowl, and their optimization.

The breeder has various choices, starting with the identification of the primary thrust of the breeding program, which may not prioritize genetic disease control by preferring to use standard procedures for that. The breeder can decide to have animals that offer resistance to pathogen establishment, growth, or dispersal, or to have stock that can tolerate the pathogen; in the latter case, the stock might then act as healthy reservoirs of infection. It is usually genetically complex and can involve a number of genes. And promoting the genes protecting stock against one disease may increase the susceptibility to others.

Unless a disease or disease vector exerts a major population pressure, e.g., ticks and enteric helminths, genetic resistance has only a marginal advantage. Industrial intensification can magnify this advantage when profit margins become slimmer. Thus, in general, it will be utilized as a disease control component along with others. But as fertility efficiency increases through artificial means such as cloning, it can only be utilized more frequently than at present.

Summary

One can summarize the whole of disease control and economics in two questions, What should we do now? and Was it worthwhile? Those questions can be answered in a variety of ways. This summary merely lays out one, briefly,[69] utilizing the various components of this chapter. Because "the world is incomplete if seen from any one point of view and incoherent if seen from all points of view at once" (Prof. Richard Shwerder, Department of Psychology, University of Chicago), it recommends the construction of three mathematical models, which should be used both to better understand what is happening or is likely to happen as well as for exploring *what-if* situations revealed as the design process evolves. The word "pest" has been used because with zoonotic diseases, one sometimes has to consider vector control separate from agent or disease control; pest is used here to cover all of these dimensions, individually and collectively. Just as "All Englishmen are virtuous, when they are dead" (George Orwell, *Burmese Days*), all successful disease control programs are correct. However, it is not necessarily so.

Many an official has claimed to have stopped an epidemic for which transmission had already ceased. Some are at last succeeding, like the U.S. USDA brucellosis program, but at a cost far in excess of any benefits. Some were continued long after success, like the former U.S.S.R.'s annual livestock vaccination for anthrax. So, be cautious when selecting model programs (Fig. 6-4).

Pest Intensity
1. Determine
   a. Normal seasonal cycles
   b. Normal variances within years and between regions
   c. Polyspecies complexes of vectors and agents
   d. Environmental and management determinants of pest(s)
2. Develop and validate Mathematical/Epidemiologic Model (I) with weather, ecological, and management parameters

Quantity and Quality Losses
1. Pest dependency—frequency and intensity of the attack by the vector or agent:
   a. Which pests produce which modular losses?
   b. Critical times in relation to age and season?
   c. Livestock/host—pest interactions for pest intensity?
   d. Reservoir identification and contribution?

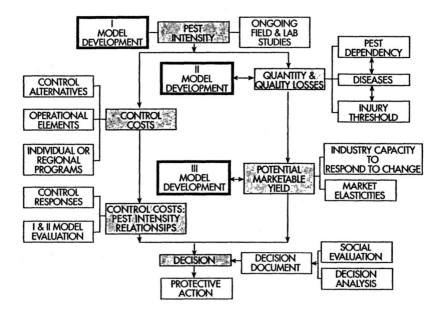

Fig. 6-4. Components of the design and development of a zoonotic disease control program.

2. Diseases—results of that attack in direct and indirect losses, the frequencies with which they will occur or can be expected, and the criteria for endemicity and epidemicity:
   a. Direct losses—(obligative and facultative vectors)
      (1) Disease agent reservoir identification and quantification
      (2) Transmission rates and thresholds
      (3) Disease losses, identification, and quantification
      (4) Specificity of losses
      (5) Control response, effects of prevention and/or vaccination on losses
   b. Indirect losses—(results of infestation or other diseases)
      (1) Identification and quantification of losses
      (2) Specificity of losses
      (3) Control response, effects of prevention and/or vaccination on losses
   c. Dependency on pest
      (1) Criticality and alternative disease sources or reservoirs
      (2) Vector threshold for endemicity
      (3) Host threshold for endemicity
      (4) Epidemic risk
3. Injury threshold—the variance of the damage
   a. Losses and injury threshold responses to pest numbers
   b. Temporal and seasonal variants
   c. Nutritional condition of host(s) affecting direct and indirect effects
   d. Host breed differences to pest, and direct and indirect effects
   e. Curative actions, cost:effects, and compensatory growth
   f. Elasticity of herd/flock operations
4. Mathematical/Production Model (II), integrating 2:a, b, and c; it might utilize Model I.

Potential Marketable Yields
1. Current yields and production systems
2. Potential production systems, both existing and under development
3. Yields at alternative levels of control within different strategies
4. Availability of extra forage/feeds, grazing, markets, management capacity
5. Elasticity of markets for animal products
6. Develop Market Model (III)

Control Costs
1. Control alternatives
   a. No control and alternative land use capability and capacity
   b. Maintain status quo
   c. Alternative control strategies

   d. Possible eradication programs
2. Operational elements of possible strategies/programs
   a. Staff availability, capability, training needs, costs, etc.
   b. Capital equipment; costs, depreciation, delivery delays and availability
   c. Variable costs: fuel, chemicals, maintenance, spares, drugs, etc.
   d. Surveillance systems and costs, report cycles and delays, etc.
   e. Disease and infestation surveillance
   f. Political modifiers
3. Within individual or regional program
   a. Social responsibility of herd/animal owners
   b. Cost sharing
   c. Economic capability of herd owners
   d. Transferability of control economics
   e. Communication needs, targets, and target response evaluation

Control Cost:Pest Intensity Relationship
1. Control curves at various pest densities at different stages, seasons, and management intensities.
2. Feasibility trials of identified potential control modules
3. Program evaluation against model predictions
4. Calculation of cost:effect ratios of possible scenarios
5. Calculation of benefit:cost ratios, internal rates of return, and net present worth
6. Sensitivity analysis of above calculations in relation to discount rates, price changes, implementation delays, cost overruns, and estimated yields
7. Elimination of least-likely solutions.

Decision
1. Social evaluation
   a. Identification of intangible costs and benefits
   b. Evaluation of social and utility costs and benefits
2. Analysis of alternatives
   a. Social benefit:cost assessment of surviving possible programs
   b. Decision and risk analyses
   c. Definition of control/eradication objectives
3. Decision document
   a. Preparation and submission of decision document
   b. Including availability of funds and financial constraints
4. Decision

Protective Action
1. Setting up
   a. Construction of control organization
   b. Initial pilot project and subsequent adjustments

    c. Funding and timetable in relation to objectives
    d. Insertion of economic and epidemiologic surveillance
2. Running
    a. Including surveillance and regular program readjustments for
    b. Program development and evolution against
    c. Target dates for reaching objectives
3. Shutting down
    a. Retrospective economic and epidemiologic evaluation of program
    b. On passing project termination date

Keep it simple. Things get complicated because one thing leads to another. Thus, it takes constant, hard work to keep a system simple. And lastly, once the program is in place, mistakes will be made. Some will be hilarious. A few will be horrific. *A la guerre, comme a la guerre.* Only noncombatants and administrators never make mistakes.

References

1. Agriculture Canada: *Food Safety Enhancement Program Implementation Manual: I Policy; II Development of HACCP Models; III Application of HACCP Models; IV FSEP Operational Guidelines.* Agriculture Canada, Ottawa, 1993.
2. Alausa O. K.: Brucellosis in Nigeria: Epidemiology and practical problems of control, ch.12 in *Human Ecology and Infectious Diseases*, eds N. A. Croll and J. H. Cross. Academic Press, pp 315-332, 1983.
3. Alonge D. O., and F. O. Ayanwale: Economic importance of bovine tuberculosis in Nigeria. *J Anim Prod Res* 4:165-170, 1984.
4. Amosson S. H., R. A. Dietrich, and R. P. Crawford: *Economic and epidemiologic analysis of U.S. bovine brucellosis programs: I Primary Report; II Model documentation, input matrices, and computer programs; III National epidemiological summaries and regional summaries of current program.* Departmental Technical Report (#86-1, #86-2, #86-3), College Station, TX, Department of Agricultural Economics, Texas A & M University, 1986.
5. Anderson R. M.: Vaccination of wildlife reservoirs. *Nature* 322:304-305, 1986.
6. Andrews L. G., and J. H. Johnston: Techniques used to assess economic, landscape and epidemiological factors affecting the eradication of bovine tuberculosis. *Proc IVth Int Symp Vet Epid Econ, Singapore*, 18-22 Nov., 1985, pp 244-246, 1986.
7. Angba A., A. Traore, and P. Fritz: Situation de la brucellose animale en Cote d'Ivoire, *Rev Elev Med Trop Pays Trop* 40:325-329, 1987.
8. Anon.: *The Rabies Reporter,* Rabies Research Unit, Wildlife Research Branch, Ontario Ministry of Natural Resources, Maple, Ontario, Nov-Dec 1990; 1(4) Jan 1991; 2(4) Mar 1992; 4(4) Feb 1994.
9. Attanasio E., and C. Palmas: Cost effectiveness analysis of echinococcosis-hydatidosis eradication project in Sardinia. *Soc Sci Med* 19:1067-1072, 1984.

10. Baer G. M., M. K. Abelseth, and J. G. Debbie: Oral vaccination of foxes against rabies. *Am J Epidemiol* 93:487-490, 1971.
11. Baer G. M.: Wildlife vaccination, chap. 16 in *The Natural History of Rabies, Vol 2*, ed G.M. Baer. New York, Academic Press, pp 261-266, 1975.
12. Barrett J. C.: *Tsetse control, land use and livestock in the development of the Zambezi Valley: some policy considerations.* Network Paper—African Livestock Policy Analysis Network, #19, International Livestock Centre for Africa, Addis Ababa, 22pp, 1989.
13. Berleant-Schiller, R.: The social and economic role of cattle in Barbuda. *Geogr Rev* 67:299-309, 1977.
14. Blancou J.: Ecology and epidemiology of fox rabies. *Rev Infect Dis* 10 (sppl 4):S606-S609, 1988.
15. Blancou J., F. A. Aubert, and M. Artois: Fox rabies, chap 13 in *The Natural History of Rabies*, ed G. M. Baer. Boca Raton, CRC Press, pp 257-290, 1991.
16. Bogel, K., A. A. Arata, H. Moegle, et al.: Recovery of reduced fox populations in rabies control. *Zbl Vet Med B* 21:401-412, 1974.
17. Bogel, K., and F. X. Meslin: Economics of human and canine rabies elimination: guidelines for programme orientation. *Bull WHO* 68:281-291, 1990.
18. Bortoletti G., F. Gabriele, V. Seu, et al.: Epidemiology of hydatid disease in Sardinia: a study of fertility of cysts in sheep. *J Helminthol* 64:212-216, 1990.
19. Bos, R.: Cost-effectiveness of environmental management for vector control in resource development projects. *Ann Soc Belg Med Trop* 71 (Suppl 1):243-255, 1991.
20. Bossert, F. W.; *Die privaten und sozialen kosten der Chagas-krankjeit (Amerikanische trypanosomiasis), diskussion und anwendung auf Brasilien, Argentinien und Bolivien.* Buchreihe, Institute fur Lateinamerikaforschung und Entwicklungszusammenarbeit an der Hochschule St. Gallen, No. 30, 398 pp, OQEH, Grusch, Switzerland; Verlag Ruegger, 1987.
21. Brierley, J. S.: *Small farming in Grenada, West Indies.* Manitoba Geographical Studies #4, Department of Geography, University of Manitoba, Winnipeg, Canada, 1974.
22. Bundy D. A. P., P. V. Arambulo, and C. L. Grey: Fascioliasis in Jamaica: Epidemiological and economic aspects of a parasite zoonosis transmitted by snails. *Bull Pan Am Health Organ* 17:243-258, 1983.
23. Camus, E., and L. Landais: Methodologie de l'evaluation sur le terrain des pertes provoquees par deux affections majeures (trypanosomose et brucellose) sur les bovins nord-ivoiriens. *Bull OIE* 83:839-847, 1981.
24. Chalker, R. B., and M. J. Blaser: A review of human salmonellosis: III Magnitude of salmonella infection in the United States. *Rev Infect Dis* 10:111-124, 1988.
25. Clarke, E.: Land tenure and the family. *Soc Econ Stud* 1:81-118, 1953.
26. Clifton-Hadley, R. S., and J. W. Wilesmith: Tuberculosis in deer: a review. *Vet Rec* 129:5-12, 1991.
27. Colmenero Castillo, J. D., F. P. Cabrera Franquelo, S Hernandez Marquez, et al.: Repercusion socioeconomica de la brucellosis humana. *Rev Clin Esp* 185(9):459-463, 1989.
28. Cooper, M. H., and A. J. Culyer: "Introduction," *Health Economics: selected*

readings, eds M.H. Cooper and A.J. Culyer. Harmondsworth, Middlesex, England, Penguin Books Ltd, pp 7-10, 1973.

29. Cordes, D. O., M. E. Carter, K. G. Townsend, et al.: Leptospirosis I: Clinical investigation of the infection in dairy cattle in the Waikato district of New Zealand. *N Z Vet J* 30:122-124, 1982.
30. Crandell, R. A.: Arctic fox rabies, chap 14 in *The Natural History of Rabies*, ed G. M.Baer. Boca Raton, CRC Press, pp 291-306, 1991.
31. Crenovich, H., and A. Zamora: Relevamiento de brucelosis en rodeos lecheros de la Cuenca Mar y Sierras: sus conclusions e implicancias. *Vet Argentina* 5:45, 425-427, 1988.
32. Czovek, L.: Az echinococcosis kartele es gazdasagi kihatasa, a karfelszamolas lehetosege. *Magy Allator Lapje* 40:195-199, 1985.
33. Dawson, F. F. F.: "A practitioner's estimate of the value of life," Chapter 14 in *Health Economics: Selected Readings*, eds M. H. Cooper and A. J. Culyer. Baltimore, Penguin Books, pp 336-356, 1973.
34. Debbie, J. G., M. K. Abelseth, and G. M. Baer: The use of commercially available vaccines for the oral vaccination of foxes against rabies. *Am J Epidemiol* 96:231-235, 1972.
35. Desmecht, M.: The present state of leptospirosis diagnosis and control, in *Current Topics in Veterinary Medicine and Animal Science*, eds W. A. Ellis and T. W. A. Little. Dordrecht, Netherlands, volume 36, pp 197-203, 1986.
36. Devaney, M. A.: New approaches to animal vaccines utilizing genetic engineering. *CRC Crit Rev Microbiol* 15(3):269-295, 1988.
37. Dietrich, R. A., S. H. Amosson, and R. P. Crawford: Economic and epidemiologic analysis of U.S. bovine brucellosis programs. *Proc US Anim Health Assoc* 89:136-149, 1985.
38. Dijkhuisen A. A., R.B. M. Huirne, and J. A. Renkema: *Modelling Animal Health Economics*, Department of Farm Management, Wageningen Agricultural University, p 6, 1991.
39. Domenech, J., J. Coulomb, and P. Lucet: La brucellose bovine en Afrique centrale: IV. Evaluation de son incidence economique et calcul du cout-benefice des operations d'assainissement. *Rev Elev Med Trop Pays Trop* 35:113-124, 1982.
40. Dransfield, R. D., B. G. Williams and R. Brightwell: Control of tsetse flies and trypanosomiasis: Myth or reality. *Parasitol Today* 7:287-291, 1991.
41. Dunlop, D. W.: Theoretical and empirical issues in benefit identification, measurement and valuation related to parasitic disease control in poor countries. *Soc Sci Med* 19:1031-1037, 1984.
42. Edwards, D.: *Report on an economic study of small farming in Jamaica*. Institute of Social and Economic Research, University College of the West Indies, Mona, Jamaica, 1961.
43. Ellis, P. R.: *An economic evaluation of the swine fever eradication programme in Great Britain: using cost-benefit analysis techniques*, Study No. 11. University of Reading, Department of Agriculture, 1972.
44. Ellis, J. E. and D. M. Swift: Stability of African pastoral ecosystems: alternate paradigms and implications for development. *J Range Manage* 41:450-459, 1988.
45. Erlewein, D. L.: Post-vaccinal rabies in a cat. *Feline Pract* 11(2):16-21, 1981.

46. Esh, J. B., J. G. Cunningham, and T. J. Wiktor: Vaccine-induced rabies in four cats. *J Am Vet Med Assoc* 180:1336-1339, 1982.

47. Farmer, F. L., J. M. Redfern, M. V. Meisch, and A. Inman: An evaluation of a community based mosquito abatement program: residents' satisfaction, economic benefits and correlates of support. *J Am Mosq Control Assoc* 5:335-338, 1989.

48. FDA: *Current Good Manufacturing Practice in Manufacturing, Packing or Holding Human Food*, 21 CFR Part 110, Industry Activities Section, Center for Food Safety and Applied Nutrition, Food and Drug Administration, Washington, D.C., US Government Printing Office, 24p, 1994.

49. FDA: *Fish and Fisheries Products Hazards and Controls Guide*, Food and Drug Administration, Washington, D.C., Draft Feb 16, 1994, pp 82-87.

50. Fine, P. E. M., and E. R. Zell: Outbreaks in highly vaccinated populations: implications for studies of vaccine performance. *Am J Epidemiol* 139:77-90, 1994.

51. Fishbein, D. B., H. J. Miranda, P. Merrill, et al.: Rabies control in the Republic of the Philippines: benefits and costs of elimination. *Vaccine* 9:581-587, 1991.

52. Ford, J.: *The role of trypanosomiasis in African ecology: a study of the tsetse fly problem.* Oxford, Clarenden Press, 1971.

53. Garcia-Carillo, C.: *Animal and human brucellosis in the Americas.* Office International des Epizooties, Paris, 299 pp, 1990.

54. Gemmell, M. A.: Australasian contributions to an understanding of the epidemiology and control of hydatid disease caused by *Echinococcus granulosus*—past, present, and future. *Int J Parasitol* 20:431-456, 1990; *erratum* 20:819, 1990.

55. Genicot, B., F. Mouligneau, and P. Lekeux: Economic and production consequences of liver fluke disease in double muscled fattening cattle. *J Vet Med*, ser B 38:203-208, 1991.

56. Gilpin, A.: *A Dictionary of Economic Terms.* Butterworths, London p 61, 1966.

57. Gittinger, J. P.: *Economic Analysis of Agricultural Projects*, 2nd ed. Baltimore, Johns Hopkins University Press, pp 480-481, 1982.

58. Goleman, D.: Hidden rules often distort ideas of risk. *The New York Times*, Tuesday, Feb 1, 1994, pp B5 and B9.

59. Gowers, Sir Ernest: *Plain Words: A guide to the use of English*, HMSO, London, (1948) 94pp; *ABC of Plain Words*, HMSO, London, 146pp (1951): now available as *The Complete Plain Words*, London, 332pp (1962).

60. Habtemariam, T., R. Howitt, R. Ruppanner, et al.: Application of linear programming model to the control of African trypanosomiasis. *Prev Vet Med* 3:1-14, 1984/5.

61. Hack, M., and A. A. Fanaroff: Outcomes of extremely immature infants—a perinatal dilemma. *N Eng J Med* 329:1649-1650, 1993.

62. Hancock, G.: *Lords of Poverty: the power, prestige, and corruption of the international aid business.* New York, Atlantic Monthly Press, 234pp, 1989.

63. Harkness, J.: *Review of conditions applied to the import of hides and skins into New Zealand.* National Agricultural Security Service Publication 91-3, Ministry of Agriculture and Fisheries, Wellington, 28pp, 1991.

64. Holmes, J. H.: Ricardo revisited: submarginal land and non-viable cattle

enterprises in the Northern Territory Gulf District. *J Rural Stud* 6:45-65, 1990.
65. Horowitz, M. M.: *Morne-Paysan: Peasant village in Martinique.* New York, Holt, Rinehart and Winston, 1967.
66. Hugh-Jones, M. E., P. R. Ellis, and M. R. Felton: *An assessment of the eradication of bovine brucellosis in England and Wales,* Study No. 19. University of Reading, Department of Agriculture and Horticulture, 1975.
67. Hugh-Jones, M., N. Barre, G. Nelson, et al.: Landsat-TM identification of *Amblyomma variegatum* (Acari: Ixodidae) habitats in Guadeloupe. *Remote Sens Environ* 40:43-55, 1992.
68. Hugh-Jones, M.: Satellite imaging as a technique for obtaining disease-related data. *Rev sci tech Off int Epiz* 10:197-204, 1991.
69. Hugh-Jones, M. E.: A systems approach to the economic assessment of disease control and eradication and a discussion of some control costs and benefits. *Prev Vet Med* 2:493-503, 1984; Steelman, C. D.: Economic thresholds in mosquito IPM programs. *Mosquito News* 39:724-729, 1979.
70. ILRAD: Controlling trypanosomiasis by reducing tsetse populations. *ILRAD Rep* 11(2):3-4, 1993.
71. Jemal, A., and M. E. Hugh-Jones: The impact of tsetse control on the health and productivity of cattle in the Diddessa valley, western Ethiopia. *Prev Vet Med*, in press.
72. Jemal, A., D. Justic, and M. E. Hugh-Jones: The estimated long term impact of tsetse control on cattle population size in the Diddessa valley, western Ethiopia. *Trop Anim Health Prod*, in press.
73. John, K. H., J. R. Stoll, and J. K. Olson: An economic assessment of the benefits of mosquito abatement in an organized mosquito control district. *J Am Mosq Control Assoc* 3:8-14, 1987.
74. Johnson, D. H., D. R. Voight, C. D. MacInnes, et al.: An aerial baiting system for the distribution of attenuated or recombinant rabies vaccines for foxes, raccoons, and skunks. *Rev Infect Dis* 10 (suppl 4):S660-S664, 1988.
75. Johnston, J.: Estimating the benefits of research to control Newcastle disease in small holder village poultry. *Agric Syst Inform Tech* 5:39-40, 1993.
76. Jones-Lee, M.: "Revealed preferences and the value of a life," Chapter 13 in *Health Economics: Selected Readings,* eds M. H. Cooper and A.J.Culyer. Baltimore, Penguin Books, 1973.
77. Jordan, A. M.: The economics of trypanosomiasis control. *Trypanosomiasis Control and African Rural Development.* OQEH, Essex, UK, Longman Group Ltd., pp 223-242, 1986.
78. Jordan, A. M.: *Trypanosomiasis control and African rural development.* Longmans, UK, 357 pp, 1986.
79. Kanyari, P. W. N., E. W. Allonby, A. J. Wilson, et al.: Some economic effects of trypanosomiasis in goats. *Trop Anim Health Prod* 15:153-160, 1983.
80. Kimsey, S. W., T. E. Carpenter, M. Pappiaoanou, et al.: Benefit cost analysis of bubonic plague surveillance and control at two camp grounds in California, USA. *J Med Entomol* 22:499-506, 1985.
81. Kindred, T. P.: Epidemiology versus risk assessment, *Proc XCVII Annu Meet US Anim Health Assoc,* Las Vegas, Oct 23-29, 1993, pp 435-440, 1994.
82. Kindred, T. P.: An overview of risk assessment, *Proc XCVII Annu Meet US*

Anim Health Assoc, Las Vegas, Oct 23-29, 1993, pp 205-209, 1994.

83. Klassen-van den Berg, J.A., and J.A. van Langen: Twee scenario's over levensverlenging. Enkele maatschappelijke gevolgen van een hogere levensverwachting. *Tijdschr Gerontol Geriatr* 21:217-221, 1990.

84. Landefeld, J. S., and E. P. Seskin: The economic value of life: linking theory to practice. *Am J Public Health* 72:555-566, 1982.

85. Lawson, J. R., M. G. Roberts, M. A. Gemmell et al.: Population dynamics in echinococcosis and cystercercosis: economic assessment of control strategies for *Echinococcus granulosus, Taenia ovis* and *T. hydatigena*. *Parasitol* 97:177-191, 1988.

86. Leech, F. B., M. P. Vessey, W. D. Macrae, et al.: *Brucellosis in the British Dairy Herd*, MAFF Animal Disease Survey Report No.4, H.M.S.O., London, 1964.

87. Lefevre, P.-C., J. Blancou, L. Dedieu, et al.: Field diagnostic kits: a solution for developing countries? *Rev sci tech Off int Epiz* 12:451-460, 1993.

88. Livingstone, P.G.: An economic approach to tuberculosis control in cattle given a wildlife reservoir of the disease. *Proc IVth Int Symp Vet and Econ, Singapore*, 18-22 Nov., 1985, pp 247-249, 1986.

89. Loaharanu, P., and S. Sornmani: Preliminary estimates of economic impact of liver fluke infection in Thailand and the feasibility of irradiation as a control measure. *Southeast Asian J Trop Med Public Health* 22 Suppl:384-390, 1991.

90. MacInnes, C. D.: Control of wildlife rabies: the Americas, chap 17 in *Rabies*, eds J. B. Cambell and K. M. Charlton. Boston, Kluwer Academic Publishers, pp 381-405, 1988.

91. MacInnes, C. D., R. R. Tinline, D. R. Voigt, et al.: Planning for rabies control in Ontario. *Rev Inf Dis* 10 (suppl 4):S665-S669, 1988.

92. Mauskopfe, J. A., and M. T. French: Estimating the value of avoiding morbidity and mortality from foodborne illnesses. *Risk Anal* 11:619-631, 1991.

93. McCapes, R. H., B. I. Osburn, and H. Riemann: Safety of foods of animal origin: Model for elimination of Salmonella contamination of turkey meat. *J Am Vet Med Assoc* 199:875-880, 1991.

94. McDaniels, T. L.: Comparing expressed and revealed preferences for risk reduction: different hazards and question frames. *Risk Anal* 8:593-604, 1988.

95. McInerney, J. P.: Bovine tuberculosis and badgers—technical, economic and political aspects of a disease control programme. *J Agric Soc*, Univ College of Wales 67:136-167, 1986.

96. McInerney, J. P.: The economic analysis of livestock diseases: the developing framework, Proc V ISVEE, Copenhagen, 25-29 July, 1988, *Acta Vet Scand* Suppl 84:66-74, 1988.

97. Morris, R. S., R. L. Sanson, J. S. Mckenzie, et al.: Decision support systems in animal health, in *Proc Soc Vet Epi & Prev Med*, Exeter, 31 March-2 April, 1993, pp 188-199, 1993.

98. Muller, J.: The effect of fox reduction on the occurrence of rabies. Observations from two outbreaks of rabies in Denmark. *Bull Off Int Epiz* 75:763-776, 1971.

99. Nader, E .J. and H. Husberg: Estimacion de perdidas de produccion por tuberculosis enun rodeo leche. *Rev Med Vet (Buenos Aires)* 69:36-43, 1988.

100. NRC.: *Improving Risk Communication*, Committee on Risk Perception & Communication, Commission on Behavioural and Social Sciences and

Education, Commission on Physical Sciences, Mathematics, and Resources, National Research Council; National Academy Press, Washington, D.C., pp 321-322, 1989.

101. NRC.: *Risk Assessment in the Federal Government: Managing the Process*, Committee on the Institutional Means for Assessment of Risks to Public Health, Commission on Life Sciences, National Research Council, National Academy Press, Washington, D.C., p 3, 1993.

102. O'Connor, R., A. Conway, and M. Murphy.: *Study of socio-economic impediments to bovine tuberculosis eradication.* Eradication of Animal Disease Board, Dept of Agriculture, Food & Forestry, Dublin 2, Irish Republic, 215 pp, 1993.

103. Oleksyuk, I.I., and E. A. Markovich: Para-allergic reactions to tuberculin in cattle and their economic significance. *Veterinariya (Kiev)* 65:57-59, 1990.

104. Olivera Filho, A. M.: Cost-effectiveness analysis in Chagas' disease vector's control interventions. *Mem Inst Oswaldo Cruz* 84 (Suppl IV):409-417, 1989.

105. Paton, W. M.: A computer-driven chronic disease recording system: advantages for producers and researchers. *Agric Systems Inform Tech* 5:13-15, 1993.

106. Pedersen, K. M., A. Alban, and B. Danneskiold-Samsoe: Oversigt over okonomiske analysetyper i sundhedsokonomien. *Ugeskr Laeger* 152:144-148, 1990.

107. Perry, B. D., P. Lessard, R. A. I. Norval, et al.: Climate, vegetation and the distribution of *Rhipicephalus appendiculatus* in Africa. *Parasitology Today* 6:100-114, 1990.

108. Phillips, M., A. Mills, and C. Dye: *Guidelines for cost-effectiveness analysis of vector control*, PEEM Secretariat, World Health Organization, Geneva, WHO/CWS/93.6, 1993.

109. Power, A. P. and B. A. Watts: *The badger control policy: an economic assessment.* Government Economic Service Working Paper No. 69, Ministry of Agriculture, Fisheries & Food, London, 41pp, 1987.

110. Prost, A., and N. Prescott: Cost-effectiveness of blindness prevention by the onchocerciasis control programme in Upper Volta. *Bull WHO* 62:795-802, 1984.

111. Purchase, H.G ., and E. F. Schultz: The economics of Marek's disease control in the United States. *World's Poultry Sci J* 34:198-204, 1978.

112. Putt, S. N. H., J. Leslie, and L. Williams: The economics of trypanosomiasis control in western Zambia. *Acta Vet Scand* Suppl 84:394-397, 1988.

113. Reid, H. W.: Management and health of farmed deer. *Current topics in Veterinary Medicine 48. A Seminar in the Commission of the European Communities Programme of Coordination of Research in Animal Husbandry*, December 10-11, 1987, Dordrecht, Netherlands; Kluwer Academic Publishers, 206pp, 1988.

114. Respaldiza Cardenosa, E., R. A. Gomez, and M. J. Rodriquez: Poblete et al Valoracion economica de la echinococcosis hidatica en los animales. *Hygia Pecor* 3:25-42, 1981.

115. Richardson, B. C.: *Caribbean Migrants: Environmental and human survival on St. Kitts and Nevis.* Knoxville, The University of Tennessee Press, 1983.

116. Roberts, T.: The economics of selected foodborne diseases, in *Economics of Animal Diseases*, eds E.C. Mather and J.B. Kaneene, Michigan State University, Agric. Exp. StationNo.12267, pp.303-322, 1987.

117. Roberts, T.: Human illness costs of foodborne bacteria. *Am J Ag Econ*

71:468-474, 1989.

118. Roberts, T.: A survey of estimated risks of human illness and costs of microbial foodborne disease. *J Agribus* 9:5-23, 1991.

119. Roberts, T.: A retrospective assessment of human health protection benefits from removal of tuberculous beef. *J Food Prot* 49:293-298, 1986.

120. Rogers, D. J., and S. E. Randolph: A review of density-dependent processes in tsetse populations. *Insect Sci Appl* 5:397-402, 1984.

121. Samuelson, P.: *Economics*, 11th ed, New York, McGraw-Hill, p 3, 1980.

122. Saravi M. A., R. Molinari, E. H. Soria, et al.: Serological and bacteriological diagnosis, and reproductive consequences of an outbreak of porcine leptospirosis caused by a member of the *pomona* serogroup. *Rev Sci Tech, OIE* 8:697-718, 1989.

123. Schelling, T. C.: "The value of preventing death," Chapter 12 in *Health Economics: Selected Readings*, eds M. H. Cooper and A. J. Culyer. Baltimore, Penguin Books, pp 295-321, 1973.

124. Schepers, J. A., and A. A. DijBalkhuisen: The economics of mastitis and mastitis control in dairy cattle: a critical analysis of estimates published since 1970. *Prev Vet Med* 10:213-224, 1991.

125. Schneider, L. G., J. H. Cox, W. W. Muller, et al.: Current oral rabies vaccination in Europe: an interim balance. *Rev Infect Dis* 10 (suppl 4):S654-S659, 1988.

126. Schofield, C. J., and J. C. P. Dias: A cost-benefit analysis of Chagas disease control. *Mem Inst Oswaldo Cruz* 86(3):285-295, 1991.

127. Selwyn, P., and S. Hathaway: A study of the prevalence and economic significance of diseases and defects of slaughtered farmed deer. *N Z Vet J* 38:94-97, 1990.

128. Sergeant, E. S. G.: Leptospirosis vaccination in beef cattle: use of decision tree analysis. *N Z Vet J* 40:62-65, 1992.

129. Shaw, A. P. M.: A spreadsheet model for the economic analysis of tsetse control operations benefitting cattle production. *Insect Sci Appl* 11:449-453, 1990.

130. Shaw, A. P. M.: Comparative analysis of the costs and benefits of alternative disease control strategies: vector control versus human case finding and treatment. *Ann Soc Belg Med Trop* 69 (Suppl. 1):237-253, 1989.

131. Shepherd, A. A., B. H. Simpson, and R. M. Davidson: An economic evaluation of the New Zealand bovine brucellosis eradication scheme, *Proc II Int Symp Vet Epid Econ*, 7-11 May, 1979, Canberra pp 443-447, 1980 [see also *Bull OIE* 92:331-338, 1980].

132. Silveira, A. C., and T. Sakamoto: Importancia medico-social de doenca de Chagas no Brasil e de seu control. *Rev Bras Malariol Doencas Trop* 35:127-134, 1983.

133. Smith, J. S., and G. M. Baer. Epizootiology of rabies: the Americas, chap 12 in *Rabies*, eds J.B. Cambell and K.M. Charlton, Boston, Kluwer Academic Publishers, pp 267-299, 1988.

134. Smith, G. C., and S. Harris: Rabies in urban foxes (*Vulpes vulpes*) in Britain: the use of a spatial stochastic simulation model to examine the pattern of spread and evaluate the efficacy of different control regimes. *Phil Trans Roy Soc*

Lond (B) Biol Sci 334:1271, 459-479, 1991.

135. Sockett, P. N., and J. A. Roberts: The social and economic impact of salmonellosis: A report of a national survey in England and Wales of laboratory confirmed salmonella infections. *Epidemiol Infect* 107:335-347, 1991.

136. Soule, C., J. Dupouy-Camet, T. Ancelle, et al.: La trichinellose: une zoonose en evolution. Off Int Epiz, Paris, 292 pp, 1991.

137. Southwood, T. R. E.: Habitat, the templet for ecological studies? *J Anim Ecol* 46:337-365, 1977.

138. Stoneham, G., and J. Johnston: *The Australian brucellosis and tuberculosis eradication campaign: an economic evaluation of options for finalising the campaign in northern Australia*. Occasional Paper No. 97, Bureau of Agricultural Economics, Canberra, Australia, 112pp, 1987.

139. Tabel, H., A. H. Corner, W. A. Webster, et al.: History and epizootiology of rabies in Canada. *Can Vet J* 15:271-281, 1974.

140. Thompson, R. C. A., and C. E. Allsop: *Hydatidosis: veterinary perspectives and annotated bibliography*. Wallingford, UK, CAB International, 1988.

141. Tinline, R. R.: Persistence of rabies in wildlife, chap 13 in *Rabies*, eds J. B Cambell and K. M. Charlton, Boston, Kluwer Academic Publishers, pp 301-322, 1988.

142. Todd, E. C.: Costs of acute bacterial foodborne disease in Canada and the United States. *Int J Food Microbiol* 9:313-326, 1989.

143. Uhaa, I. J., V. M. Dato, F. E. Sorhage, et al.: Benefits and costs of using an orally absorbed vaccine to control rabies in raccoons. *J Am Vet Med Assoc* 201:1873-1882, 1992.

144. Vagstrom, I., L. L. Neese, and R. Gudding: Economic analysis of vaccination applied to ovine listeriosis. *Vet Rec* 128:183-185, 1991.

145. Voigt, D. R., R. R. Tinline, and L. H. Broekoven: A spatial simulation model for rabies control, in *Population Dynamics of Rabies in Wildlife*, ed P. J. Bacon. New York, Academic Press, pp 311-349, 1985.

146. Wandeler, A. I.: Oral vaccination of wildlife, chap 27 in *The Natural History of Rabies*, ed G. M. Baer, Boca Raton, CRC Press, pp 485-503, 1991.

147. Wandeler, A., J. Muller, G. Wachendorfer, et al:. Rabies in wild carnivores in central Europe. *Zbl Vet Med B* 21:765-773, 1974.

148. Wandeler, A. I., A. Kappeler, and R. Hauser: Oral immunization of wildlife against rabies: concept and first field experiments. *Rev Infect Dis* 10 (suppl 4): S649-S653, 1988.

149. WHO: *Report of the IV WHO Consultation on oral immunization of dogs against rabies*. Geneva 14-15 June, 1993, WHO/Rab.Res./93.42, World Health Organization, Geneva, Switzerland, 17pp, 1993.

150. WHO: Fox Rabies. Prophylaxis of fox rabies: a cost-benefit study. *WHO Weekly Epidemiol Rec* 64 (25):189-192, 1989.

151. Williams, B. G., R.D. Dransfield, R. Brightwell, and R. J. Rogers: Trypanosomiasis: Where are we now? *Health Policy & Planning* 8:85-93, 1993.

152. Wilson, A. J., G. M. Gatuta, A. R. Njogu, et al.: A simple epidemiological method for animal trypanosomiasis to provide relevant data for effective financial decision-making. *Vet Parasitol* 20:261-274, 1986.

153. Wilson, A. J., A. R. Njogu, G. Gatuta, et al.: An economic study on the use of

chemotherapy to control trypanosomiasis in cattle on Galana Ranch, Kenya, *Proceedings of XVII Meeting of the International Scientific Council for Trypanosomiasis Research and Control,* Arusha, Tanzania, 19-24 October, 1981; Organization of African Unity, Scientific, Technical and Research Commission, Nairobi, Kenya, pp 306-317, 1983.

154. Wilson, C. R. and J. S. Remington: What can be done to prevent congenital toxoplasmosis? *Am J Obstet Gynecol* 138:357-63, 1980; modified by Roberts, T. *ibid,* 1987.

155. Wyble, M. L., and D. C. Huffman: *Economics of brucellosis eradication and prevention programs for Louisiana beef herds,* Research Report No. 672, 38 pp, Department of Agricultural Economics and Agribusiness, Louisiana Agricultural Experiment Station, Louisiana State University Agricultural Center, Baton Rouge, 1987.

156. Zhilinskii, A. G., R. G. Bahirov, and A. V. Zen'kov: (Economic losses from bovine tuberculosis in the Belorussian Republic of the USSR.) *Vet Nauka Proizvod* 24:20-24, 1986.

157. Zhunushov, A. T., and V. I. Kim: Epidemiological and economic effectiveness of control measures for bovine brucellosis. *Veterinariya,* Moscow 2:35-37, 1991.

SECTION IV

Synopses

7

PARASITIC ZOONOSES

ARTHROPOD INFECTIONS

DISEASE: Pentastomid Infection

AGENT
  Linguatula serrata, Armillifer spp. (*A. armillatus, A. grandis, A. monilifor-mis*)

RECOGNITION
  Syndrome: Human: *L. serrata*; irritation of throat, larynx, and/or nose sometimes accompanied by dyspnea, vomiting, lacrimation, and headache. Self-limiting in a day to 1-3 weeks. *Armillifer* spp.; usually asymptomatic but may produce pneumonia or peritonitis.
  Animal: nasal discharge and sneezing in definitive host (carnivores). Subclinical in intermediate host.
  Incubation period: 1/2 hour (*Linguatula*).
  Case fatality rate: None. Self-limiting.
  Confirmatory tests: Microscopic examination of saliva or nasal secretions to identify larval stage of parasite.
  Occurrence: Dogs are primary definitive host; sheep and goats are major intermediate hosts. *Linguatula:* worldwide. *A. armillatus* and *A. grandis* are African species, *A. moniliformis* is Asian.
  Transmission: *Linguatula:* ova in feces or nasal discharge from infected dogs are ingested by sheep, goats, or humans.

Armillifer: Adults are in snakes. Intermediate hosts (including humans) ingest ova in water or raw snake meat.

CONTROL AND PREVENTION
Individual/herd: Treatment usually not indicated unless worm located in anterior chamber of eye, in which case surgical removal is required. Severe respiratory syndrome caused by invasion of many *L. serrata* larvae ("halzoun") can be alleviated by use of antihistamines. Avoid contact with dog feces. Boil drinking water. Cook snake meat.
Local/community: Prevent feeding of raw viscera of sheep or goats to dogs.
National/international: None.

NEMATODE INFECTIONS

DISEASE: Angiostrongyliasis

AGENT
Angiostrongylus cantonensis, Angiostrongylus costaricensis

RECOGNITION
Syndrome: Human: Abdominal form—moderate fever, abdominal pain, anorexia, vomiting, diarrhea. With invasion of central nervous system (most common)—headache, stiff neck and back, paresthesia. Animal: Primarily subclinical. With heavy infection, rats may have lymphadenopathy and respiratory distress.
Incubation period: 1-3 weeks.
Case fatality rate: Low.
Confirmatory tests: Presumptive; eosinophilic pleocytosis (25-100% eosinophils) in cerebrospinal fluid. Confirmatory; occasionally worms appear in spinal fluid (or eye).
Occurrence: *A. cantonensis*: Pacific islands and Southeast Asia. A few cases have been reported in Cuba. *A. costaricensis*: Western Hemisphere.
Transmission: Ingestion of intermediate hosts (snails, slugs, planaria) or paratenic hosts (fish, land crabs).

CONTROL AND PREVENTION

Individual/herd: No treatment except surgical removal of abdominal mass. Avoid eating greens possibly contaminated by intermediate hosts without first washing and cooking. Cook paratenic hosts before eating.

Local/community: Rodent control. Education regarding transmission and necessity for avoiding food contaminated by intermediate hosts and cooking paratenic hosts.

National/international: None.

DISEASE: Anisakiasis

AGENT

Anisakis marina, other members of family Anisakidae

RECOGNITION

Syndrome: Human: Signs limited to people after second exposure. Febrile gastrointestinal disease, acute onset, occult blood in feces. Animal: In fish—hepatosis, weight loss, death. In marine mammals—gastritis from ulcers produced by parasite in gastric mucosa.

Incubation period: 4 hours-10 days.

Case fatality rate: Deaths may occur from peritonitis following intestinal perforation by larvae.

Confirmatory tests: Recognition of larvae imbedded in gastrointestinal wall of tissue removed surgically, or observed by gastroscopic examination.

Occurrence: Most cases observed in northern Europe and Japan among 20- to 40-year-old males with a history of eating raw, pickled, or lightly salted fish or squid. A few cases have been reported in North America.

Transmission: Ingestion of infective larvae in uncooked or inadequately treated marine fish, usually herring or squid. Dolphins and porpoises are the usual definitive hosts. After ova hatch they are eaten by an intermediate fish host and encyst in intestinal wall.

CONTROL AND PREVENTION

Individual/herd: Treat by resecting damaged gut wall and administering antibiotics for secondary infections. Larvae may be removed from stomach with gastrofiberscope in cases with short incubation. Gut and salt fish immediately after catching. Cook or freeze fish.

Local/community: Require appropriate handling/treatment of commercial fish catch.

National/international: None.

DISEASE: Ascariasis

AGENT
Ascaris suum

RECOGNITION
Syndrome: Human: Initially, respiratory distress, coughing, and fever associated with pulmonary migration of larvae. Intestinal phase usually mild unless parasite load is heavy, in which case there may be colic, vomiting, and diarrhea.
Animal: Same as human.
Incubation period: 2 weeks until the respiratory phase begins; 2 months until the intestinal phase.
Case fatality rate: Very low unless a massive infection produces bowel obstruction, or adult worms migrate to the peritoneal cavity, upper respiratory tract, or invade the liver or pancreas and obstruct ducts.
Confirmatory tests: Microscopic examination of fresh feces for ova of *A. suum* (Ova are not present in feces during the 2-month prepatent period).
Occurrence: Most common in warm, humid climates. Swine are the normal reservoir. The prevalence in swine varies with the level of care and ranges from 20%-70%. Infection is most common among children and persons working with swine. A related organism, *Lagochilascaris minor*, normally found in clouded leopards, has been reported as the cause of subcutaneous abscesses in humans. *Parascaris equorum* and *Neoascaris vitulorum* can cause visceral larva migrans in humans.
Transmission: Ingestion of ova in contaminated soil or on fresh vegetables.

CONTROL AND PREVENTION
Individual/herd: Treat with albendazole, mebendazole, or pyrantel pamoate. Proper personal hygiene.
Local/community: Sanitary disposal of swine feces. Steam clean concrete runs. Treat sows with ascaricide before farrowing.
National/international: None.

DISEASE: Capillariasis

AGENT
Capillaria hepatica, hepatic form; *Capillaria philippinensis*, intestinal form; *Capillaria aerophila*, pulmonary form

RECOGNITION

Syndrome: Human: Hepatic—hepatomegaly, splenomegaly, intermittent fever, nausea, vomiting, diarrhea, edema, and ascites. Intestinal—abdominal pain, intermittent diarrhea, weight loss. Pulmonary—asthmatic breathing, cough, fever, mucoid or bloody expectoration.

Animal: Same as human.

Incubation period: 3-4 weeks.

Case fatality rate: Approximately 10%. Higher if untreated.

Confirmatory tests: Hepatic: Microscopic examination of liver biopsy for ova of *C. hepatica*. Intestinal: Microscopic examination of fresh feces for ova, larvae, or adults of *C. philippinensis*. Pulmonary: Microscopic examination of sputum and feces for ova of *C. aerophila*.

Occurrence: Hepatic: Worldwide. Rats are major reservoir, but also present in many species of domestic and wild mammals. Intestinal: Southeast Asia (Philippines and Thailand). Reservoirs may be birds and fish. Pulmonary: Cases reported from Russia and Middle East. Reservoirs are dogs, cats, foxes, and other carnivores.

Transmission: Hepatic and pulmonary: Ingestion of soil contaminated with ova or infective larvae. Intestinal: Ingestion of raw or undercooked fish containing infective larvae.

CONTROL AND PREVENTION

Individual/herd: Intestinal and pulmonary: Treat with mebendazole. Hepatic and pulmonary: Prevent ingestion of soil potentially contaminated with ova or larvae. (Particularly important around silver fox farms.) Intestinal: Prevent ingestion of raw or undercooked fish.

Local/community: Hepatic: Institute effective rodent control program. Prevent dogs and cats from eating rodents. Intestinal: Treat cases with mebendazole and educate public about neccesity of cooking fish. Pulmonary: Treat cases with mebendazole. For all forms: Institute proper fecal waste disposal system.

National/international: None

DISEASE: Cutaneous Larva Migrans

AGENT

Ancylostoma braziliense. Rarely, *Ancylostoma caninum*, *Uncinaria stenocephala*, *Bunostomum phlebotomum*, or *Strongyloides stercoralis* ("larva currens")

RECOGNITION

> **Syndrome:** Human: Papules at site of entry. Highly pruritic, erythematous, serpentine lesions, commonly accompanied by secondary bacterial infection resulting from scratching.
>
> Animal: Primarily a disease of young animals. Anemia, diarrhea, malabsorption. In severe cases, prostration and death.
>
> **Incubation period:** 2-3 days.
>
> **Mortality rate:** Self-limiting in several weeks to months.
>
> **Confirmatory tests:** Clinical diagnosis is based on syndrome. Results of skin biopsies are not reliable.
>
> **Occurrence:** Most prevalent in areas with warm, moist climate and sandy soil.
>
> **Transmission:** Direct contact with filariform larvae in soil contaminated with feces from dogs or cats. Most common in children and in adults with frequent soil contact, such as construction workers, gardeners and sun bathers on sandy beaches. Autoinfection can occur in persons infected with *S. stercoralis*.

CONTROL AND PREVENTION

> **Individual/herd:** Treat with thiabendazole, antipruritics, and sedatives. Antibiotics may be indicated to control secondary infection. Protective clothing when working in contact with soil potentially contaminated with dog or cat feces. Periodioc anthelmintic treatment of dogs and cats.
>
> **Local/community:** Elimination of strays. Prohibition of dogs and cats on playgrounds and beaches.
>
> **National/international:** None.

DISEASE: Dioctophymiasis

AGENT

> *Dioctophyma renale*

RECOGNITION

> **Syndrome:** Human: Renal dysfunction, hematuria, renal colic.
> Animal: Same as human.
>
> **Incubation period:** 3-6 months.
>
> **Case fatality rate:** If person is healthy and only one kidney is involved (which is usual), the case fatality rate is low. If the person is debilitated, or both kidneys are involved, the prognosis is poor.
>
> **Confirmatory tests:** Microscopic examination of urine for ova of *D. renale*. If the parasite is in the abdominal cavity, or if it is a male

(normally only one worm is present), no ova will be seen in urine and diagnosis can only be made by laparotomy.

Occurrence: Worldwide. Carnivores are the reservoir. The life cycle involves a free-living aquatic annelid. Fish, frogs, and crawfish can serve as paratenic hosts.

Transmission: Ingestion of the undercooked or raw mesentery or liver of infected fish, frogs, or crawfish.

CONTROL AND PREVENTION

Individual/herd: Treat by surgical removal. Cook freshwater fish, frogs, and crawfish before eating.

Local/community: Educate public about method of transmission. Abstain from feeding raw freshwater fish, frogs, or crawfish to carnivores.

National/international: None.

DISEASE: Dracunculiasis

AGENT

Dracunculus medinensis, Dracunculus insignis

RECOGNITION

Syndrome: Human: Prepatent period asymptomatic. Parasite erupts from blister most commonly located on lower extremity. Fever, nausea, diarrhea, and generalized urticaria precede formation of blister by several hours. Signs abate after blister ruptures, but sepsis is common in lesion.

Animal: Same as human.

Incubation period: 8-14 months.

Case fatality rate: Low, unless severe secondary bacterial infection develops. Duration of disability is approximately one year.

Confirmatory tests: Parasite can only be identified after it appears but, in endemic areas, the hypersensitization reaction that immediately precedes the patent infection is usually sufficient for presumptive diagnosis. Larvae may be present in discharge from lesion.

Occurrence: Primarily in western Africa and western India. Small foci exist in the Mideast and Pakistan. Dogs are the major nonhuman host, but cats, bovines, equines, wild ungulates, and nonhuman primates may also harbor the parasite. A few cases of infection with *D. insignis*, a parasite of dogs, wild carnivores, and raccoons have been reported in the eastern United States.

Transmission: When infected host enters water, the adult worm releases larvae which are ingested by the intermediate host, copepods of the genus *Cyclops*. Definitive host is infected when copepods are ingested with drinking water.

CONTROL AND PREVENTION

Individual/herd: Treat with niridazole, diethylcarbamazine. Frequent flushing of exposed worm until parturition is completed, then remove worm through opening in skin. Great care must be exercised to avoid breaking the worm because secondary bacterial infection along the worm tunnel is common. Boil or filter potentially contaminated drinking water. Chlorine or iodine will destroy the copepods.

Local/community: Educate public regarding method of transmission. Eliminate step wells and provide safe water sources. Treat infected people to hasten removal of adult worm.

National/international: None.

DISEASE: Filariasis

AGENT

Brugia malayi, Dirofilaria spp.(*D. immitis, D. tenuis, D. repens*), *Loa loa, Onchocerca* spp.(*O. volvulus, O. cervicalis*), *Dipetalonema* spp.(*D. perstans, D. streptocerca*)

RECOGNITION

Syndrome: Human: Most infections produce painful subcutaneous swellings. *B. malayi* produces lymphangitis, lymphadenitis, orchitis, and fever. *D. immitis* produces "coin" lung lesions (visible on radiographs) that are usually asymptomatic.

Animal: *B. malayi*—unknown. *D. immitis* (dog)—fatique after moderate exercise, cough, ascites. *Onchocerca* and *Dipetalonema* infections usually subclinical.

Incubation period: 8-9 month prepatent period.

Case fatality rate: Low.

Confirmatory tests: For *B. malayi*: microscopic examination of blood for presence of microfilaria. Also test paired sera for complement fixation, hemagglutination and immunofluorescent antibodies. Radiology for *D. immitis* infection. Because humans are aberrant hosts for other filariae, and adults do not reproduce, microfilariae will not be seen in blood.

Occurrence: *B. malayi*: Southeast Asia. Others are worldwide. The primary reservoirs of *B. malayi* are monkeys, cats, and wild carnivores. Dogs and wild canids are primary reservoir for *D. immitis*.

Others utilize mainly wild animals.

Transmission: By many genera of anopheline and culicine mosquitoes. *B. malayi* utilizes primarily *Mansonia* spp. *Onchocerca* is transmitted by the female blackfly (*Simulium* spp.) rather than mosquitoes.

CONTROL AND PREVENTION

Individual/herd: Treat with diethylcarbamazine. Mosquito repellents and screens.

Local/community: Institute vector control program. For *D. immitis*, treat dogs with diethylcarbamazine or ivermectin.

National/international: None.

DISEASE: Strongyloidiasis

AGENT

Strongyloides spp. (*S. stercoralis, S. fuellborni, S. ransomi, S. ratti, S. westeri, S. procyonis, S. myopotami*)

RECOGNITION

Syndrome: Human: Usually asymptomatic. Pruritis at point of entry. Coughing during lung migration. Nausea, vomiting, abdominal pain, tenesmus, and weight loss during intestinal phase.

Animal: In young dogs syndrome parallels that of humans.

Incubation period: 2-4 weeks until larvae appear in feces.

Case fatality rate: Low.

Confirmatory tests: Microscopic examination of fresh feces for motile rhabditiform larvae with *S. stercoralis* infection, ova with *S. fuellborni* infection.

Occurrence: Common in warm, moist climates. Reservoir for *S. stercoralis* includes humans, dogs, foxes, cats, and nonhuman primates. Reservoir for *S. fuellborni* is in nonhuman primates. Other reservoirs include *S. ratti* in rodents, *S. westeri* in equines, and *S. procyonis* in raccoons.

Transmission: Only female parasite is infective. Larvae penetrate skin in contact with fecal-contaminated soil. Interhuman transmission is more common than from animals such as dogs or cats. Autoinfection is possible, especially among immunocompromised individuals.

CONTROL AND PREVENTION

Individual/herd: Treat with thiabendazole or mebendazole.

Local/community: Treat infected animals. Institute proper disposal of human and animal fecal waste. Prevent fecal contamination of

playground soil.
National/international: None.

DISEASE: Thelaziasis

AGENT
Thelazia spp., especially *T. callipaeda, T. californiensis*

RECOGNITION
Syndrome: Human: Conjunctivitis, photophobia, lacrimation. Corneal
scarring may follow prolonged infection.
Animal: Same as human.
Incubation period: 2-6 weeks.
Case fatality rate: None.
Confirmatory tests: Microscopic identification of parasite after removal
from eye.
Occurrence: Worldwide. Primary reservoirs for *T. callipaeda* are canids.
Many mammals (deer, lagomorphs) serve as reservoirs for *T.
californiensis*.
Transmission: Flies that feed on the lacrimal secretion of infected hosts
serve as intermediate hosts and vectors.

CONTROL AND PREVENTION
Individual/herd: Remove worm from conjunctival sac.
Local/community: Education regarding method of transmission. Fly
control.
National/international: None.

DISEASE: Trichinosis

AGENT
Trichinella spp., primarily *T. spiralis*

RECOGNITION
Syndrome: Human: Ranges from asymptomatic to mild febrile reaction
to myalgia, diarrhea, ocular pain, palpebral edema, myocardial
failure, CNS disturbance, and death. Prognosis is infective dose
related.
Animal: Usually subclinical.
Incubation period: 5-15 days, average 10 days.

Case fatality rate: Low.

Confirmatory tests: Paired sera for complement fixation, indirect fluorescent antibody, ELISA, or bentonite flocculation testing. Muscle biopsy for microscopic identification of larvae.

Occurrence: Worldwide. Reservoir exists in rats, swine, dogs, cats, and many wild animals. (Meat of bears and seals has been important for human exposure.) The trichinellae have been divided into eight distinct gene pools (each given tentative species names). Most are associated with a specific host species or geographic region. Isolations from humans, however, have been primarily *T. spiralis.*

Transmission: Ingestion of raw or undercooked meat containing viable larvae of *T. spiralis.* Larvae mature in intestine and, when adults, mate and produce larvae that penetrate intestinal wall.

CONTROL AND PREVENTION

Individual/herd: Treat with thiabendazole and corticosteroids. Cook or freeze to kill larvae in all meat from potentially infected sources (pork, pork products, bears, and seals) before eating.

Local/community: Sanitary disposal of garbage. Cook all garbage fed to swine. Rodent control.

National/international: None.

DISEASE: Trichostrongyliasis

AGENT

Trichostrongylus spp., *Haemonchus contortus, Ostertagia* spp.

RECOGNITION

Syndrome: Human: Usually asymptomatic. Occasionally diarrhea, abdominal pain, anorexia, weight loss.

Animal: Normally only a disease of young animals. Diarrhea, weight loss, emaciation, anemia, and death.

Incubation period: 3 weeks

Case fatality rate: None.

Confirmatory tests: Microscopic examination of fresh feces for ova.

Occurrence: Worldwide. Most cases reported in Asia and the Middle East. Reservoir is among domestic and wild herbivores, especially ruminants.

Transmission: Ingestion of larvae on vegetation contaminated with feces of infected animals. In some areas of world, transmission is fecal-oral when preparing manure for use as fuel.

CONTROL AND PREVENTION

Individual/herd: Treat with pyrantel pamoate. Personal hygiene—wash hands after handling manure.

Local/community: Cook vegetables potentially contaminated with feces of infected animals. Treat infected animals. Utilize pasture management.

National/international: None.

DISEASE: Visceral Larva Migrans

AGENT

Toxocara canis, Toxocara cati, Baylisascaris procyonis, Gnathostoma spinigerum

RECOGNITION

Syndrome: Human: Usually mild. Heavy infection may produce fever, cough, skin rash. If eye is involved, it may simulate retinoblastoma with strabismus and blindness.

Animal: Usually only among young. Diarrhea, vomiting, pneumonitis, and general malaise.

Incubation period: Weeks to months.

Case fatality rate: Low.

Confirmatory tests: Paired sera for ELISA, complement fixation, indirect hemagglutination. Liver biopsy for microscopic identification of larvae.

Occurrence: Worldwide. Primarily a childhood disease. Reservoirs of *T. canis* are dogs and wild canids and of *T. cati* cats and wild felids. The reservoir of *B. procyonis* is the raccoon.

Transmission: Ingestion of larvae in dirt or percutaneous from poultices. *G. spinigerum* is transmitted by ingestion of undercooked fish, poultry, or meat.

CONTROL AND PREVENTION

Individual/herd: Treat with diethylcarbamazine. Personal hygiene.

Local/community: Prevent contamination of soil with dog and cat feces. Treat dogs and cats beginning at 3 weeks of age. Avoid contact with raccoon feces. Cook meat, fish, and poultry before eating.

National/international: None.

CESTODE INFECTIONS

DISEASE: Diphyllobothriasis

AGENT
Diphyllobothrium spp. In humans, primarily *D. latum*

RECOGNITION
Syndrome: Human: Often asymptomatic with occasional segments in feces as only sign of infection. Approximately 50% of infections are associated with diarrhea, anorexia, nausea, vomiting, and weight loss. A craving for salt is common. Occasionally a macrocytic, hyperchromic anemia develops as a result of the parasite competing with the host for vitamin B12.
Animal: Usually subclinical.
Incubation period: 3-6 weeks.
Case fatality rate: Low, unless pernicious anemia develops and reduces ability to cope with subsequent stressors.
Confirmatory tests: Microscopic examination of fresh feces for ova or segments of *D. latum*, or related species.
Occurrence: Worldwide. Most prevalent where social customs include ingestion of raw fish. Adult worms may be found in dogs and cats as well as fish-eating wild mammals such as foxes, wolves, and bears.
Transmission: Consumption of raw or undercooked fish that have ingested infected copepods and have plerocercoid larvae in their musculature or organs. Pike, salmon, trout, and perch are the major source for humans. The copepods become infected with the procercoid stage when infected mammals defecate in water.

CONTROL AND PREVENTION
Individual/herd: Treat with niclosamide, quinacrine, or praziquantel. In endemic areas, heat fish to 56°C/132°F for 5 minutes, or freeze at −10°C/14°F for 48 hours.
Local/community: Educate public regarding method of transmission. Institute proper fecal waste disposal.
National/international: None.

DISEASE: Dipylidiasis

AGENT
Dipylidium caninum

RECOGNITION
Syndrome: Human: Varies from asymptomatic discharge of proglottids to anal pruritis, colic, diarrhea, and ascites.
Animal: Usually subclinical. Anal pruritis, proglottids on hair of rear legs and tail.
Incubation period: Up to 1 month.
Case fatality rate: Normally, not fatal. Rarely, a severe sensitization will occur in children resulting in urticaria, fever, and convulsions.
Confirmatory tests: Examination of fresh feces on transparent adhesive tape applied to perianal area for segments of *D. caninum*.
Occurrence: Worldwide. Primarily in young children at crawling age having close contact with dogs or cats.
Transmission: Ingestion of an intermediate host (*Ctenocephalides canis*, the dog flea, or *Ctenocephalides felis*, the cat flea) containing the infective cysticercoid stage of the tapeworm.

CONTROL AND PREVENTION
Individual/herd: Treat affected children with niclosamide. Periodic treatment of pet dogs or cats with a taenicide to eliminate tapeworms, combined with the elimination of fleas and their eggs and larvae from pets and households.
Local/community: Education of pet owners regarding the method of transmission and the need for periodic treatment of pets to eliminate internal and external parasites.
National/international: None.

DISEASE: Echinococcosis/Hydatidosis

AGENT
Echinococcus spp. (*E. granulosus, E. multilocularis, E. oligarthrus, E. vogeli*)

RECOGNITION
Syndrome: Human: Varies with organ infected; most commonly the liver. Many infections asymptomatic and only discovered during surgery or necropsy. Clinical signs may include hepatomegaly,

ascites, swollen abdomen, or dull abdominal pain. Rupture of cyst formed in liver may produce anaphylaxis.

Animal: Usually subclinical in definitive and nonhuman intermediate hosts.

Incubation period: Months to years before illness ensues.

Case fatality rate: Very high; 50%-75%. Even with successful surgical removal of cyst, recovery takes several months.

Confirmatory tests: Radiographic or ultrasonographic observation of space occupying lesion. Hemmagglutination, immunofluorescence, immunoelectrophoresis, or ELISA testing of serum. (Serologic tests may be negative, if cyst has never leaked, contains no scolices, or is dead.) Confirm by microscopic examination of tissues (obtained during surgery) for free scolices or daughter cells.

Occurrence: *E. multilocularis* (alveolar form), rural areas of the northern hemisphere. *E. granulosus* (unilocular or cystic form), the Mediterranean coast, Middle East, southern South America, southern Russia, northern Africa, Australia, and New Zealand. *E. vogeli* (polycystic form), South America. No confirmed human cases from *E. oligarthrus*.

Transmission: Dogs and wild canids are the primary definitive hosts for *E. granulosus*. The natural definitive hosts of *E. multilocularis* are foxes, but dogs and cats, feeding on rodents (intermediate hosts), can also be infected. *E. oligarthrus* is normally a parasite of wild felids and *E. vogeli* of wild canids and rodents. Humans or other intermediate hosts (domestic and wild ungulates, rodents) are infected by ingestion of dog feces or by eating food contaminated with dog feces. Children are most often infected because of poor personal hygiene.

CONTROL AND PREVENTION

Individual/herd: Treatment is surgical extirpation of the cyst or cysts. Mebendazole may produce some regression of cysts, if surgery is not feasible. Educate public regarding method of transmission, and institute good personal hygiene. Wash food potentially contaminated with dog feces.

Local/community: Prevent dogs from eating the viscera of ungulates or rodents. Treat dogs with praziquantel or niclosamide. Eliminate stray dogs.

National/international: Dogs entering a country in which hydatidosis has been eradicated should be quarantined and treated before entry.

DISEASE: Hymenolepiasis

AGENT

Hymenolepis spp. (*H. nana, H. diminuta*)

RECOGNITION

Syndrome: Human: Primarily in children. Frequently asymptomatic. With heavy infestation—nausea, anorexia, vomiting, and diarrhea. *H. nana* may produce allergic signs and central nervous system disturbances ranging from restlessness to convulsions.
Animal: Usually benign.
Incubation period: Prepatent period, 2-4 weeks.
Case fatality rate: None.
Confirmatory tests: Fecal examination for presence of ova. False-negative results are common, therefore repeat testing may be required.
Occurrence: Worldwide.
Transmission: *H. nana*: Usually direct human fecal-oral route, but ova may be ingested in rodent feces. Autoinfection may occur. *H. diminuta*: Ingestion of arthropod (e.g., beetles in flour) intermediate host that has been infected by ingestion of rodent feces.

CONTROL AND PREVENTION

Individual/herd: Treat with praziquantel. Maintain good personal hygiene.
Local/community: Rodent control. Prevent contamination of human food with rodent feces.
National/international: None.

DISEASE: *Mesocestoides* Infection

AGENT

Mesocestoides spp. (*M. lineatus, M. variabilis*)

RECOGNITION

Syndrome: Human: abdominal pain, anorexia, diarrhea.
Animal: Definitive host (dogs, cats)—subclinical. Intermediate host (amphibians, reptiles, birds, mammals)—peritonitis, ascites.
Incubation period: Prepatent period 2-3 weeks.
Case fatality rate: None.
Confirmatory tests: Microscopic examination of fresh feces for presence of ova or proglottids.

Occurrence: Rare. Worldwide.

Transmission: Ingestion of raw or undercooked meat from secondary intermediate host containing larval form.

CONTROL AND PREVENTION

Individual/herd: Treat with niclosamide.

Local/community: Prevent ingestion of raw or undercooked meat (frogs, snakes, birds, squirrels).

National/international: None.

DISEASE: Raillietiniasis

AGENT

Raillietina spp. (More than 200 species in birds and mammals)

RECOGNITION

Syndrome: Human: Usually asymptomatic. More severely affected individuals may have diarrhea, headache, anorexia, and suffer weight loss.

Animal: Usually subclinical. Intestinal nodules in poultry.

Incubation period: Unknown.

Case fatality rate: Low.

Confirmatory tests: Microscopic examination of fresh feces for presence of proglottids.

Occurrence: Worldwide. Actual disease most common in children. Rodents are primary reservoir.

Transmission: Ingestion of arthropod (ant, beetle, cockroach, fly) intermediate host containing infective cysticercoid.

CONTROL AND PREVENTION

Individual/herd: Treat with quinacrine or mebendazole.

Local/community: Arthropod and rodent control. Instruct population regarding method of transmission.

National/international: None.

DISEASE: Sparganosis

AGENT

Spirometra spp. (*S. erinacei-europaei, S. mansoni, S. mansonoides, S. proliferum, S. theileri*)

RECOGNITION
> **Syndrome:** Human: Pruritic tender nodule around parasite in subcutis. Severe inflammation if parasite dies in situ. Ocular sparganosis produces intense pain, lacrymation, lagophthalmus, and corneal ulceration.
> Animal: Dogs, usually subclinical. Cats may have weight loss and be irritable.
>
> **Incubation period:** 3 weeks to 1 year.
>
> **Case fatality rate:** Low.
>
> **Confirmatory tests:** Identification of parasite in subcutaneous tissues after surgical removal.
>
> **Occurrence:** Worldwide. Common parasite of canids and cats.
>
> **Transmission:** Requires two intermediate hosts—a copepod and then a vertebrate. Infection of humans can occur in three ways: ingestion of an infected copepod in water contaminated with dog or cat feces, ingestion of raw or undercooked meat containing the plerocercoid stage, or direct contact with the plerocercoid in meat being used as a poultice.

CONTROL AND PREVENTION
> **Individual/herd:** Treat by surgical removal.
>
> **Local/community:** Education regarding method of transmission, with particular emphasis on hazard of meat poultices. Cook meat from possibly infected secondary intermediate hosts. Treat drinking water to kill copepods.
>
> **National/international:** None.

DISEASE: Taeniasis

AGENT
> *Taenia* spp. (*T. saginata, T. solium.* Occasionally *T. ovis T. hydatigena, T. taeniaeformis*)

RECOGNITION
> **Syndrome:** Human: Usually asymptomatic. May produce digestive disturbances, abdominal pain, anorexia. Infection with the larval stage of *T. solium* (cysticercosis) can produce severe response which will vary depending upon location of organisms (brain—neurologic signs, heart—may be fatal).
> Animal: Usually subclinical. Heavy infections can produce gastroenteritis and weight loss, particularly in young animals.

Incubation period: 8-14 weeks.

Case fatality rate: Low except for cysticercosis, which is high without treatment.

Confirmatory tests: Microscopic identification of proglottids from feces or ova from tape applied to anal area. Species identification can be confirmed after scolex is retrieved following deworming (*T. solium* has hooklets; *T. saginata* does not). Cysticercosis can be diagnosed by radiography or microscopic examination of excised cyst.

Occurrence: Worldwide. Most common where beef or pork is eaten raw or undercooked. *T. solium* is most common in developing countries.

Transmission: Ingestion of cysticerci in raw or undercooked beef or pork. *T. solium* can be transmitted by ingestion of ova (cysticercosis). Cysticerci develop in cows (*T. saginata*) or pigs (*T. solium*) 2-3 months after ingesting embryophores from feces of infected humans. The cysticerci of *T. ovis* and *T. hydatigena* are found in sheep and goats, and *T. taeniaeformis* in rodents.

CONTROL AND PREVENTION

Individual/herd: Treat with niclosamide, praziquantel, or quinacrine hydrochloride. Mebendazole may be effective for cysticercosis. Cook meat thoroughly.

Local/community: Prevent contamination of swine or cattle feed with human fecal waste.

National/international: None.

TREMATODE INFECTIONS—GASTROINTESTINAL

DISEASE: Amphistomiasis

AGENT
Gastrodiscoides hominis

RECOGNITION
Syndrome: Human: Usually subclinical. Mucoid diarrhea if parasites are numerous.

Animal: Similar to humans.

Incubation period: Unknown.

Case fatality rate: None.

Confirmatory tests: Microscopic examination of fresh feces for ova of

G. hominis or identification of expelled flukes following treatment.

Occurrence: Asia and Guyana. Reservoirs are humans, pigs, deer, rodents, and nonhuman primates. Pigs are the primary reservoir.

Transmission: Ingestion of metacercariae on plants growing in water contaminated with feces of infected pigs (usually) or humans. Cercariae develop in planorbid snails.

CONTROL AND PREVENTION

Individual/herd: Treat with tetrachlorethylene. Avoid eating uncooked aquatic plants in endemic areas.

Local/community: Treat infected pigs. Prevent contamination of water containing edible plants. Education regarding method of transmission.

National/international: None.

DISEASE: Echinostomiasis

AGENT

Echinostoma spp. (*E. ilocanum, E. malayanum*), for mammals; *Echinostoma* spp. (*E. lindoense, E. revolutum*), *Echinoparyphium recurvatum, Echinochasmus perfoliatus, Hypoderaeum conoideum,* for birds

RECOGNITION

Syndrome: Human: Usually asymptomatic. With heavy parasite load— colic and diarrhea.

Animal: Same as human.

Incubation period: 2-3 weeks.

Case fatality rate: None.

Confirmatory tests: Microscopic examination of fresh feces for ova of *Echinostoma* spp.

Occurrence: Asia and the Philippines. Reservoirs are humans, dogs, cats, some wild animals, birds, and reptiles.

Transmission: Ingestion of one of the two intermediate hosts which may be (uncooked) planorbid snails or fish containing encysted metacercariae, or from water contaminated with feces of infected humans or animals.

CONTROL AND PREVENTION

Individual/herd: Treat with tetrachlorethylene. Avoid eating uncooked fish or planorbid snails in endemic areas.

Local/community: Education regarding method of transmission.

National/international: None.

DISEASE: Fasciolopsiasis

AGENT

Fasciolopsis buski

RECOGNITION

Syndrome: Human: Diarrhea, vomiting, anorexia. Edema of face, abdomen, or legs. Ascites from toxic metabolites of parasite. With very heavy parasite load, intestinal obstruction may occur.
Animal: Usually subclinical, but a heavy parasite load can mimic the human syndrome.

Incubation period: 1-2 months.

Case fatality rate: Low.

Confirmatory tests: Microscopic examination of fresh feces for ova of *F. buski*.

Occurrence: Southeast Asia. Reservoirs are humans and pigs. Dogs may be infected.

Transmission: Ingestion of uncooked aquatic plants with encysted metacercariae from eggs voided into water by infected humans or pigs. Cercariae develop in planorbid snails.

CONTROL AND PREVENTION

Individual/herd: Treat with tetrachlorethylene. Avoid eating uncooked aquatic plants in endemic areas.

Local/community: Education regarding method of transmission. Mass chemotherapy of infected humans and pigs. Proper human and swine fecal waste disposal.

National/international: None.

DISEASE: Heterophydiasis

AGENT

Heterophyes spp. (*Het. heterophyes, Het. continua*), *Haplorchis* spp. (*H. pumilio, H. taichui, H. yokogawai*)

RECOGNITION

Syndrome: Human: Usually asymptomatic. Heavy load of parasites may produce abdominal pain and mucoid diarrhea.
Animal: Same as human.

Incubation period: Unknown.

Case fatality rate: None.

Confirmatory tests: Microscopic examination of fresh feces for ova of heterophyid flukes.

Occurrence: Asia, Pacific islands, Australia, Mediterranean. Reservoirs are humans, domestic and wild carnivores, and fish-eating birds.

Transmission: Ingestion of uncooked freshwater, brackish, or saltwater fish (primarily mullet) containing encysted metacercariae of heterophyid flukes. Cercaria develop in snails living in water contaminated with feces of infected host animals.

CONTROL AND PREVENTION

Individual/herd: Treat with tetrachlorethylene. Avoid eating uncooked fish in endemic areas.

Local/community: Prevent fecal contamination of fish ponds. Avoid feeding raw fish to cats and dogs in endemic areas.

National/international: None.

DISEASE: Metagonimiasis

AGENT

Metagonimus yokogawai

RECOGNITION

Syndrome: Human: Often asymptomatic. May produce mucoid diarrhea. Animal: Same as human.

Incubation period: Unknown.

Case fatality rate: None.

Confirmatory tests: Microscopic examination of fresh feces for ova of *M. yokogawai.*

Occurrence: Asia. Human cases have been reported in Spain. Reservoirs are humans, dogs, cats, mice, and fish-eating birds.

Transmission: Ingestion of uncooked fish (especially trout) with metacercariae encysted on undersurface of scales. Cercariae develop in snails living in water contaminated with feces of infected host animals.

CONTROL AND PREVENTION

Individual/herd: Treat with tetrachlorethylene. Avoid eating uncooked fish in endemic areas.

Local/community: Prevent fecal contamination of fish ponds. Education regarding method of transmission.

National/international: None.

TREMATODE INFECTIONS—LIVER

DISEASE: Clonorchiasis

AGENT
Clonorchis sinensis

RECOGNITION
Syndrome: Human: Asymptomatic in light infection. Fever, diarrhea, anorexia. Icterus and hepatomegaly may occur, if bile ducts become obstructed.
Animal: Same as human. Carcinoma of bile duct may develop in cats and dogs.
Incubation period: Variable. Up to 1 month.
Case fatality rate: Low.
Confirmatory tests: Microscopic examination of fresh feces or bile for ova of *C. sinensis*.
Occurrence: Southeast Asia. Reservoirs are humans, dogs, cats, pigs, and rats.
Transmission: Cercariae develop in primary intermediate hosts (snails) inhabiting water contaminated with feces of infected animal definitive hosts. Cercariae emerge from the snail and attach to a second intermediate host, one of several species of freshwater fish or snails, in which they develop into metacercariae. Humans are infected by ingestion of raw secondary intermediate hosts.

CONTROL AND PREVENTION
Individual/herd: Treat with bithionol or praziquantel. Cook freshwater fish in endemic areas.
Local/community: Education regarding method of transmission. Prevent fecal contamination of fish ponds. Snail control.
National/international: None.

DISEASE: Dicroceliasis

AGENT
Dicrocelium spp. (*D. dendriticum, D. hospes*)

RECOGNITION
> **Syndrome:** Human: Usually asymptomatic. Colic, diarrhea, flatulence. Animal: With heavy parasite burden, weight loss, anemia, edema.
> **Incubation period:** 7 weeks.
> **Case fatality rate:** Low.
> **Confirmatory tests:** Microscopic examination of fresh feces for presence of ova of *Dicrocelium* spp. A false-positive result may occur if the patient recently consumed the liver of an infected animal. (Ova will appear in feces without infection).
> **Occurrence:** Worldwide. Reservoir cattle, sheep, other herbivores.
> **Transmission:** Ingestion of metacercariae in ants. Cercariae develop in land snails inhabiting pasture contaminated with feces of infected herbivores. Ants become infected when feeding on snails.

CONTROL AND PREVENTION
> **Individual/herd:** Treat with bithionol or praziquantel. Avoid chewing on plants in endemic areas. Treat infected herbivores with hetolin or thiabendazole.
> **Local/community:** Education regarding method of transmission. Control snails with molluscicides.
> **National/international:** None.

DISEASE: Fascioliasis

AGENT
> *Fasciola* spp. (*F. hepatica, F. gigantica*)

RECOGNITION
> **Syndrome:** Human: Often asymptomatic. Abdominal pain, diarrhea, icterus. With a chronic infection, toxemia. Laryngopharyngitis ("halzoun") may occur following ingestion of raw infected liver. Animal: Hepatic necrosis, weight loss, ascites, death.
> **Incubation period:** Variable. 6-16 weeks.
> **Case fatality rate:** Low.
> **Confirmatory tests:** Microscopic examination of feces or bile for *Fasciola* spp. ova. False-positive results will occur if patient recently consumed liver from an infected animal. During early stages of infection, eggs will not be present, therefore serum for ELISA testing should be collected.
> **Occurrence:** *F. hepatica* is worldwide. Human infection with *F. gigantica* has been reported in Africa, Asia, and Hawaii. Reservoirs are cattle, sheep, and other herbivores.

Transmission: Ingestion of aquatic plants with encysted metacercariae. Cercariae develop in snails inhabiting water contaminated with feces of infected herbivores. Halzoun results from eating raw liver from infected animals.

CONTROL AND PREVENTION

Individual/herd: Treat people with bithionol or praziquantel. Treat infected herbivores with triclabendazole. Avoid eating aquatic plants without first cooking in endemic areas. Cook liver from herbivores in endemic areas.

Local/community: Education regarding method of transmission. Eliminate snail intermediate hosts.

National/international: None.

DISEASE: Opisthorchiasis

AGENT
Opisthorchis spp. (*O. felineus, O. viverrini*), *Amphimerus pseudofelineus*

RECOGNITION

Syndrome: Human: Varies from asymptomatic to fever and icterus. Animal: Same as human.

Incubation period: Unknown.

Case fatality rate: Low.

Confirmatory tests: Microscopic examination of feces or bile for ova. Serum for ELISA testing.

Occurrence: Europe and Asia. Reservoirs are humans, pigs, and fish-eating carnivores (otters, seals, foxes, etc).

Transmission: Ingestion of uncooked freshwater fish containing metacercariae. Cercariae develop in snails inhabiting water contaminated with feces from infected host animals.

CONTROL AND PREVENTION

Individual/herd: Treat with bithionol or praziquantel. Avoid eating uncooked fish in endemic areas.

Local/community: Education regarding method of transmission. Prevent fecal contamination of freshwater fish ponds. Snail control.

National/international: None.

TREMATODE INFECTIONS—LUNG/PHARYNGEAL

DISEASE: Clinostomiasis

AGENT
Clinostomum complenatum

RECOGNITION
Syndrome: Human: Sporadic cases, often asymptomatic. Cough, pharyngitis.
Animal: Unknown.
Incubation period: Unknown.
Case fatality rate: None.
Confirmatory tests: Microscopic examination of fresh feces for presence of ova of *C. complenatum.* Adult flukes may occasionally be found in oral cavity.
Occurrence: Japan, Middle East. Reservoir is in fish-eating birds and some reptiles.
Transmission: Ingestion of raw freshwater fish harvested in water contaminated with feces of infected host animals.

CONTROL AND PREVENTION
Individual/herd: Treat with bithionol, niclofolan, or praziquantel. Avoid eating raw, freshwater fish in endemic areas.
Local/community: Education regarding method of transmission.
National/international: None.

DISEASE: Paragonimiasis

AGENT
Paragonimus spp. (*P. westermani,* possibly other species)

RECOGNITION
Syndrome: Human: Often asymptomatic. Cough, hemoptysis. Central nervous system disturbances, if brain is invaded.
Animal: Cough, dyspnea in dogs.
Incubation period: Long (weeks) and variable.
Case fatality rate: Low, unless ectopic localization of parasite occurs.
Confirmatory tests: Microscopic examination of feces or sputum for ova

of *Paragonimus* spp. Paired sera for complement fixation or indirect hemagglutination testing. Intradermal skin test.

Occurrence: Southeast Asia, Philippines, Africa, Pacific coast of South America. Reservoirs are humans, canids, felids, pigs, and wild carnivores.

Transmission: Ingestion of freshwater crustaceans containing metacercariae. Cercariae develop in snails inhabiting ponds contaminated with feces or sputum of infected host animals.

CONTROL AND PREVENTION

Individual/herd: Treat with bithionol, praziquantel, or niclofolan. Cook crustaceans gathered in potentially contaminated water, before eating.

Local/community: Education regarding method of transmission. Proper fecal waste disposal. Eliminate stray dogs and cats. Snail control.

National/international: None.

DISEASE: Schistosomiasis

AGENT

Schistosoma spp. (*S. mansoni, S. japonicum, S. hematobium*)

RECOGNITION

Syndrome: Human: Pruritis from larvae entering through skin. Syndrome varies from subclinical to fever and hepatosplenomegaly. *S. mansoni* and *S. japonicum* produce colitis; *S. hematobium* produces a self-limiting cystitis and hematuria.

Animal: With heavy burden of parasites, diarrhea, dehydration, anorexia, and weight loss. Recovery is usually spontaneous.

Incubation period: 4-6 weeks.

Case fatality rate: Low.

Confirmatory tests: Microscopic examination for ova of *Schistosoma* spp. in feces, urine, or biopsy specimens. Paired sera for ELISA, or indirect fluorescent antibody testing.

Occurrence: *S. mansoni* in Africa, South America, and the Caribbean. Reservoirs are primarily humans and rodents. *S. japonicum* in Southeast Asia. Reservoir is primarily humans but also found in dogs, cats, pigs, cattle, rodents, and nonhuman primates. *S. hematobium* in Africa and the Middle East. Reservoir is almost completely humans.

Transmission: Ova are passed into water in urine or feces and develop into larvae (miracidiae), which penetrate into the snail intermediate host. Larvae develop into cercariae in the snail intermediate hosts, escape and penetrate the skin of human and other definitive hosts, and develop into schistosomula. After a period of time in the lungs and liver, they reach the intestine (*S. mansoni* and *S. japonicum*) or urinary bladder (*S. hematobium*).

CONTROL AND PREVENTION
Individual/herd: Treat with praziquantel. Wear rubber boots, if wading in water is required in endemic areas.

Local/community: Education regarding method of transmission. Sanitary disposal of fecal and urinary waste. Mass therapy of infected individuals. Snail control.

National/international: None.

PROTOZOAN INFECTIONS

DISEASE: Amebiasis

AGENT
Entamoeba spp. (*E. histolytica, E. polecki*)

RECOGNITION
Syndrome: Human: Most infections are asymptomatic. Clinical manifestations vary from intermittent periods of mucoid or bloody diarrhea to severe dysentery accompanied by pyrexia. With hepatic invasion, hepatomegaly, and abdominal pain.
Animal: Usually subclinical, but colitis and diarrhea can occur, particularly in nonhuman primates.

Incubation period: 2-4 weeks, but infections may be subclinical for several months before signs appear.

Case fatality rate: In severe cases, and with hepatic abscessation—up to 100% without treatment.

Confirmatory tests: Microscopic examination of fresh feces from diarrheic patients for trophozoites or cysts in feces of asymptomatic individuals. Treatment with an amebicide is diagnostic when clinical signs are reduced. Radiology and/or test serum by hemagglutination for evidence of extraintestinal infection.

Occurrence: Worldwide but most common in tropical areas with poor sanitation. Common in nonhuman primates, especially in Asia and

Africa. *E. polecki* is a parasite of swine.

Transmission: Ingestion of food or water contaminated with cysts from asymptomatic individuals. (Trophozoites, passed by acute cases, are too fragile to survive outside the host.)

CONTROL AND PREVENTION

Individual/herd: Treat infected individuals with metronidazole. Personal hygiene should include thorough cooking of food and treatment of water with iodine to destroy cysts.

Local/community: Water purification. Proper fecal waste disposal. Education regarding method of transmission, particularly for food handlers.

National/international: None.

DISEASE: Balantidiasis

AGENT
Balantidium coli

RECOGNITION

Syndrome: Human: Colic, tenesmus, nausea, vomiting, diarrhea. In severe cases—anorexia, bloody dysentery, and weakness. Infection is often asymptomatic.

Animal: Usually subclinical.

Incubation period: Unknown. Probably 3-4 days.

Case fatality rate: Low. Humans are usually quite resistant to infection unless debilitated, in which case disease may be fatal.

Confirmatory tests: Microscopic examination of fresh feces from diarrheic patients for trophozoites or cysts in feces of asymptomatic individuals. Trophozoites may be found in material obtained by sigmoidoscopy.

Occurrence: Worldwide. Swine, as well as rats, dogs, and nonhuman primates serve as major sources of infection for humans.

Transmission: Consumption of water or vegetables contaminated with feces from infected animals. Direct fecal-oral transmission of cysts from asymptomatic humans.

CONTROL AND PREVENTION

Individual/herd: Treat with metronidazole. Personal hygiene should include thorough cooking of food and boiling of water possibly contaminated with pig feces.

Local/community: Treat infected humans with metronidazole. Filter drinking water through diatomaceous earth to remove cysts. Chlorine is ineffective in killing cysts, therefore, if filtration of potentially contaminated water is impossible, drinking water should be treated with iodine or boiled.

National/international: None.

DISEASE: Cryptosporidiosis

AGENT
    Cryptosporidium spp. (*C. parvum*, possibly others)

RECOGNITION
    Syndrome: Human: Abdominal pain, nausea, watery diarrhea lasting 3-4 days. In immunodeficient or immunosuppressed people, the disease is severe, with persistent diarrhea (6-25 evacuations per day) and maladsorption of nutrients.
    Animal: Normally a clinical disease only among young. Gastroenteritis and diarrhea in ruminants. A respiratory syndrome among chicken and turkey poults.
    Incubation period: 3-7 days.
    Case fatality rate: In normal persons the disease is self-limiting. In immunocompromised individuals, disease is severe and case fatality rate may be high.
    Confirmatory tests: Microscopic examination of fresh feces for the identification of oocysts.
    Occurrence: Worldwide. Common in domestic livestock and birds. Found in 1%-5% of gastroenteritis patients.
    Transmission: Oocysts are infective when passed in feces. Not species specific (strain from one animal can infect many other species). Fecal-oral transmission from infected animals or humans.

CONTROL AND PREVENTION
    Individual/herd: At present there is no effective treatment. Good personal hygiene. Immunocompromised individuals should avoid contact with diarrheic animals or people.
    Local/community: Proper fecal waste disposal. Education of public, particularly the immunocompromised, regarding the method of transmission and potential danger associated with infection.
    National/international: None.

DISEASE: Giardiasis

AGENT
Giardia lamblia (intestinalis)

RECOGNITION
Syndrome: Human: Usually subclinical. Abdominal pain, bloating, diarrhea, steatorrhea, fatigue, weight loss. Sometimes nausea and vomiting will occur.
Animal: Same as human.
Incubation period: 1-4 weeks.
Case fatality rate: None.
Confirmatory tests: Microscopic examination of feces for presence of cysts or trophozoites of *G. lamblia.* False-negative results are common, therefore repeat 3 times before accepting negative results.
Occurrence: Worldwide. The most common intestinal parasitic infection in the developed world. Prevalence very high in areas with poor sanitation and in institutions. Human infections usually originate from other humans but may result from contact with dogs, cats, rodents, beavers, or nonhuman primates.
Transmission: Ingestion of cysts (trophozoites are too fragile to survive outside host) on food, or by direct fecal-oral transfer. Commonly waterborne, including municipal outbreaks.

CONTROL AND PREVENTION
Individual/herd: Treat with quinacrine or metranidazole. Practice good personal hygiene. Cook food thoroughly. Boil water. Chlorine treatment of water will not kill cysts; iodine will.
Local/community: Sanitary disposal of fecal waste. Filter municipal drinking water.
National/international: None.

DISEASE: Leishmaniasis

AGENT
Leishmania spp.; *L. mexicana, L. braziliensis,* cutaneous (New World); *L. tropica, L. major, L. aethiopica, L. donovani,* cutaneous (Old World); *L. donovani,* visceral

RECOGNITION
Syndrome: Human: Cutaneous—erythematous papule on exposed

portions of body which develops into a slowly healing ulcer. Visceral—Progressive weakness, intermittent fever, splenomegaly, anorexia, weight loss, hair loss, bleeding from gums and mucous membranes.

Animal: frequently subclinical. Skin lesions have been observed on dogs and horses.

Incubation period: Cutaneous—Usually 2-6 weeks but may extend to 10 years. Visceral—2-4 months but may extend to several years.

Case fatality rate: Old World type usually not fatal but New World type may result in face lesions involving mucocutaneous junction with secondary bacterial infection resulting in death.

Visceral: if untreated is usually fatal.

Confirmatory tests: Cutaneous: biopsy of ulcer edge to examine microscopically for the organism. Visceral: microscopic examination of blood or bone marrow aspirate for organism or culture to reveal Leishman-Donovan bodies, ELISA test of paired sera.

Occurrence: Cutaneous: Old World: Africa, Asia, southern Europe. New World: Latin America, southern United States.

Visceral: Asia, Africa, Europe, Latin America.

Transmission: Phlebotomine (sand) flies transmit from reservoir hosts, which are primarily humans or dogs and other canids for the visceral type and wild rodents for the cutaneous type.

CONTROL AND PREVENTION

Individual/herd: Treat with pentavalent antimony compounds. Use of repellents and screening.

Local/community: Vector control. Elimination of infected dogs (treatment usually ineffective).

National/international: None.

DISEASE: Malaria

AGENT

Plasmodium spp. (*P. cynomolgi, P. knowlesi, P. inui, P. schwetzi, P. simium, P. brazilianum, P. eylesi*)

RECOGNITION

Syndrome: Human: cyclical febrile periods accompanied by chills, sweating, and headache.

Animal: with the exception of *P. brazilianum*, which can be fatal, most infections of nonhuman primates are mild versions of the human form.

Incubation period: Usually 10-30 days, sometimes several months.

Case fatality rate: None. Recovery is spontaneous.

Confirmatory tests: Microscopic examination of Giemsa-stained thick blood smear for presence of parasite.

Occurrence: Rare. Africa, Asia, Latin America.

Transmission: By anopheline mosquitoes.

CONTROL AND PREVENTION

Individual/herd: Treat with chloroquine or amodiaquine. Use repellents. Chemoprophylaxis for human malarias will be effective.

Local/community: Mosquito control, screening.

National/international: None.

DISEASE: Piroplasmosis

AGENT

Babesia spp. (*B. bovis, B. divergens, B. microti*)

RECOGNITION

Syndrome: Human: Commonly subclinical. Fever, headache, malaise, myalgia, hemolytic anemia, hemoglobinuria. Severe in splenecto-mized individuals. May be fatal.

Animal: Fever, anorexia, hemolytic anemia, icterus.

Incubation period: 1-12 months.

Case fatality rate: Low.

Confirmatory tests: Test paired sera by indirect hemagglutination or fluorescent antibody. Microscopic examination of thin blood smear for parasite in RBCs.

Occurrence: Worldwide. In the United States mainly in the Northeast. Primary reservoir of species affecting humans is in rodents, but bovines may also serve as reservoir of infection.

Transmission: Transmitted primarily by the bite of the nymphal stage of ixodid ticks. Transovarial and transstadial transmission of *Babesia* spp. exists among many species of these ticks.

CONTROL AND PREVENTION

Individual/herd: Treat with chloroquine or pentamidine. Tick repellents.

Local/community: Tick control. Rodent control.

National/international: Importation of bovines from endemic areas into areas free of bovine babesiosis is usually restricted, varying from complete prohibition to quarantine and blood testing to ensure freedom from infection.

DISEASE: *Pneumocystis* Infection

AGENT
Pneumocystis carinii

RECOGNITION
Syndrome: Human: Asymptomatic infection common among immuno-competent individuals. Cough, dyspnea, cyanosis. Self-limiting except in debilitated children or immunosuppressed individuals among whom the syndrome will be severe and often fatal.
Animal: Usually subclinical, but interstitial pneumonia may develop if animal is debilitated or stressed.
Incubation period: 1-2 months.
Case fatality rate: Usually fatal in immunosuppressed without treatment.
Confirmatory tests: Radiography usually reveals bilateral interstitial pneumonia. Examine lung aspirate or tracheal mucus for organism after staining with Giemsa, Gomori, or toluidine blue O.
Occurrence: Worldwide. Humans are the primary reservoir, but many animals, especially rodent species, harbor the organism.
Transmission: Uncertain. Assumed to be airborne.

CONTROL AND PREVENTION
Individual/herd: Treat with trimethoprim, sulfamethoxazole, or pentami-dine.
Local/community: Isolation of severely affected patients. Rodent control.
National/international: None.

DISEASE: Sarcocystosis

AGENT
Sarcocystis spp. (*S. hominis[bovihominis], S. suihominis*)

RECOGNITION
Syndrome: Human: Intestinal phase—usually asymptomatic. May have nausea, diarrhea, malaise. The tissue phase is rare and also usually asymptomatic, but severely affected individuals may have fever, weight loss, and myositis.

Animal: Usually subclinical in adults but may cause abortion. High case fatality rate among young calves and pigs.

Incubation period: 2 weeks.

Case fatality rate: Low.

Confirmatory tests: Microscopic examination of feces for presence of oocysts, or muscle biopsy of intermediate hosts for cysts.

Occurrence: Worldwide. Cysts are found in striated muscles of mammalian intermediate hosts (cattle, swine); oocysts in intestines of definitive hosts (humans).

Transmission: Ingestion of cysts in raw or undercooked beef or pork or ingestion of oocysts in feces of definitive hosts.

CONTROL AND PREVENTION

Individual/herd: Treat with sulfonamides. Cook meat. Institute good personal hygiene.

Local/community: Prevent human fecal contamination of livestock feed.

National/international: None.

DISEASE: Toxoplasmosis

AGENT

Toxoplasma gondii

RECOGNITION

Syndrome: Human: Usually asymptomatic. Infection can produce fever, lymphadenopathy, lymphomatosis. If severe—myalgia, pneumonitis, CNS disturbances. Infection during pregnancy can produce chorioretinitis, hydrocephaly, or microcephaly in fetus or fetal death. Dormant infection can be reactivated in immunosuppressed individuals.

Animal: Infection usually subclinical, except abortion is common among sheep and swine. Fever and CNS signs in dogs and cats.

Incubation period: 1-4 weeks, usually 7-14 days.

Case fatality rate: Low except for prenatal and neonatal infection or among immunosuppressed.

Confirmatory tests: Paired sera for Sabin-Feldman, indirect fluorescent antibody, complement fixation, indirect hemagglutination, or ELISA testing. Many individuals become infected and infection rate increases with age so paired sera are required.

Occurrence: Worldwide. Reservoir is among cats. Intermediate hosts include most species of birds and mammals.

Transmission: Cats excrete oocysts for about 10 days when first infected.

Intermediate hosts are infected by ingesting oocysts from soil or vegetables contaminated by cat feces, or ingesting bradyzoites in undercooked meat from infected animals. If newly infected host is pregnant, transplacental infection can occur. Most primary infections occur as the result of eating undercooked meat. Some cases have been associated with drinking raw milk.

CONTROL AND PREVENTION
Individual/herd: Treat with pyrimethamine and sulfa. Cook meat, and pasteurize milk. Avoid contact with cat feces or soil contaminated with cat feces.

Local/community: Education regarding mechanism of transmission and need for adequate cooking of meat. Avoid feeding cats raw meat.

National/international: None.

DISEASE: Trypanosomiasis, African

AGENT
Trypanosoma brucei var. *gambiense, Trypanosoma brucei* var. *rhodesiense*

RECOGNITION
Syndrome: Human: Chancre at site of fly bite. Fever, headache, lymphadenopathy, anemia. In later stages—somnolence ("sleeping sickness").

Animal: Usually subclinical. In cattle—lacrimation, anorexia, anemia, and weight loss may occur.

Incubation period: *T. rhodesiense*—1-3 weeks. *T. gambiense*—longer, perhaps years.

Case fatality rate: Approaches 100% without treatment.

Confirmatory tests: Microscopic examination of lymph from nodes and of buffy coat of blood for presence of the parasite. May be found in CNS fluid in later stages of infection. Paired sera for ELISA, complement fixation, and fluorescent antibody testing.

Occurrence: Tropical Africa. *T. rhodesiense* in upland savannas, *T. gambiense* in rain forests. Reservoirs are humans, wild game, and domestic cattle.

Transmission: *Glossina* spp. (tsetse) flies are the biological vector. Mechanical transmission by mouth parts of other biting flies can occur. Carnivores can acquire infection by ingestion of infected carcasses.

CONTROL AND PREVENTION

Individual/herd: Treat with pentamidine, suramin, or melarsoprol. Chemoprophylaxis with these products will be effective against *T. gambiense* but cannot be relied upon against *T. rhodesiense*.

Local/community: Eliminate breeding places of tsetse flies. Mass chemotherapy of infected humans. Provide education regarding method of transmission.

National/international: None.

DISEASE: Trypanosomiasis, American

AGENT

Trypanosoma cruzi

RECOGNITION

Syndrome: Human: Often asymptomatic. Inflammation at site of bite. Fever, malaise, lymphadenopathy, hepatosplenomegaly, unilateral palpebral edema, myocarditis, meningoencephalitis. Chronic form may produce megaesophagus and megacolon.

Animal: Subclinical in wild animals, but syndrome in dogs parallels that in humans.

Incubation period: 1-5 weeks. 30-40 days, if infection derives from blood transfusion.

Case fatality rate: 10%.

Confirmatory tests: Microscopic examination of blood for parasite. Paired sera for ELISA, complement fixation, indirect fluorescent and agglutination testing. Identify parasite by xenodiagnosis (bug fed on patient's blood).

Occurrence: Western hemisphere. South and Central America, Mexico. Reservoirs are humans, wild (armadillos, opossums, rabbits, rodents) and domestic animals, especially dogs and cats. Most human cases are in children.

Transmission: Contamination of bite wound with feces from infected triatomid bugs of the family Reduviidae ("assassin bugs") during feeding. Also by blood transfusion and prenatal transmission.

CONTROL AND PREVENTION

Individual/herd: Treat with Nifurtimox (Bayer 2502), aminoquinalone. Utilize insect repellents.

Local/community: Education regarding method of transmission. Vermin control. Screen blood donors.

National/international: None.

8

FUNGAL, BACTERIAL, SPIROCHAETAL, AND RICKETTSIAL ZOONOSES

FUNGAL INFECTIONS

DISEASE: Dermatomycosis

AGENT
> *Microsporum canis, Trichophyton mentagrophytes, Trichophyton verrucosum,* animal reservoir; other species involving human or soil reservoir

RECOGNITION
> **Syndrome:** Human: Lesions occur on human head or body, and on most species, are circular or annular because of central healing. Usually scaling or hair loss or breakage, occasional itching. Sometimes erythema, induration, crusting, or suppuration occurs. May be confused with many allergic, hormonal, or other infectious conditions.
>
> Animal: Most mammalian species susceptible; lesions similar to those in humans.
>
> **Incubation period:** 4-14 days.
>
> **Case fatality rate:** Insignificant. Confirmatory tests: Microscopic examination of KOH-treated scrapings from edge of lesion, observe lesion under ultraviolet light (*Microsporum*), culture.
>
> **Occurrence:** *M. canis* more common in young. Cats, dogs usual source of *M. canis* infection whereas cattle, horses most common source of

T. mentagrophytes. More common in warm, humid climate. Skin irritation, crowding, and debilitation predispose.

Transmission: Direct contact of skin with infected individual or indirect contact with fomites such as saddle blankets and brushes. Agent may survive months on fomites if dry, cool, shaded.

CONTROL AND PREVENTION
Individual/herd: Treat human cases with griseofulvin orally if persistent infection. Clip and clean around lesion and treat with antimycotic locally. Clean and disinfect fomites. Practice good sanitation.
Local/community: Before pets are kept in nursing homes or other institutions, examine for evidence of dermatomycosis.
National/international: None

BACTERIAL INFECTIONS

DISEASE: Anthrax

AGENT
Bacillus anthracis

RECOGNITION
Syndrome: Human: Cutaneous: most common, cutaneous pruritic macule, becomes edematous, vesiculates, then necrotic with black central scar; Pulmonary: febrile respiratory tract disease, mild onset, then sudden onset of second stage with dyspnea, sweating, cyanosis, and death with 24 hours; Intestinal: febrile gastrointestinal disease. Animal: Affects domestic and wild ruminants (cattle, goats, sheep), horses, and swine.
Incubation period: Cutaneous, 1-7 days; pulmonary, 1-5 days; intestinal, 12 hours-5 days.
Case fatality rate: If untreated, cutaneous 5%-20%, pulmonary 100%, and intestinal 50%.
Confirmatory tests: Gram or Giemsa stain, Ascoli precipitin test, culture blood or tissue. Radiographic evidence of mediastinal widening in pulmonary cases.
Occurrence: Worldwide, particularly in areas of alkaline soil subject to flooding. Occurs in dry, warm periods after heavy rains, frequently

recurring on same pasture. Seen in occupations handling livestock or wool.

Transmission: Usually, by direct contact with infected animal. Also, by ingestion of undercooked meat or, occasionally, by inhalation of spores in wool from infected ruminants. Spores are found in bone meal, soil, water, and on vegetation. Some arthropods, such as horseflies, may be involved in animal-to-animal spread. Spores form readily when vegetative form is exposed to air, are long-lived, and are very resistant to environmental extremes and disinfectants.

CONTROL AND PREVENTION

Individual/herd: Treat with penicillin; tetracyclines or erythromycin effective if treated early. Vaccinate livestock in endemic areas. Vaccination may be considered for high-risk occupations. Avoid necropsy of (suspected) infected carcasses beyond collection of blood specimen. Dispose of carcass by deep burial or burning.

Local/community: Control dust in industries handling wool or hides. Wash and disinfect wool/hair from endemic areas (10% formalin, 5% lye). Prevent livestock movement from affected premises during outbreak.

National/international: Require sterilization of imported bone meal.

DISEASE: Arizona Infection

AGENT

Salmonella arizona

RECOGNITION

Syndrome: Human: Diarrhea most common. Many subclinical infections. Septicemia in immunosuppressed.

Animal: Most isolates from reptiles and birds, but all species probably susceptible. Reduced hatchability and production in poultry. Poults and chicks have weakness, anorexia, and shivering. Outbreaks in turkeys, chicks, and canaries with up to 60% mortality rate.

Incubation period: 6-72 hours, usually 12-36 hours.

Case fatality rate: Insignificant, except for young, aged, immunodeficient, or debilitated.

Confirmatory tests: Culture of feces or affected tissue.

Occurrence: Worldwide. Associated with ingestion of desiccated rattlesnake meat as folk medicine. Young at greatest risk. Stress may cause recrudescence in carriers.

Transmission: Fecal-oral, with some egg spread. Long-term (years) intestinal carriers. Agent can survive months in soil, feed, and water.

CONTROL AND PREVENTION

Individual/herd: Supportive treatment. Prevent infection with good hygiene, sanitation, and fumigation of hatching eggs.

Local/community: Educate ethnic groups regarding hazards associated with ingestion of potentially contaminated folk medicines.

National/international: None.

DISEASE: Botulism

AGENT

Clostridium botulinum. Toxin types A, B, E, F, and G affect people; A-D affect horses; C, D affect cattle; C affects sheep; A, C, and E affect birds; C and E affect mink.

RECOGNITION

Syndrome: Human: Nausea, vomiting, sometimes constipation followed by toxic effects on the central nervous system (ptosis, blurred or double vision, dizziness, dysphagia, blurred speech, muscle weakness, respiratory paralysis).

Animal: Deaths occur in wild waterfowl, cattle, chickens, horses, mink, pheasants, and sheep.

Incubation period: 4 hours-4 days.

Case fatality rate: Incubation, severity, and prognosis related to toxin dose. If incubation is short, prognosis is very poor.

Confirmatory tests: Test suspect food or patient serum for specific toxin by mouse protection, hemagglutination inhibition, or indirect fluorescent antibody.

Occurrence: Worldwide. Principal reservoirs are soil and intestinal flora of herbivores and fish. Type E toxin associated with fish and marine mammals. Infant botulism, associated with use of contaminated honey in formula, results from multiplication and toxin formation in the intestine.

Transmission: Ingestion of toxin.

CONTROL AND PREVENTION

Individual/herd: Treat patients immediately with polyvalent antitoxin. Provide respiratory support. Properly preserve food contaminated by soil or intestinal flora to prevent anaerobic replication and toxin production. Heat (boil 3 minutes) preserved foods likely to contain toxins (fruits and vegetables with pH >4.5, certain fish, and meat products) to destroy heat-labile toxin before eating. To prevent disease in animals: prevent herbivores from eating carrion (rodent carcasses in forage, bovine pica); do not feed spoiled meat to mink; prevent birds and mink from eating sarcophagous insect larvae in which toxin concentrates.

Local/community: Educate community regarding proper home food preservation, especially canning to destroy spores, and the use of home-preserved foods.

National/international: None.

DISEASE: Brucellosis

AGENT
Brucella spp. (*B. abortus, B. canis, B. melitensis, B. suis*), multiple biotypes. Humans resistant to infection with *B. neotomae* and *B. ovis*.

RECOGNITION
Syndrome: Human: Gradual onset, febrile systemic disease without rash, undulating fever, chills, sweating, headache, myalgia, fatigue, backache, weakness, malaise, weight loss; long convalescence; often chronic with relapses following stress; arthritic, cardiac, and emotional complications. Human disease most often severe when infected with *B. melitensis,* less frequently severe in decreasing order when infected with *B. suis, B. abortus,* and *B. canis.*

Animal: Syndromes include abortion, weak newborn, reduced milk yield, retained placenta, orchitis, spondylitis, salpingitis, testicular atrophy. Most susceptible bovine is pregnant female. Many inapparent infections in all susceptible species. Also occurs in some regions among sheep, reindeer, camels, elk, and bison. Fistulous withers or poll evil seen in horses in contact with infected cattle.

Incubation period: 1 week-several months. Varies inversely with stage of gestation in cattle.

Case fatality rate: <1%.

Confirmatory tests: Test paired sera by agglutination or complement-fixation. Cultural examination of acute blood or lesions (include placenta, fetus, milk, or semen). Biotyping is aid in epidemiologic studies.

Occurrence: Worldwide. Occupational in livestock farmers, veterinarians, diagnostic laboratory workers. Major reservoirs are cattle (*B. abortus*), dogs (*B. canis*), goats (*B. melitensis*), and swine (*B. suis*).

Infection persists for lifetime in animals.

Transmission: Contact with infected tissues or fluids, usually placental. Ingestion of raw milk or dairy products (e.g., soft cheeses). Airborne under abattoir or laboratory conditions. Can penetrate intact skin or mucous membranes. Venereal in swine and dogs. Agent resists environmental stresses. Strain 19 vaccine pathogenic for humans.

CONTROL AND PREVENTION

Individual/herd: Treat human patients with tetracyclines (also dihydro-streptomycin in severe cases) for 3-4 weeks. Add animals to herd or breed to animals from known uninfected premises only. Segregate parturient females. Shorten breeding season to limit time when susceptible animals are available. Use serologic surveillance, remove infected animals. Use strain 19 or 45/20 vaccine in heifer calves, Rev 1 in goats and sheep. Cook meat. Wear protective clothing.

Local/community: Pasteurize milk and dairy products. Eradicate infection in domestic animal reservoir. Control airflow in abattoirs and laboratories.

National/international: None.

DISEASE: Campylobacteriosis

AGENT

Campylobacter spp. (*C. fetus* ssp. *intestinalis, C. jejuni*), multiple serotypes

RECOGNITION

Syndrome: Human: Systemic form (*C. fetus*): variable onset, chills, sweats, fever (repeated episodes, 1-2 days in adults, up to 12 days in children), cough, headache, meningitic signs (usually premature neonatal infants), weight loss, inappetence, vomiting, diarrhea in infants and children, abortion in latter half of pregnancy. Enteric form (*C. jejuni*): acute diarrhea—some with visible blood, fever, abdominal pain, vomiting; may have headache, malaise, myalgia; course 7-10 days; meningitis unusual complication.

Animal: *C. fetus:* Abortion, as well as embryonic death and resorption in sheep, cattle, other ruminants, dogs. *C. jejuni:* Diarrhea in calves and puppies, abortion in sheep.

Incubation period: *C. jejuni:* 1-10 days, usually 2-5 days; *C. fetus:* unknown.

Case fatality rate: *C. jejuni:* typically benign enteritis, risk with unusual systemic complications (<1%); *C. fetus:* up to 50% in premature infants, prognosis good in older persons unless complicated by underlying disease (e.g., AIDS).

Confirmatory tests: Culture feces (enteric), blood (febrile), cerebrospinal fluid, aborted fetus, or bile (*C. jejuni*). Test paired sera by agglutination or indirect hemagglutination. Lack of detectable response not uncommon.

Occurrence: Worldwide. *C. fetus:* Unusual in people; stress (pregnancy), debilitation, impaired immune response predispose. *C. jejuni:* Very common, is leading cause of human diarrheal illness in many areas. Large outbreaks associated with contaminated milk, municipal water supply.

Transmission: Ingestion of food, raw milk, or water contaminated by intestinal or biliary (*C. jejuni*) carriers. Contact with household pets (especially immature). Transplacental to fetus if bacteremia. Several ruminant species, dogs, swine, domestic and wild birds are reservoirs of *C. jejuni*, whereas *C. fetus* found principally in sheep and cattle. People may be carriers of either species.

CONTROL AND PREVENTION

Individual/herd: Treat patients with systemic infection with ampicillin or dihydrostreptomycin for 4 weeks; if severe enteric illness, treat 10 days with gentamicin or erythromycin. Dispose of aborted fetuses and placentas promptly. Use proper hygiene and cooking of meat and poultry. Keep pets with diarrhea away from children. Immunize cattle and sheep to prevent abortion (does not prevent carrier).

Local/community: Pasteurize milk.

National/international: None.

DISEASE: Cat Scratch Disease

AGENT
Rochalimaea henselae (presumptive evidence)

RECOGNITION
Syndrome: Human: Usually benign and nonrecurring, beginning with erythematous papule at inoculation site, then unilateral regional lymphadenopathy, usually painful, often suppurative. Mild fever, infrequent chills, malaise, anorexia, myalgia, nausea. Occasional manifestations: palpebral conjunctivitis, encephalopathy, meningitis, osteolytic lesions, granulomatous hepatitis, pneumonia.

Animal: No signs of illness in cats.

Incubation period: 3-14 days.

Case fatality rate: Insignificant.

Confirmatory tests: Test paired sera by ELISA or indirect fluorescent antibody. Skin test antigen prepared from heated pus is no longer recommended.

Occurrence: Worldwide. Usually in children during cool months. Direct contact with immature cats or cat-associated fomites involved in skin trauma. Familial clusters occur infrequently. In immunocompromised individuals, may become systemic or recurrent.

Transmission: Usually follows cat scratch or bite, occasionally other skin injuries. Cat is reservoir; infection may persist for several months.

CONTROL AND PREVENTION

Individual/herd: Supportive treatment. Aspiration, but not incision, of suppurative nodes. Thoroughly cleanse all cat scratches or bites and prevent cats from contacting open wounds. Immunocompromised persons should avoid young cats.

Local/community: None.

National/international: None.

DISEASE: Clostridial Histotoxic Infection

AGENT

Clostridium spp. (*C. bifermentans (sordellii), C. fallax, C. histolyticum, C. novyi, C. septicum;* and especially *C. perfringens,* type A)

RECOGNITION

Syndrome: Human: Posttraumatic forms (in increasing clinical severity): (1) Simple contamination has watery, brown, foul exudate from wound. (2) Anaerobic cellulitis has gas in cutaneous tissue without pain, edema, or discoloration. (3) Anaerobic myonecrosis (true gas gangrene) has sudden increasing local pain, thin hemorrhagic exudate, edema, swelling, toxemia, shock, eventually gas appearance. (4) Uterine form has sudden onset, acute course, local pain, dysuria, uterine myonecrosis. Nontraumatic forms: (1) Idiopathic gas gangrene, as in true gas gangrene, likely originates at site of healed wound with focal necrosis. (2) Infected vascular gangrene has gas, foul odor in ischemic tissues (usually extremities).

Animal: Malignant edema in cattle, sheep, and horses; hepatic necrosis (black disease) in sheep; gangrenous cellulitis and hepatic necrosis in chickens. Liver flukes produce hepatic necrosis permitting clostridial replication.

Incubation period: Posttraumatic forms: <3 days, usually <24 hours. Nontraumatic forms: Unknown.

Case fatality rate: Prognosis good to poor, depending on extent of necrosis and tissue affected.

Confirmatory tests: Test lesion material by direct fluorescent antibody, immunoprecipitin or anaerobic culture.

Occurrence: Worldwide. Trauma, ischemic tissue (including hepatic necrosis in animals) predispose.

Transmission: Wound contact with intestinal flora (often patient's own), soil, or dust; contaminated vehicle (penetrating nail, etc.).

CONTROL AND PREVENTION

Individual/herd: To treat, debride and drain wound, amputate ischemic tissue, administer penicillin or erythromycin parenterally and in wound; polyvalent clostridial antitoxin; hyperbaric oxygen therapy. To prevent, promptly treat wounds, prevent tissue ischemia (frostbite, etc.). Immunize calves and lambs with polyvalent formolized culture bacterin. Control liver flukes in sheep.

Local/community: None.

National/international: None.

DISEASE: *Clostridium Perfringens* Food Poisoning

AGENT

Clostridium perfringens, commonly type A, types C and D unusual. (See clostridial histotoxic infection.)

RECOGNITION

Syndrome: Human: Sudden onset, nausea, diarrhea, cramps, gas formation with distention of large and small bowel, afebrile, rarely vomiting. Necrotic enteritis (type C), or gastroenteritis (type D).

Animal: Types A-E produce enterotoxemia and other syndromes in young and adult cattle and sheep, the frequency of disease in relation to toxin type varying by age, species, and geographic region.

Incubation period: 5-24 hours, usually 10-12 hours.

Case fatality rate: Usually benign, may be fatal in debilitated individuals.

Confirmatory tests: Microscopic examination (presumptive) and quantitative culture (confirmatory, $>10^5$/gm) of suspect food or patient feces ($>10^6$/gm). Serotyping has been a useful epidemiologic tool in some areas.

Occurrence: Worldwide. Reservoir is soil, source of food contamination usually intestinal flora of herbivores. Restaurant and institutional outbreaks associated with improper cooking and storage of meat foods.

Transmission: Ingestion of large numbers of viable vegetative organisms in food.

CONTROL AND PREVENTION

Individual/herd: Supportive treatment. Vaccinate pregnant ewes and nursing lambs with polyvalent toxoid.

Local/community: Initially, thoroughly cook foods containing meat to destroy vegetative (often heat-resistant) cells. Rapidly cool and refrigerate food if not to be eaten immediately. Reheat stored foods rapidly.

National/international: None.

DISEASE: Colibacillosis

AGENT

Escherichia coli, multiple somatic (O), capsular (K), and flagellar (H) antigens. Some strains produce heat-labile (LT) and/or heat-stable (ST) enterotoxins.

RECOGNITION

Syndrome: Human: Diarrhea, which may be complicated by other syndromes often associated with certain specific serotypes, e.g., hemolytic uremic syndrome (O157:H7). Enteroinvasive strains cause fever, dysentery. Enterotoxigenic strains may cause dehydration and shock. Enterohemorrhagic strains may cause HUS, hemorrhagic colitis, or thrombotic thrombocytopenic purpura (TTP).

Animal: In livestock, causes abortion, mastitis; diarrhea in young. In poultry, causes septicemia, chronic respiratory disease, synovitis, pericarditis, salpingitis.

Incubation period: 0.5-5 days, usually 12-72 hours.

Case fatality rate: May be high in neonates with diarrhea, otherwise low unless underlying disease or develops nonenteric syndrome such as HUS or TTP with brain damage.

Confirmatory tests: Culture of fresh feces (diarrhea) or acute blood (systemic). Serotyping aids in identifying potentially pathogenic strains as well as the possible source.

Occurrence: Worldwide. More common with poor hygiene, fecal-contaminated raw or undercooked food.

Transmission: Ingestion via fecal-oral cycle; often foodborne. Normal inhabitant of the intestinal tract of vertebrates; many serotypes are species-specific. Most transmission human-to-human but animal reservoirs important for spread via milk and meat. Not all strains are pathogenic; fairly resistant to environmental stress.

CONTROL AND PREVENTION
Individual/herd: Treat patients with diarrhea symptomatically or with neomycin if severe; if systemic, administer antibiotic such as ampicillin. Practice good personal hygiene. Thoroughly cook food.
Local/community: Practice good food sanitation; prevent fecal contamination. Pasteurize milk.
National/international: None.

DISEASE: Corynebacterial Infection

AGENT
Corynebacterium spp. (*C. equi, C. hemolyticum, C. pseudotuberculosis, C. pyogenes, C. ulcerans*)

RECOGNITION
Syndromes (observed by agent species): Human: Fever, chest pain, cough, lung cavitation, abscesses (*C. equi*). Sore throat, pharyngitis, purulent skin wounds (*C. hemolyticum*). Sudden onset, painful lymph nodes, occasionally mild fever, malaise, and pneumonitis (*C. pseudotuberculosis*). Septicemia; pharyngitis; tonsillitis; pleural effusion; ulcerative vulvovaginitis with pruritis, swelling, dyspareunia (*C. pyogenes*). Sore throat, acute tonsillitis, atypical diphtheria, occasionally with pseudomembrane (*C. ulcerans*).
Animal: Seasonal prevalence (late summer to fall) of equine abscess syndrome—ulcerative lymphangitis (hind legs) or abscesses of ventral torso (pectoral, abdominal) (*C. pseudotuberculosis*) and bovine summer mastitis (*C. pyogenes*). Other diseases include: bovine mastitis (*C. pseudotuberculosis, C. ulcerans*), suppurative pneumonia in foals (*C. equi*), ovine pneumonia (*C. hemolyticum*), localized or disseminated abscesses in various species (*C. pyogenes*), and ovine suppurative lymphadenitis (*C. pseudotuberculosis*).
Incubation period: Unknown.
Case fatality rate: Uncertain, greater risk among individuals with decreased resistance. If treated, prognosis usually good.
Confirmatory tests: Aerobic culture of lesion material.
Occurrence: Essentially worldwide (although significant geographic differences in frequency of animal cases reported). Number of human cases reported too few to establish a geographic pattern. Wounds (including arthropod bite) or any condition decreasing

resistance predispose.

Transmission: Usually endogenous from skin or mucous membrane flora via trauma or inhalation; infrequently contact or droplet spread from lesions or carriers. *C. equi, C. pseudotuberculosis, C. pyogenes* common infections among domestic animals; *C. hemolyticum, C. ulcerans* occur infrequently; people more frequent source of latter two. Human-to-cow spread suggested in instances of bovine mastitis from *C. ulcerans* with resulting amplification and common-source spread to people by ingestion of raw milk.

CONTROL AND PREVENTION

Individual/herd: Treat patients with erythromycin or tetracyclines; curettage and drainage; diphtheria antitoxin if *C. ulcerans.* Prevent skin (hand) wounds among sheep shearers and other occupations handling livestock. Trim livestock hooves carefully to avoid penetrating vasculature. Control biting flies where equine abscess syndrome occurs. Promptly cleanse wounds.

Local/community: Pasteurize milk.

National/international: None.

DISEASE: Dermatophilosis

AGENT

Dermatophilus congolensis

RECOGNITION

Syndrome: Human: Afebrile, acute to chronic pustular to exudative dermatitis.

Animal: Affects many domestic and wild mammals, particularly ruminants.

Incubation period: <7 days.

Case fatality rate: Insignificant. Prognosis good.

Confirmatory tests: Microscopic and cultural examination of lesion material.

Occurrence: Worldwide in temperate and warmer regions, with frequency of spread and severity of lesions increasing during warm, wet weather.

Transmission: Direct contact, as lesions are only identified source. Trauma and biting arthropods believed to aid in spread.

CONTROL AND PREVENTION

Individual/herd: Treat with dihydrostreptomycin. May have reinfection, as there is no effective immunity. Avoid contact with lesions. Keep skin dry and intact by reducing trauma and biting arthropods. Control ticks on livestock, shear affected sheep last, burn affected wool.

Local/community: None.

National/international: None.

DISEASE: Erysipeloid

AGENT

Erysipelothrix rhusiopathiae

RECOGNITION

Syndrome: Human: If localized, usually on the hands; a slightly raised, nonpitting, dark erythematous cutaneous zone slowly progressing peripherally; severe burning pain, sometimes intense itching, seldom desquamation; occasionally forms serosanguinous vesicles. If generalized, fever, malaise, myalgia, headache.

Animal: Characteristic rhomboid (diamond) skin disease in swine and dolphins; arthritis in sheep and swine; cyanosis (blue comb) and widespread hemorrhages in adult male turkeys.

Incubation period: 1-7 days.

Case fatality rate: Insignificant. Prognosis good.

Confirmatory tests: Culture lesion material (if localized) or blood (if generalized). Repeat blood culture if subacute or chronic endocarditis suspected. In people, differentiate skin lesions from erysipelas caused by Group A *Streptococcus pyogenes*.

Occurrence: Worldwide, principally occupational among those handling fish, swine/pork, or poultry. Skin wounds, particularly on the hands, predispose.

Transmission: Direct contact with: pharyngeal or intestinal lymphoid tissue or feces of carrier animals, particularly swine and rats; lesions, particularly skin; surface slime of fish; contaminated vehicles, including soil exposed to infected animals.

CONTROL AND PREVENTION

Individual/herd: Treat with penicillin until erythema disappears (2-10 days) to avoid systemic involvement. Prevent skin wounds; wear gloves while handling fish and meat; cleanse skin wounds promptly; control rodents; immunize swine and turkeys.

Local/community: Prevent movement of animals from premises where cases are occurring.

National/international: None.

DISEASE: Glanders

AGENT
Pseudomonas mallei

RECOGNITION
Syndrome: Human: Febrile systemic disease without rash, prostration, death 7-10 days.

Animal: Maintained in equines only, in which acute pulmonary and acute to chronic cutaneous (purulent lymphangitis) forms occur. Occasionally seen in canids and felids, cases reported in small ruminants.

Incubation period: Usually 1-14 days.

Case fatality rate: Prognosis poor if untreated.

Confirmatory tests: Use blood or local lesion material in direct fluorescent antibody test. Differentiate culturally from *Pseudomonas pseudomallei*. Test paired sera by agglutination, complement-fixation, indirect hemagglutination, or indirect fluorescent antibody. Use mallein in intrapalpebral test to detect infected equines.

Occurrence: Endemic foci limited to eastern Mediterranean and Asia. Human cases from equine contact in endemic areas. Seasonal and other stress factors (foaling, heavy work) predispose to equine recrudescence.

Transmission: Infectious discharges spread agent by contact, droplet, and vehicle. Carnivores infected by ingestion of infected flesh.

CONTROL AND PREVENTION
Individual/herd: Isolate patients, and treat with sulfadiazine or tetracyclines for 10 days, repeated with 10 day rest interval. No immunity to reinfection. If endemic, test equines for slaughter.

Local/community: Dispose of infected carcasses to avoid contact with scavenging carnivores.

National/international: Test equines from endemic regions before allowing entry.

DISEASE: Leprosy

AGENT
Mycobacterium leprae

RECOGNITION

Syndrome: Human: In endemic areas, many subclinical infections exist. Range of clinical response from tuberculoid (paucibacillary) to lepromatous (multi-bacillary active). Clinically, begins as indeterminate form with small, flat, hypopigmented patches which may be anesthetic. These may regress or develop into tuberculoid form with one or several roughly circular lesions with raised edges or lepromatous form with numerous, diffuse skin lesions, thickening of the ears and lips, and madarosis. A third form, borderline, is intermediate between the tuberculoid and lepromatous forms and may progress into either of the "polar" forms. Because of nerve damage a dropped foot or clawed hand may be present. Wounds resulting from loss of heat or touch sensation are common.

Animal: Naturally acquired infections have been found in armadillos in the southern United States as well as in a few primates from West Africa.

Incubation period: Indeterminate: 6 months->10 years, usually 3-4 years; tuberculoid: 4 years; lepromatous: 8 years.

Case fatality rate: 1%-2%. Fatalities are usually the result of secondary complications or from erythema nodosum leprosum, the "reaction" seen in borderline and lepromatous cases.

Confirmatory tests: Microscopic examination of lesion material, although in tuberculoid may be difficult to find organisms. In lepromatous form, organisms are easily isolated from lymphoid organs, respiratory tract, and the skin. A very sensitive ELISA test has been developed recently.

Occurrence: In the past century, infection has been eliminated from much of the temperate world so that the remaining endemic areas of human leprosy, except for China and Korea, are in the tropics.

Transmission: Human-to-human only route of major significance. Prolonged close contact, such as with infected member of household, important. Inhalation and through broken skin most likely. Childhood exposure greatest risk. Significance of interspecies transmission uncertain.

CONTROL AND PREVENTION

Individual/herd: Treat patients with dapsone, rifampicin, clofazimine, often in combination, for 6 weeks and monitor for 2 years. Surgically correct deformities and treat ulcers locally.

Local/community: Active case detection and health education in endemic areas. BCG vaccination possibly protective in affected households.

National/international: None.

DISEASE: Listeriosis

AGENT
Listeria monocytogenes (7 serotypes and 14 subtypes)

RECOGNITION
Syndrome: Human: Usually subclinical; clinically, most often in neonates. Febrile systemic, neurologic, or respiratory tract disease; may include meningoencephalitis, abortion, endocarditis, conjunctivitis, pustular cutaneous lesions.
Animal: Especially ruminants, encephalitis, septicemia, fetal death, and abortion.

Incubation period: Uncertain, probably a few days-3 weeks. Possibly carrier with period of latent infection.

Case fatality rate: 30%-50% in neonates. Prognosis poor in untreated advanced cases of meningoencephalitis or the aged.

Confirmatory tests: Culture cerebrospinal fluid, blood, brain, or fetal tissues and fluids. Serotype identification useful epidemiologically.

Occurrence: Worldwide, infecting many mammals and birds. Also isolated from ticks and fish. Common in ruminants fed poor quality silage (high pH), debilitated persons, alcoholics. Foodborne outbreaks associated with dairy products.

Transmission: Vertical, either transplacental after maternal primary infection or milkborne, including human; ingestion, dairy products source of human outbreaks; direct contact, particularly among health professionals and abattoir workers. Shed in feces and milk of carriers. Agent persists for months in soil, silage, sewage, and manure.

CONTROL AND PREVENTION
Individual/herd: Treat with penicillin or ampicillin and tetracyclines (if >8 years) or erythromycin. Feed only good quality silage; control rodents; practice good sanitation and personal hygiene during parturition, especially with abortion; thoroughly clean vegetables; adequately cook meat; do not consume raw milk or dairy products.

Local/community: Assure adequate pasteurization of milk and dairy products as well as prevent postpasteurization contamination. Avoid use of manure, sludge, or silage as fertilizer on vegetables.

National/international: None.

DISEASE: Pasteurellosis

AGENT
> *Pasteurella* spp. (*P. haemolytica, P. multocida, P. pneumotropica, P. ureae*)

RECOGNITION
> **Syndrome:** Human: Wound infection: Local redness, swelling, severe pain; occasionally mild fever and regional lymph node swelling. Upper respiratory tract syndromes: usually after some form of head trauma; may result in conjunctivitis, sinusitis, otitis media, meningitis, brain abscess. Lower respiratory tract syndromes: bronchiectasis, pneumonitis, empyema, pneumonia. Abdominal or pelvic infection: Syndrome associated with organ affected (e.g., cystitis, pyelonephritis, appendicitis, metritis, vaginitis). Septicemia: Infrequent; fever, generalized signs; may be associated with endocarditis, liver abscess, osteomyelitis.
> Animal: Pneumonia ("shipping fever" in cattle, "snuffles" in rabbits), septicemia (avian cholera, hemorrhagic septicemia in ruminants), mastitis.
>
> **Incubation period:** Wound infections <24 hours, others unknown.
>
> **Case fatality rate:** Low in localized wound infection, risk increases greatly if generalized or patient aged or debilitated.
>
> **Confirmatory tests:** Microscopic examination (presumptive) and culture (confirmatory) of lesion material (exudate, sputum) or blood (septicemia). Serologic tests of limited value because of frequent lack of host response and variations in agent antigenic array.
>
> **Occurrence:** Worldwide. Trauma (animal bite or scratch, surgical incision, head injury), any condition decreasing resistance predispose. *P. multocida* most common in all syndromes, *P. pneumotropica* and *P. haemolytica* less frequent, *P. ureae* infrequent nonwound-associated only (meningitis, pneumonia).
>
> **Transmission:** Animal (especially dog or cat) bite or scratch. Endogenous from upper respiratory flora (*P. multocida* widely distributed among birds and mammals, including humans; *P. haemolytica* principally in ruminants; *P. pneumotropica* mainly in rodents, occasionally cats, dogs, humans; people only known *P. ureae* reservoir). Inhalation; wound contamination from infected tissue; ingestion (especially fecal contamination among birds).

CONTROL AND PREVENTION
> **Individual/herd:** Treat patients with penicillin. Surgical excision (e.g., lung) or drainage of affected tissue often needed. Promptly cleanse wounds. Avoid animal bites and scratches. Adequately ventilate

poultry houses to reduce dust-laden aerosols. Immunize cattle and poultry to reduce disease severity.

Local/community: Dog population control/leash law.

National/international: None.

DISEASE: Plague

AGENT
Yersinia pestis

RECOGNITION
Syndrome: Human: Bubonic: febrile lymphadenopathy, meningitic signs; Pneumonic: febrile respiratory tract disease, sputum mucoid to bright red; Septicemic: febrile systemic disease without rash, vascular collapse, and sometimes hemorrhagic rash.

Animal: Camels, domestic cats, susceptible rodents, and lagomorphs may become ill and die in endemic areas.

Incubation period: 2-6 days.

Case fatality rate: If untreated, 60% among bubonic cases, 95% among pneumonic-septicemic cases.

Confirmatory tests: Culture or direct fluorescent antibody test of lymph node aspirate, blood, or sputum. Examine mammalian (cat, rabbit, rodent) spleen or bone marrow. Test paired sera by complement-fixation or indirect hemagglutination.

Occurrence: Agent persists in Africa, the Americas, and Asia where it is maintained in sylvatic foci involving flea-wild rodent-flea cycles. Commingling of infected wild rodents with domestic rats may initiate an urban cycle of flea-domestic rat-flea spread.

Transmission: Bite from infective flea is essential in maintenance cycles and is usual source of human bubonic infection. Infectious sputum is important source in human-to-human spread of pneumonic plague epidemics. Occasionally, is spread by direct contact (animal to human) or ingestion of infected carcass (animal to animal).

CONTROL AND PREVENTION
Individual/herd: Isolate patient and treat with dihydrostreptomycin and tetracyclines for 21 days to avoid relapse. Immunization among high-risk groups offers partial protection.

Local/community: First, control domestic rat fleas, then control domestic rats. Wild rodent flea control is feasible in selected endemic or epidemic recreational areas.

National/international: Prevent movement of infected rats and their fleas via ships and other carriers from endemic areas.

DISEASE: Rat-Bite Fever

AGENT
Streptobacillus moniliformis, Haverhill disease; *Spirillum minus*, Sodoku

RECOGNITION
Syndrome: Human: Haverhill: High fever, chills, headache, backache, disturbances of consciousness, vomiting, sore throat, myalgia. Sodoku: Nonsuppurative indurated swelling at bite wound with regional lymphatic involvement, followed in less than a day with fever, chills, tachycardia, digestive upset, myalgia, arthralgia, headaches; sometimes central nervous system involvement; skin eruptions 1-2 days later; relapses may occur for years.
Animal: Haverhill: Arthritis in turkeys; dieoffs in mice. Sodoku: Disease not reported in animals.
Incubation period: Haverhill: 2-14 days; Sodoku: 1 week-2 months.
Case fatality rate: Up to 10% in untreated, prognosis good in treated.
Confirmatory tests: Microscopic examination of lesion material to observe agent. Isolate agent from acute blood or lesion material.
Occurrence: Worldwide, usually sporadic. Respiratory carrier rats principal known reservoir of both agents.
Transmission: Rat bite. One outbreak of Haverhill disease associated with ingestion of contaminated raw milk.

CONTROL AND PREVENTION
Individual/herd: Disinfect bite wounds. Treat patients with penicillin.
Local/community: Control rats. Protect against occupationally associated rat bites. Haverhill: prevent food contamination with rat excreta.
National/international: None.

DISEASE: Salmonellosis

AGENT
Salmonella spp. (approximately 2,000 serotypes)

RECOGNITION
Syndrome: Human: Most infections subclinical. Usual clinical signs are diarrhea, vomiting, low-grade fever. Sometimes progresses to dehydration, prostration, death, especially in very young or very old. Septic syndrome (enteric fever) has high-spiking fever, septicemia, splenomegaly, headache. Focal infection may occur in any organ

independently of septic fever; usually abscess or inflammation in lung, heart, kidney, periosteum, joints, meninges.

Animal: Diarrhea is usual clinical sign. Causes abortion in cows, sheep, horses.

Incubation period: 6-72 hours, usually 12-36.

Case fatality rate: 1%-2% with most serotypes, particular risk in very young, aged, and debilitated.

Confirmatory tests: Culture feces, affected tissue, or fluid. Bacteriophage typing aids in epidemiologic investigation. Agglutination test of serum useful only in serotypes producing enteric fever (e.g., *S. typhi* in humans; *S. pullorum, S. gallinarum* in poultry). Differentiate from gastroenteritis caused by *Shigella* spp., *Clostridium perfringens*, *Escherichia coli*, enteroviruses, various parasites.

Occurrence: Worldwide. Most animals susceptible to infection. Disease most frequent in stressed individuals. Often occurs in outbreaks.

Transmission: Ingestion, usually through variations of the fecal-oral cycle, exception *S. dublin* in raw milk from cow with udder infection. Fecal excretion commonly varies from a few days to weeks. In a few instances (e.g., *S. typhi*) may shed for life. Some infections persist for years in bone marrow or lymph nodes, then relapse after stress (See Arizona Infection). Penetrates eggshell (e.g., *S. enteritidis*). Most serotypes have broad host spectrum. Arthropods (e.g., flies) occasional mechanical vectors. Agent fairly resistant to drying; susceptible to heat, sunlight, most disinfectants; resists freezing; can survive months in inanimate environment under proper conditions.

CONTROL AND PREVENTION

Individual/herd: Treat patients symptomatically, including fluids and electrolytes. Use ampicillin or amoxicillin only when bacteremia or infection localized other than in intestine. Antibiotic therapy of enteric infection may prolong carrier state. Sanitation very important. Cook food thoroughly. Control rodents, birds, insects. Practice personal hygiene. Avoid stress. Use *Salmonella*-free feed for livestock, poultry, and pets. Adequately heat meat, bone, and fish meal to be used in animal feed. Obtain hatching eggs from *Salmonella*-free flocks.

Local/community: Pasteurize milk. Prohibit sale of pet turtles and other *Salmonella* carriers. Educate food handlers.

National/international: None.

DISEASE: Shigellosis

AGENT

Shigella spp. (*S. sonnei*; multiple serotypes of S. boydii, *S. dysenteriae, S. flexneri*)

RECOGNITION

Syndrome: Human: Bloody diarrhea, tenesmus, fever, nausea.
Animal: Diarrhea seen in nonhuman primates.

Incubation period: 1-4 days.

Case fatality rate: Insignificant, except may be up to 20% for debilitated and immunodeficient.

Confirmatory tests: Immediate aerobic culture of fresh feces.

Occurrence: Worldwide. Usually children. People primary hosts; nonhuman primates frequently infected, and pigs and dogs occasionally infected, then can reinfect people. Carriers may excrete up to 3 months. Agent sensitive to heat and chemicals; survives best under high humidity, low temperature and lighting.

Transmission: Via fecal-oral route with some mechanical vectors (e.g., flies).

CONTROL AND PREVENTION

Individual/herd: Treat patients supportively with fluids and electrolytes; ampicillin, trimethoprim/sulfamethoxazole, tetracyclines. Personal hygiene.

Local/community: Good sanitation practices, fly control.

National/international: None.

DISEASE: Staphylococcosis

AGENT

Staphylococcus aureus, 6 enterotoxin types, A-F; multiple bacteriophage types, groups I-IV and miscellaneous

RECOGNITION

Syndrome: Human: Predominantly subclinical infections. Gastroenteritis (enterotoxin food poisoning): sudden onset, salivation, nausea, abdominal cramps, vomiting, diarrhea; prostration common. Suppuration: in any tissue, but usually skin (impetigo, boils), lung (pneumonia), mammae (mastitis or abscess), endocardium, or periosteum. Toxic epidermal necrosis: noninflammatory separation of epidermis, especially in newborn.

Animal: Outbreaks of suppuration with high fatality rate in rabbits and hares. Important cause of bovine mastitis.

Incubation period: Gastroenteritis: 0.5-7 hours, usually 2-4 hours. Suppuration: 4-10 days.

Case fatality rate: Gastroenteritis: deaths only in the debilitated or those with cardiac problems. Suppuration: unusual, following septicemia.

Confirmatory tests: Culture lesion material (suppuration) or vomitus, feces, and food (gastroenteritis). Demonstrate enterotoxin if food poisoning. Bacteriophage typing and antibiogram are epidemiologic aids.

Occurrence: Worldwide. All species susceptible to infection, but enterotoxin-associated gastroenteritis unusual in species other than man. Greatest risk of suppuration in neonates, new mothers, the debilitated, surgical patients, those on extended steroid or antibiotic therapy. Poor personal hygiene predisposes.

Transmission: Carried in intestinal tract, nares, and skin as part of normal flora. Gastroenteritis: usually by ingestion of heat-stable toxin preformed in food, but toxin may form in intestine of severely stressed or heavily exposed person. Suppuration: direct contact or fomites; airborne common (hospital problem); infective dose fairly high in most healthy subjects. Interspecies transmission occurs but is infrequent. Agent resistant to environmental factors.

CONTROL AND PREVENTION

Individual/herd: Patient therapy: gastroenteritis—supportive, self-limiting in a few hours; suppuration—antibiotics, after sensitivity testing. Practice personal hygiene. Ensure aseptic surgery. Use antibiotics judiciously. Cover draining lesions. Use triple dye (brilliant green, proflavine hemisulfate, crystal violet) on umbilicus of newborn.

Local/community: Ensure proper food hygiene. Constantly control food temperature. Pasteurize milk. Detect and eliminate reservoir in outbreaks.

National/international: None.

DISEASE: Streptococcosis

AGENT

Streptococcus spp., Lancefield groups A (*S. pyogenes*), B (*S. agalactiae*), C (*S. equi*), D (*S. bovis*), F, G, H, L, and M

RECOGNITION

Syndrome: Human: Suppurative disease, septicemia, pneumonia, puerperal fever, endocarditis, arthritis, rash (scarlet fever), pharyngitis, impetigo. Rheumatic fever or nephritis delayed sequelae of group A. Group B important in neonatal infection.
Animal: Bovine mastitis and equine abortion.

Incubation period: 1-3 days.

Case fatality rate: 20%-50% in neonates, increasing with immaturity and earlier age at onset.

Confirmatory tests: Culture lesion material and hemolysin test isolate. Lancefield grouping or CAMP test may be epidemiologic aid.

Occurrence: Worldwide. Neonates, immunocompromised individuals at greatest risk. Crowding, poor hygiene, hot humid climates, skin trauma predispose.

Transmission: Inhalation, direct contact, ingestion. Interspecies spread uncommon; most frequent with groups A, B, and D. Upper respiratory tract, intestinal, vaginal, skin, udder carriers.

CONTROL AND PREVENTION

Individual/herd: Treat patients with penicillin or erythromycin (if patient penicillin-sensitive). Practice personal hygiene. Culture human pharyngitis and treat group A infections promptly to prevent delayed sequelae. Screen pregnant women for group B genital carriage so can initiate newborn therapy. Use bacterins against *S. equi* in foals. Avoid crowding.

Local/community: Pasteurize milk.

National/international: None.

DISEASE: Tetanus

AGENT

Clostridium tetani

RECOGNITION

Syndrome: Human: Intermittent to continuous tonic muscular spasms (usually descending), terminal asphyxia.
Animal: Muscular spasms, especially in horses, calves, and lambs.

Incubation period: Few days-several weeks, mean 10 days.

Case fatality rate: 30%-90%, varying with age, length of incubation, and treatment.

Confirmatory tests: Laboratory confirmation often impossible. Wound tissue for mouse protection or direct fluorescent antibody or anaerobic culture.

Occurrence: Worldwide. People and horses at greatest risk; less often in cattle, sheep, swine; seldom in dogs, turkeys. Wounds predispose, particularly those inducing anaerobic conditions.

Transmission: Wound contamination by spores from soil reservoir or intestinal flora of people and especially herbivores. Sporulation and replication occur under anaerobic conditions, producing toxin. Toxin passage to the CNS seems to be enhanced through absorption by peripheral nerves.

CONTROL AND PREVENTION

Individual/herd: Treat patients with tetanus immune globulin (TIG) or tetanus antitoxin, penicillin, respiratory support, muscle relaxants, and tetanus toxoid concurrently. To prevent in people and horses, administer toxoid. Cleanse wounds thoroughly, using toxoid booster or antitoxin as appropriate whenever deep wounds occur. Ensure aseptic surgery. Apply antiseptic (iodine) to newborn umbilicus, tail stump of docked lamb, and castration wound of colt or lamb.

Local/community: Promote prophylactic immunization.

National/international: None.

DISEASE: Tuberculosis

AGENT

Mycobacterium spp. (*M. africanum, M. avium, M. bovis, M. tuberculosis*)

RECOGNITION

Syndrome: Human: Pulmonary: Productive cough, fever, weight loss, fatigue, night sweats, chest pain, hemoptysis. Extrapulmonary: cervical lymphadenitis (scrofula), meningitis, osteomyelitis, pericarditis; also associated with infection of most other organs. Typically, encapsulated inflammatory nodules (tubercles) with epithelioid and giant cells surrounding caseous or liquefied center. *M. avium* typically produces tubercle lesions in birds only; in mammals, lesions usually slight (regional lymphadenitis) or absent (stimulates tuberculin reactivity).

Animal: Cattle: pulmonary (*M. bovis*)—cough, weight loss, decreased milk production. Swine: extrapulmonary (*M. avium*)—pharyngeal, mesenteric lymphadenitis.

Incubation period: 4-12 weeks for observable lesion (e.g., lung nodule) or significant tuberculin reaction. Although the greatest risk is within 1-2 years, it may be decades before progressive disease evident.

Case fatality rate: Severe outcome more likely with primary infection in young or immunodeficient (e.g., AIDS).

Confirmatory tests: Direct microscopic examination (presumptive) and aerobic culture of lesion material (pus, sputum).

Occurrence: Worldwide. Crowding and any condition decreasing resistance (particularly lung damage, AIDS) predispose. Prevalence increases with age. Less than 100 human cases *M. avium* infection confirmed, occasionally associated with bovine mastitis. *M. africanum,* related to *M. bovis,* causes disease in people; nonhuman host distribution still uncertain (cases reported in zoo primates).

Transmission: Primarily inhalation of infectious droplets or droplet nuclei from pulmonary lesion. Also ingestion, particularly raw milk from cow with mammary lesion. People are reservoir and main source for *M. tuberculosis*; cattle for *M. bovis.* Wide range of mammalian species infected from mammalian reservoirs, but parrot only bird known to be infected. Dogs and primates infected particularly from exposure to human infections. Infected badgers involved in persistence of *M. bovis* in United Kingdom; opossums similarly involved in New Zealand. *M. avium* spread, especially to swine, by ingestion of food or water contaminated by feces from shedder birds.

CONTROL AND PREVENTION

Individual/herd: Prolonged therapy (several months) with isoniazid, dihydrostreptomycin, ethambutol, rifampicin, pyrazinamide. Prognosis good with proper therapy in people and cattle (*M. bovis* highly sensitive). *M. avium* infection is the exception, highly resistant to antibiotics; surgical excision of affected lymph nodes may be needed.

Local/community: Pasteurize milk. Immunize high-risk groups with BCG. Find cases with use of tuberculin test (cattle, people, primates). Slaughter tuberculin reactor cattle. Depopulate tuberculous poultry flocks. Screen radiographically tuberculin-positive people.

National/international: None.

DISEASE: Tularemia

AGENT

Francisella tularensis, Jellison types A and B

RECOGNITION

Syndrome: Human: Associated primarily with portal of entry. Skin exposure most common: sudden onset of fever, chills, headache, and malaise with necrotizing ulcer at site and regional lymphadenitis (ulceroglandular). Ingestion: results in necrotizing lesions of upper gastrointestinal tract, angina, vomiting, and diarrhea (typhoidal). Inhalation: results in pneumonia. Conjunctiva unusual: ulcerated papule on lower eyelid and regional lymphadenitis (oculo-glandular).

Animal: Outbreaks/dieoffs seen in sheep, rabbits, beavers, foxes, muskrats, occasionally hares.

Incubation period: 1-10 days, usually 3-5.

Case fatality rate: If untreated, up to 10% for infection with Jellison type A whereas negligible with type B.

Confirmatory tests: Culture or fluorescent antibody test blood, sputum, exudates, scrapings, or regional lymph nodes. Test paired sera by agglutination. Cross-reactivity with *Brucella*.

Occurrence: Many species of arthropods, birds, and mammals naturally infected in Europe, North America, China, Iran, Japan, Russia, Thailand, and Tunisia. Jellison type A associated with lagomorphs, type B associated with rodents. Occupational/recreational peaks in spring and fall, principally from tick exposure.

Transmission: Potential modes quite varied, including direct contact of unbroken skin with blood or tissues of infected animals; tick or other arthropod bites; ingestion of meat or water; inhalation of dust or fluid aerosol; bite of infected animal. Small mammals, such as rabbits and muskrats, are major reservoirs; and ticks are principal vector.

CONTROL AND PREVENTION

Individual/herd: Treat with dihydrostreptomycin, and tetracyclines (may have relapse if use latter alone as is bacteriostatic). Early therapy may greatly reduce length of illness from weeks to days. Wear protective clothing to avoid exposure to ticks, wear rubber gloves when handling wild game, and cook the meat thoroughly. Boil possibly contaminated water. Sheepshearers and fur handlers in endemic areas should wear face masks. Control ticks in public parks and campgrounds where highly endemic.

Local/community: Warn public regarding handling wild game, exposure to arthropods (especially ticks), and swimming in water frequented by wildlife in highly endemic areas. May vaccinate high-risk groups with live vaccine.

National/international: None.

DISEASE: Vibriosis

AGENT
Aeromonas hydrophila, Vibrio spp. (*V. alginolyticus, V. parahaemolyticus, V. vulnificus*)

RECOGNITION
Syndrome: Human: Gastroenteritis: diarrhea, occasionally bloody; abdominal pain, vomiting, fever. Wound infection: a variety of skin lesions, including cellulitis and necrosis, usually progressing to systemic involvement. Septicemia: systemic illness, fever, or hypotension, no wound preceding.
Animal: *A. hydrophila* common cause of septicemia in amphibia, fish, and reptiles. Pathogenicity of other species for animals uncertain.
Incubation period: 4-96 hours, usually 12-24 hours.
Case fatality rate: Septicemia: may exceed 50%; wound infection: up to 25%; gastroenteritis: fatality unusual. Risk greater in those with underlying debility, e.g. liver disease.
Confirmatory tests: Culture feces (diarrhea), blood (septicemia), or lesion material.
Occurrence: Worldwide, more often in coastal areas. More frequent in warm months in temperate regions.
Transmission: Ingestion of raw or undercooked shellfish (oysters), freshwater or marine fish. Insanitary handling practices and temperature abuse before or after cooking increase opportunity for contamination and replication. Exposure to untreated water, particularly estuarine or marine, often associated with trauma such as penetrating fish spine. Some human *A. hydrophila* infections associated with therapeutic use of medicinal leeches. Reservoirs uncertain.

CONTROL AND PREVENTION
Individual/herd: Supportive therapy, surgical debridement of wounds. Treat severely affected with tetracyclines, aminoglycosides. Cook all fish and shellfish just before consumption.
Local/community: Ensure hygiene in fish markets and kitchens.
National/international: None.

DISEASE: Yersiniosis

AGENT
Yersinia spp. (*Y. enterocolitica, Y. pseudotuberculosis*), multiple serotypes

RECOGNITION
Syndrome: Human: Acute mesenteric lymphadenitis most common syndrome (suggestive of appendicitis) with fever, abdominal tenderness, anorexia, vomiting, sometimes erythema nodosum (may occur as distinct syndrome). Enteritis with diarrhea, sometimes toxemia, dehydration. Less common forms include septicemia (often with icterus, hepatomegaly), conjunctivitis, pulmonary abscess, arthritis.

Animal: Acute septicemia or enteritis are usual epidemic forms. Chronic localized abscesses affecting various organs (liver, lung, mammary gland) and abortion seen sporadically.

Incubation period: Generally <10 days.

Case fatality rate: Generally <1%, risk increases significantly in elderly and immunocompromised.

Confirmatory tests: Culture lesion material, blood (septicemia), or feces (enteritis). Test paired sera by agglutination or indirect hemagglutination. Some serotypes cross-react with *Brucella abortus, Salmonella pullorum,* or *Yersinia pestis.*

Occurrence: Worldwide, considerable geographic differences in frequency. Known to affect many species of domestic and free-living mammals and birds (mammals and birds carriers of *Y. pseudotuberculosis*; *Y. enterocolitica* found in mammals only; humans may be carriers of either). Stress, immunosuppression, other factors decreasing resistance predispose, particularly to septicemia. Acute mesenteric adenitis most frequent in human males (5-18 years).

Transmission: Ingestion of food, including milk, or water contaminated by intestinal carriers; transplacental to fetus if primary maternal bacteremia.

CONTROL AND PREVENTION
Individual/herd: Treat patients with tetracyclines or dihydrostreptomycin.

Local/community: Prevent fecal contamination of food and drinking water. Pasteurize milk.

National/international: None.

SPIROCHAETAL INFECTIONS

DISEASE: Endemic Relapsing Fever

AGENT

Borrelia spp., identified in relation to geographic region and/or tick vector. Species in relation to region include: *B. hermsii, B. turicatae, B. parkeri, B. mazzottii, B. venezuelensis, B. brasiliensis* (Western Hemisphere); *B. duttonii, B. hispanica, B. marocana, B. persica* (Eastern Hemisphere).

RECOGNITION

Syndrome: Human: Sudden onset, high fever; headache, alternating with chills, sweating, and temperature drop; myalgia, arthralgia, sometimes petechial rash or neurologic signs (impaired vision, peripheral neuritis). Clinical course 2-9 days per episode with as many as 14 relapses up to a week apart.

Animal: Disease not reported in animals.

Incubation period: 5-15 days, usually 6-8.

Case fatality rate: 2%-5%, greater risk if untreated.

Confirmatory tests: Microscopic examination and culture of acute blood.

Occurrence: Worldwide except for Pacific (Australia, New Zealand, Oceania). Usually sporadic. Soft tick (*Ornithodoros* spp.) vectors generally adapted to life in nests, burrows, and dwellings. Spirochaetemia occurs in many wild and domestic mammalian hosts of *Ornithodoros* spp.

Transmission: Principally tick bite, usually at night; occasionally by contact with tissues of infected mammal. *Borrelia-Ornithodoros* species relationship exists, ticks are host-specific. Often transovarial transmission. All tick stages feeding on blood (larvae, nymphs, adults,) are infective.

CONTROL AND PREVENTION

Individual/herd: Treat patients with tetracyclines or penicillin. Prevent tick bite.

Local/community: Eliminate ticks and their harborage in and around dwellings.

National/international: None.

DISEASE: Leptospirosis

AGENT
Leptospira interrogans (20 serogroups, 170 serovars)

RECOGNITION
Syndrome: Human: Typically, febrile systemic disease without rash, aseptic meningitis; may include icterus, renal insufficiency.
Animal: Often subclinical, but may cause abortion and other clinical signs in dogs, horses, ruminants, and swine.
Incubation period: May be 2-30 days, usually 7-12.
Case fatality rate: <1%-20%, depending on severity of disease especially with hepatorenal involvement. More severe in relation to factors increasing host susceptibility (age) and infection with certain serovars.
Confirmatory tests: Culture of blood, kidney, urine. Test paired sera by microscopic or plate agglutination.
Occurrence: Worldwide, with greater frequency during warmer months in temperate climates. Reservoirs among many domestic and wild mammalian species. Regional and species variations in distribution of serovars.
Transmission: Contact with urine from carrier animals either directly or in water, penetrates mucous membrane or abraded skin; droplet; rarely ingestion; venereal in swine and rodents. Carrier state in maintenance hosts persists for a few months in cattle to a lifetime in rodents. Leptospires are susceptible to drying, heat, acidity, and most common disinfectants.

CONTROL AND PREVENTION
Individual/herd: If patient treated early, dihydrostreptomycin, tetracyclines, or penicillin are effective clinically; only dihydrostreptomycin eliminates shedding. Provide pasture drainage; protect water supply from animal contamination; test herd additions; treat domestic animal carriers; segregate species; remove wildlife and rodent harborage; wear protective clothing; vaccinate animals at high risk (people limited to few hyperendemic areas, e.g. rice fields in Italy); practice personal hygiene.
Local/community: Chlorinate swimming areas (pools) or exclude animals (ponds, streams).
National/international: None.

DISEASE: Lyme Disease

AGENT
Borrelia burgdorferi

RECOGNITION

Syndrome: Human: Two stages: Early—Erythema chronicum migrans (ECM); fever, regional lymphadenopathy, malaise, myalgia may accompany. Late—arthritis, especially large joints, which may persist for years; neurologic (meningitis, encephalitis, retinitis) or cardiac involvement.

Animal: Fever and arthritis in dogs and horses.

Incubation period: 3-32 days for appearance of ECM after tick bite; late stage sequelae appear a few weeks to several months later.

Case fatality rate: No deaths reported. Usually benign with ECM, but risk increases greatly with cardiac or neurologic involvement or infection in fetus or neonate.

Confirmatory tests: Microscopic examination of acute blood (presumptive for *Borrelia*). Test paired sera by indirect fluorescent antibody or enzyme-linked immunoabsorbent assay; however some reduction in serologic response may occur in patients with early antibiotic therapy. Some serologic cross-reactivity with relapsing fever.

Occurrence: Australia, Europe, North America, Russia. Primarily during warm months when ticks are active. Risk of infection associated primarily with entry into woodland habitats where tick vectors found. Field rodents, lagomorphs, and deer are major reservoirs.

Transmission: Bite of ixodid (*Ixodes* spp.) tick; transstadial transmission, no transovarial. Regional differences in tick vector species and stage (i.e., larva, nymph, adult) of major importance in relation to mammalian host preferences (e.g., rodents, large domestic and free-living mammals, dogs, people). Larvae cannot transmit. Most human cases from bite of nymphs; adults prefer deer. Transplacental transmission occurs. Although agent shed in urine of many species, including people, significance in spread uncertain.

CONTROL AND PREVENTION

Individual/herd: Treat patients with tetracyclines or penicillin. Examine dog for ticks and remove them carefully. Use tick repellents and protective clothing when entering tick habitat.

Local/community: Control ticks through use of insecticides and brush clearance.

National/international: None.

RICKETTSIAL INFECTIONS

DISEASE: Boutonneuse Fever

AGENT
Rickettsia conori, member of spotted fever group

RECOGNITION
Syndrome: Human: Characteristic ulcer with black, necrotic center at site of tick bite usually present before onset of other clinical signs. Abrupt onset of fever, arthralgia, myalgia, severe headache, and regional lymphadenitis. Erythematous rash followed by maculopapular rash on forearms, which spreads over entire body. Differentiate from measles, meningitis, typhoid.
Animal: Disease recognized in humans only.
Incubation period: 5-7 days.
Case fatality rate: Usually <3%, greater risk in aged and debilitated.
Confirmatory tests: Test paired sera by Weil-Felix (presumptive), complement-fixation, microagglutination, or mouse toxin-neutralization.
Occurrence: Africa, India, areas surrounding Black, Caspian, and Mediterranean seas. In temperate areas, primarily in warmer months. Outbreaks seen occasionally in tourists to endemic areas. May be introduced to new areas by tick-infested dogs brought from endemic areas. Ticks, dogs, lagomorphs, and many rodents are natural reservoirs.
Transmission: Spread by tick bite, especially dog tick, or inoculating wound or conjunctiva with material from crushed ticks. Transovarial in ticks.

CONTROL AND PREVENTION
Individual/herd: Rapid recovery with tetracycline treatment. Control ticks on dogs and in dwellings.
Local/community: Control stray dogs and rodents.
National/international: None.

DISEASE: Murine Typhus

AGENT
   Rickettsia typhi (R. mooseri), member of typhus group

RECOGNITION
   Syndrome: Human: Fever, chills, headache, and generalized myalgia. Macular rash begins on abdomen about the fifth day and quickly becomes generalized except soles, palms, and face. Cough, nausea, vomiting, and delirium are common. Differentiate from other rickettsioses, typhoid, measles, scarlet fever, relapsing fever, malaria, and yellow fever.
   Animal: Disease not reported in animals.
   Incubation period: 6-14 days.
   Case fatality rate: About 2%, only in aged.
   Confirmatory tests: Test paired sera by complement-fixation, agglutination, or indirect fluorescent antibody. Isolate agent from acute blood.
   Occurrence: Worldwide in natural hosts, *Rattus rattus, R. norvegicus.* Also found in *Didelphis marsupialis.* Often seasonal, in late summer and fall.
   Transmission: Typically, feces of infected rat fleas entering bite or scratch wound. Also may be from *Ctenocephalides felis* from infected opossums. Fleas are infective for life.

CONTROL AND PREVENTION
   Individual/herd: Treat patients 14 days with tetracyclines.
   Local/community: Use insecticides in rodent runways and burrows, then rodenticides. Eliminate rodent food and harborage. Ratproof buildings.
   National/international: None.

DISEASE: North Asian Tick Typhus

AGENT
   Rickettsia sibirica, member of spotted fever group

RECOGNITION
   Syndrome: Human: Sudden onset, high fever, malaise, weakness, chills, myalgia, anorexia, primary tick bite lesion, and regional lymphadenitis. Roseate or papular rash appears a few days later on extensor

surfaces of limbs, spreads to trunk and buttocks. No complications or recurrences. Differentiate from tickborne encephalitides, murine typhus, louseborne typhus, typhoid, paratyphoid fever, RMSF, Omsk hemorrhagic fever, scrub typhus, hemorrhagic nephrosonephritis. Animal: Disease not reported in animals.

Incubation period: 1-13 days, usually 3-6 days.

Case fatality rate: Insignificant.

Confirmatory tests: Test paired sera by complement-fixation.

Occurrence: Russia, Mongolia, especially steppe landscapes of Central Asia, Czechoslovakia, Pakistan. European hare and many rodent species are natural reservoirs, all infections subclinical. Most cases in spring.

Transmission: Tick bite, particularly *Dermacentor* and *Haemaphysalis* spp. Infection rate in ticks may be >20%, transovarial transmission common.

CONTROL AND PREVENTION

Individual/herd: Treat patients with tetracyclines. Use protective clothing and tick repellents. Control ticks on dogs and other domestic animals that may carry adults of multi-host tick species into human habitat.

Local/community: Control ticks in parks and other areas where high risk of human exposure.

National/international: None.

DISEASE: Psittacosis

AGENT
Chlamydia psittaci

RECOGNITION

Syndrome: Human: Febrile respiratory tract disease, sudden onset, chills, cough, epistaxis, anorexia, chest pain, splenomegaly, myocarditis, relative bradycardia.

Animal: Diarrhea and pneumonitis are usual signs in birds, occasionally with high mortality rate; drop in egg production in turkeys. Some birds (e.g., finches, ricebirds) extremely susceptible; chickens resistant. Among the diseases seen in mammals, causes abortion in sheep and cattle, conjunctivitis in guinea pigs, and pneumonitis in cats.

Incubation period: 4-15 days, typically 10 days.

Case fatality rate: Usually benign (<1% if treated), but may be severe and life-threatening in elderly if untreated. Strain differences in virulence of agent; e.g., strains highly virulent for people have been isolated from seagulls and egrets in Louisiana.

Confirmatory tests: Microscopic examination of stained tissue smears. Isolation of agent from patient sputum or blood, or from avian spleen, liver, heart, intestine by mouse or cell culture inoculation. Test paired sera by complement-fixation.

Occurrence: Worldwide. Affects more than 100 avian species. In the United States, major disease problems in psittacines, turkeys, and pigeons; whereas major problem in ducks and geese in Europe. Carrier rate high in birds. Low infection rates in wild birds; increased by crowding and other stress. Poor sanitation and inadequate ventilation facilitate spread. Young are more susceptible except in humans. Occupational in persons associated with psittacines, turkey slaughter, pigeons, laboratories. Role of mammalian chlamydiae in human disease is unclear.

Transmission: Usually inhalation of agent shed from carrier animal. Main reservoirs are carrier birds that excrete agent in feces and to lesser extent in nasal secretions. Shedding is sporadic but is usually stress induced. Carrier state may persist for years. Agent survives drying, facilitating aerosol spread. Oral spread from parent to young in some avian species. Some human-to-human transmission, usually through patient's saliva. Human case reported associated with cat affected with pneumonitis.

CONTROL AND PREVENTION

Individual/herd: Treat human patients with tetracyclines for 21 days. Treat pet birds 45 days with chlortetracycline-medicated feed to eliminate infection. Treating pigeons and turkeys 3-4 weeks will reduce mortality but will not eliminate infection. Must treat entire flock and new additions because recovered birds are susceptible. Good sanitation, ventilation, management practices reduce stress and inhibit spread.

Local/community: Promote treatment of pet birds before sale.

National/international: None.

DISEASE: Q Fever

AGENT

Coxiella burnetii, phase I and II (avirulent)

RECOGNITION

Syndrome: Human: Sudden onset of fever, retrobulbar or frontal headache, chills, myalgia, sweating, weakness, malaise, pneumonitis, endocarditis; hepatitis.

Animal: In Europe, abortion, and bronchopneumonia in ruminants, elsewhere subclinical.

Incubation period: 2-4 weeks.

Case fatality rate: <1%.

Confirmatory tests: Isolate agent from acute blood or sputum. Test paired sera by complement-fixation or agglutination.

Occurrence: Worldwide. Virulence varies widely, most U.S. strains are avirulent. Ruminants primary reservoir; agent shed with placenta, less in milk. Cattle infection rate often 50%, higher in dairy herds than beef. Occupational among persons working with livestock (particularly associated with calving or lambing), abattoir workers, and personnel in biomedical diagnostic laboratories. Subclinical infection in many wild mammals.

Transmission: Primarily by inhalation; agent extremely resistant to drying and sunlight, environmental contamination during ruminant parturition. Ticks of many genera are important in spread among wildlife. Raw milk ingestion less important; direct contact with carcass or placenta least important source.

CONTROL AND PREVENTION

Individual/herd: Treat patients with tetracyclines for at least 15 days. Prognosis good, recovery often slow. Segregate livestock at parturition, and destroy placenta. A vaccine, effective in preventing infection in cattle, has been used in people at high risk but causes severe local reactions.

Local/community: Pasteurize milk at 62.9°C for 30 minutes or at 71.6°C for 15 seconds.

National/international: None.

DISEASE: Queensland Tick Typhus

AGENT

Rickettsia australis, member of spotted fever group

RECOGNITION

Syndrome: Human: Insidious onset of malaise, headache, moderate fever, flat black eschar, painful regional lymphadenopathy, rash of variable appearance. Differentiate from murine and scrub typhus.

Animal: Disease not reported in animals.

Incubation period: 7-10 days.

Case fatality rate: Insignificant.

Confirmatory tests: Isolation from acute blood. Test paired sera by complement-fixation.

Occurrence: Sporadic. Queensland, Australia. Serologic evidence that various marsupial and rodent species are reservoirs.

Transmission: Bite of ixodid ticks.

CONTROL AND PREVENTION

Individual/herd: Treat patients with tetracyclines.

Local/community: Control ticks.

National/international: None.

DISEASE: Rickettsialpox

AGENT

Rickettsia akari, member of spotted fever group

RECOGNITION

Syndrome: Human: Papule at site of bite followed in a week by sudden onset of fever, chills, photophobia, sweating, myalgia, and frontal headache. Papule later becomes vesicular, then forms dark crust. Rash appears 3-4 days after onset of fever and covers most of body. Animal: Experimental infection causes pneumonia in laboratory mice.

Incubation period: 10-24 days.

Case fatality rate: Fatalities are rare.

Confirmatory tests: Test paired sera by complement-fixation using specific antigen. Isolate agent from acute blood.

Occurrence: House mice are reservoir. Mites can transmit transovarially. An urban disease among households with mouse infestation. Recognized foci in the United States, Russia, equatorial and southern Africa, Korea.

Transmission: Bites of infected mites, *Liponyssoides sanguineus*; mite feces in wound.

CONTROL AND PREVENTION

Individual/herd: Treat patients 3-4 days with tetracyclines. Untreated patients recover in 10-14 days without sequelae. Apply miticides in home followed by mouse eradication with rodenticides and elimination of harborage. Practice good sanitation to prevent mouse reinfestation.

Local/community: None
National/international: None

DISEASE: Rocky Mountain Spotted Fever

AGENT
Rickettsia rickettsii, member of spotted fever group

RECOGNITION
Syndrome: Human: Sudden onset of frontal and occipital headache, persistent fever, chills, myalgia, weakness, conjunctival injection, flushed face, relative tachycardia. Macular rash begins on extremities a few days later, becomes petechial or even hemorrhagic, persisting for weeks.
Animal: Short, mild, febrile illness in dogs.
Incubation period: 2-14 days.
Case fatality rate: 20% in untreated cases, increases with age.
Confirmatory tests: Isolate agent from acute blood. Test paired sera by complement-fixation (preferably with purified antigen), indirect hemagglutination, or indirect microfluorescent antibody.
Occurrence: Much of the Western Hemisphere. May-September in most endemic areas of the United States. Rural or suburban illness, usually seen in persons with outdoor occupation or recreation, and owners of tick-infested dogs. Tick exposure usual. Has been marked increase in number of cases reported. Dogs important in transporting ticks to people. Numerous small mammals are reservoirs.
Transmission: Usually bites from ticks that have attached 10-20 hours (*R. rickettsii* is avirulent in starving ticks and requires 37^0C, usually through feeding, for reactivation); sometimes skin contamination with tick feces or crushed ticks. Many tick species serve as vectors (1%-13% infected) or reservoirs with lifetime infection as well as transstadial and transovarial transmission.

CONTROL AND PREVENTION
Individual/herd: Treat patients with tetracyclines, improvement within 24-48 hours, continue until afebrile at least 24 hours. Prompt treatment prevents fatalities. Supportive therapy to combat increased capillary permeability and liver damage. Tick surveillance on dogs and humans. Use repellents and careful tick removal.
Local/community: Control ticks through use of insecticides and brush clearance. Reduce small mammal reservoir populations.
National/international: None.

DISEASE: Scrub Typhus

AGENT
Rickettsia tsutsugamushi, multiple antigenic strains

RECOGNITION
Syndrome: Human: Sudden onset of fever, chills, severe headache, malaise, cough, conjunctival injection, generalized lymphadenopathy, pneumonitis. Often primary lesion at site of mite bite. Initial papule becomes multilocular vesicle, then flat black eschar. Second week, macular rash appears on trunk; may remain only a few hours or extend to limbs and persist for days. Differentiate from North Asian tick typhus.
Animal: Generally subclinical in naturally infected animals.
Incubation period: 6-21 days.
Case fatality rate: May reach 60% in older untreated cases whereas almost none in treated.
Confirmatory tests: Culture agent from acute blood. Test paired sera by complement-fixation, or indirect fluorescent antibody.
Occurrence: China, Japan, Southwest Pacific to Siberia and Pakistan. Cases sporadic, more frequent in rural populations. Many small mammal species, especially rodents, are infected.
Transmission: Only by bite of larval mite (*Leptotrombidium* spp.). Other stages do not feed on mammals. The mite species varies with ecosystem and foci tend to be quite circumscribed. Transovarial transmission occurs.

CONTROL AND PREVENTION
Individual/herd: Treat patients with tetracyclines; effective but relapses common unless re-treated beginning on sixth day after terminating first course. Untreated cases may develop deafness, delirium, pneumonitis, encephalitis, cardiac failure. Use mite repellents.
Local/community: Use miticides, rodent control, vegetation clearing.
National/international: None.

9

VIRAL ZOONOSES

Acronyms of Viral Diseases and Tests

AHF: Argentine hemorrhagic fever
BHF: Bolivian hemorrhagic fever
BPS: Bovine papular stomatitis
CCHF: Crimean-Congo hemorrhagic fever
CF: Complement fixation
CP: Cowpox
EEE: Eastern equine encephalitis
EHF: Ebola hemorrhagic fever
ELISA: Enzyme-linked immunosorbent assay
EMC: Encephalomyocarditis
FA: Fluorescent antibody
HA, HB, HC, HD, HE: Viral hepatitis types A, B, C, D, E
HI: Hemagglutination inhibition
HPS: Hantavirus pulmonary syndrome
IFA: Indirect immunofluorescence
JBE: Japanese encephalitis
KFD: Kyasanur Forest disease
LCM: Lymphocytic choriomeningitis
LF: Lassa fever
MVE: Murray Valley encephalitis
ND: Newcastle disease
NSD: Nairobi sheep disease
OHF: Omsk hemorrhagic fever
PCR: Polymerase chain reaction
RIA: Radioimmunoassay
RSSE: Russian spring-summer encephalitis

RVF: Rift Valley fever
SLE: St. Louis encephalitis
SN: Serum neutralization
VEE: Venezuelan equine encephalitis
WEE: Western equine encephalitis
WNF: West Nile fever
WSL: Wesselsbron disease
YF: Yellow fever

VIRAL DISEASES

DISEASE: Argentine Hemorrhagic Fever (AHF)

AGENT
Junin virus; RNA virus, genus *Arenavirus,* family Arenaviridae

RECOGNITION
  Syndrome: Human: Gradual onset of fever, malaise, headache, muscular
    and back aches, retro-orbital pain, conjunctival congestion, and
    gastrointestinal signs. Petechiae appear on the skin and palate, and
    axillary and inguinal lymphadenopathies develop. CNS signs,
    hypotension, and bradycardia develop on about day 4, and hemor-
    rhagic manifestations appear several days later. Bleeding gums and
    epistaxis are most common, although in severe cases hematemesis,
    melena, hemoptysis, or hematuria may occur. Usually, rapid
    improvement occurs after the second week and recovery is complete
    in 1-3 months. However, profuse hemorrhages, pronounced
    neurologic signs, and shock may appear 8-12 days after onset of
    fever, and most of these cases are fatal. Superimposed bacterial
    infections also contribute to mortality.
    Animal: Field rodents with subclinical infections are reservoirs.
  Incubation period: 6-16 days.
  Case fatality rate: 10%-30%.
  Confirmatory tests: Virus isolation requires several weeks. Immunohisto-
    chemical techniques (e.g., immunoperoxidase staining of cell
    culture) can detect viral antigen within a few days. Serologic tests
    are CF, SN, IFA, and ELISA.
  Occurrence: Widespread throughout the Argentine pampas, with most
    cases occurring in a large area west-southwest of Uruguay. Out-

breaks occur annually, and the area where they are recognized is expanding. Male agricultural workers are most often affected.

Transmission: Virus in excreta from rodents most likely transmitted to humans via aerosols, contaminated food or water, or directly inoculated into broken skin. Although interhuman transmission may occur, it is not regarded as contagious.

CONTROL AND PREVENTION

Individual/herd: Immune plasma is effective in treating severe cases. A live attenuated vaccine is available. When caring for patients, general hygienic precautions are sufficient to prevent interhuman transmission.

Local/community: None. Field rodent hosts do not frequent human habitation.

National/international: None.

DISEASE: Bolivian Hemorrhagic Fever (BHF)

AGENT

Machupo virus; RNA virus, genus *Arenavirus,* family Arenaviridae

RECOGNITION

Syndrome: Human: Very similar to AHF. Insidious onset of fever, headache, chills, and conjunctivitis. Hemorrhages (including gingival, nasal, gastrointestinal, and uterine) occur in about one-third of cases between day 4 and 6. A period of hypotension follows a few days later and is a main cause of death. CNS signs, usually tremors but sometimes convulsions and coma, are frequently seen. Survivors experience prolonged convalescence.

Animal: *Calomys callosus,* a hamsterlike rodent, is reservoir in which disease is mild to subclinical, but causing abortion among chronically infected females.

Incubation period: About 2 weeks.

Case fatality rate: 20%-30%.

Confirmatory tests: Virus isolation from febrile patients, or serologic tests (CF, plaque-neutralization in cell culture, IFA) on paired sera.

Occurrence: Outbreaks occurred in northeast Bolivia from 1959 until 1971. No cases have been reported since 1975.

Transmission: By contact with reservoir rodents or their excreta. The rodents occur in the savannahs and fields, but will also enter houses, where they may contaminate food or water. Nosocomial spread by contact with secretions from affected patients may occur.

CONTROL AND PREVENTION

Individual/herd: Avoid contact with rodents and their excreta.

Local/community: Rodent control to eliminate *C. callosus* from homes and peridomestic habitats.

National/international: None.

DISEASE: Bovine Papular Stomatitis (BPS)

AGENT

DNA virus, genus *Parapoxvirus,* family Poxviridae; closely related to contagious ecthyma virus

RECOGNITION

Syndrome: Human: Manifests as a cutaneous nodule or papule 3-8 mm in diameter at the site of virus entry, usually on a finger or hand. The lesion persists for about a month, gradually decreasing in size. No systemic signs in humans.

Animal: Only affects cattle, characterized by proliferative ulcers around the lips and on mucous membranes of the mouth. Lesions begin as small, hyperemic spots and rapidly progress into ulcerous papules that last for a few days to a few weeks. Although the course is generally mild, it may last for several months. Most animals experience only slight fever and little difficulty in grazing, but some develop diarrhea, hypersalivation, and teat lesions.

Incubation period: In humans, 3-8 days.

Case fatality rate: None.

Confirmatory tests: Resembles several, more severe, diseases of cattle, such as foot-and-mouth disease and vesicular stomatitis, and it is important to differentiate among these. May isolate virus, or demonstrate by electron microscopy of lesions.

Occurrence: In cattle, worldwide distribution most often affecting young animals. Only a few confirmed cases of human infection. Because of the minimal lesions, many may go unreported.

Transmission: Direct and indirect contact spread of the virus between animals. Humans are infected from handling or examining infected cattle, the virus usually entering the body through cuts or scratches on the hand.

CONTROL AND PREVENTION

Individual/herd: Because BPS is of minimal economic significance, no control measures are necessary for cattle. Human infection can be prevented by the use of gloves, hand washing, and general caution when working with infected animals.

Local/community: None.
National/international: None.

DISEASE: California (LaCrosse) Encephalitis

AGENT
   RNA virus, genus *Bunyavirus* (group CAL), family Bunyaviridae

RECOGNITION
   Syndrome: Human: Onset is characterized by fever, cephalgia, nausea
      and vomiting, and nuchal rigidity. Lethargy, convulsions, and other
      neurologic signs develop in severe cases on about day 3 and persist
      for approximately a week. Subclinical infection is much more
      common than clinical cases.
      Animal: No known clinical disease in animals.
   Incubation period: About 5-15 days.
   Case fatality rate: Low.
   Confirmatory tests: Serologic tests (HI, CF, SN) are used.
   Occurrence: Occurs mainly in children under 15 years of age, predomi-
      nantly in the eastern and central United States, primarily in
      summer.
   Transmission: Mosquitoborne. Chipmunks and squirrels are reservoirs
      and amplifiers of the virus. The main vector is *Aedes triseratus,* a
      forest-breeding mosquito in whose eggs the virus overwinters, thus
      serving as a reservoir.

CONTROL AND PREVENTION
   Individual/herd: Avoid mosquito bites by use of protective clothing and
      chemical repellents, especially in wooded areas. Screen dwellings
      and use mosquito netting around beds. Spray campsites with
      insecticides.
   Local/community: None.
   National/international: None.

DISEASE: Colorado Tick Fever (CTF)

AGENT
   RNA virus, genus *Orbivirus,* family Reoviridae

RECOGNITION

Syndrome: Human: Sudden onset of fever, chills, headache, retro-ocular pain, and myalgia. Typically, characterized by a few days of illness followed by a few days of remission, then recurrence of illness, which may worsen over several cycles. Young children may occasionally develop hemorrhages, encephalitis, or myocarditis, but the disease is generally milder in adults.

Animal: No clinical signs occur in animals.

Incubation period: 3-6 days.

Case fatality rate: Very low.

Confirmatory tests: Virus isolation, detection of antigen in erythrocytes by FA, or serologic tests (CF, SN), however antibodies do not appear for at least 2 weeks after onset.

Occurrence: Throughout the range of vector ticks in the mountainous western United States and Canada, but more than 80% of cases from Colorado and Wyoming. Occurs in spring and summer when ticks are active.

Transmission: To humans by the bite of adult *Dermacentor andersoni* ticks. The main reservoirs are least chipmunks and golden-mantled ground squirrels, which are hosts to the immature stages of the ticks.

CONTROL AND PREVENTION

Individual/herd: Prevent tick bites by avoiding tick-infested areas whenever possible. When entering tick-infested areas, protective clothing should be worn and chemical repellents used, and the body should be inspected periodically. Any attached ticks should be carefully removed to avoid crushing and to avoid leaving mouth parts in the wound.

Local/community: None.

National/international: None.

DISEASE: Contagious Ecthyma

AGENT

DNA virus, genus *Parapoxvirus,* family Poxviridae; closely related to bovine papular stomatitis

RECOGNITION

Syndrome: Human: Characterized by a (usually) single maculopapular or pustular lesion at the site of virus entry, most often on the hands, arms, or face. The papule is painful and gradually becomes a firm, weeping nodule. Regional lymphadenitis may also occur. Usually, healing is complete in 2-4 weeks, but occasional cases progress into a more widespread cutaneous eruption. Disseminated disease may occur, as well as severe ocular lesions.

Animal: Sheep, goats, domestic camels, and wild ungulates (deer and reindeer) are the reservoir, most infections occurring in young animals. Lesions begin as papules on the skin, eyelids, ears, lips, and nostrils, and progress into vesicles and pustules. Numerous confluent sores cause severe pain and may interfere with the animals' eating. Teats and udders may be affected in females nursing infected young. Although morbidity is often high, mortality is low and usually results from secondary bacterial infection or fly larvae infestation.

Incubation period: In humans, 3-7 days; in sheep and goats, 2-3 days.

Case fatality rate: Humans, none; sheep and goats, low.

Confirmatory tests: In humans, visualize virus particles by electron microscopy of affected tissue or isolate virus. Detect antigen by CF test or demonstrate specific antibody using agar gel diffusion or SN. In domestic animals, clinical signs and history sufficient to establish diagnosis.

Occurrence: Throughout the world wherever sheep and goats are raised. It is an occupational disease of sheep handlers, veterinarians, and abattoir workers, with most cases reported in New Zealand.

Transmission: Direct contact with lesions or mucous membranes of infected animals, or by transfer of the virus via contaminated knives, shears, or other fomites. The live (virulent) vaccine used to protect sheep is also a source of human infection.

CONTROL AND PREVENTION

Individual/herd: A crude live vaccine made from pulverized scabs is used to immunize newborn lambs in endemic areas. Recently, an effective attenuated vaccine has been developed. Persons handling infected animals or administering vaccine should protect the hands by wearing gloves and washing as soon as possible after exposure.

Local/community: None.

National/international: None.

DISEASE: Cowpox (CP)

AGENT

DNA virus, genus *Orthopoxvirus*, family Poxviridae

RECOGNITION

Syndrome: Human: Characterized by lesions at the site of inoculation (usually the hands), and progress from macular, through papular and vesicular stages, to pustule formation. Fever, lymphadenitis, and edema near the lesions may also occur.

Animal: Affects cattle, and has been reported in domestic cats and in felines in zoos. In cattle, onset is characterized by a mild febrile period during which papules appear on the teats. These progress to vesicles, then pustules; when the pustules rupture they leave raw, ulcerated areas that take about a month to heal. CP is similar in domestic cats, with dermal lesions that vary from red, hairless, well-circumscribed areas to ulcerated or purulent spots. Occasionally ulcers may appear on the tongue or lips, and respiratory signs, such as nasal discharge and dyspnea, may develop. Cheetahs have severe respiratory disease.

Incubation period: 3-7 days in humans and cattle.

Case fatality rate: None in humans and cattle; may be high in cats, especially zoo species, if the respiratory tract is affected.

Confirmatory tests: Because CP indistinguishable from vaccinia virus serologically, virus isolation is essential to confirm. Lesion material examined by electron microscopy to detect virions.

Occurrence: Rare, only reported from Great Britain and western Europe.

Transmission: The reservoir is unknown; source of cattle infection is unknown, possibly rodents; humans are infected from the same source or from exposure to affected cattle. In domestic cats, lesions usually develop near a bite wound, possibly sustained while hunting. Infections in zoo felines have been traced to white rats used as feed.

CONTROL AND PREVENTION

Individual/herd: Wear gloves and practice good hygiene when handling infected animals.

Local/community: None.

National/international: None.

DISEASE: Crimean-Congo Hemorrhagic Fever (CCHF)

AGENT

RNA virus, genus *Nairovirus* (group CON), family Bunyaviridae

RECOGNITION

Syndrome: Human: Typically, sudden onset, with high fever and chills, headache, dizziness, and myalgia. Gastrointestinal signs, such as abdominal pain, nausea, vomiting, and diarrhea, are commonly seen, as is bradycardia. The face and neck may be flushed, and the conjunctivae congested. Fever lasts 5-12 days, with hemorrhage beginning about day 4. Bleeding from the nose, gums, kidneys, and gastric mucosa are the most frequent manifestations, and petechiae in the mouth and skin may also be seen. Death usually results from shock caused by blood loss, or from neurologic complications or pulmonary hemorrhage. The hemorrhagic phase continues for some 10-15 days. Patients who survive experience extreme weakness, sweating, headache, and malaise; vision and hearing impairment, loss of memory, and respiratory dysfunction may also occur. Sequelae are not permanent, but may persist for a year or more. Less severe illnesses, with only mild fever and no hemorrhaging, may outnumber the hemorrhagic cases, and subclinical infections occur.

Animal: Subclinical viremia in cattle and sheep.

Incubation period: 3-7 days.

Case fatality rate: 2%-50%.

Confirmatory tests: Virus isolation from acutely ill patients or from autopsy specimens, or various serologic tests (e.g., ELISA).

Occurrence: Usually sporadic cases scattered throughout Eurasia and Africa, generally from June to September, the period of maximal vector activity. The virus has been isolated from southern Europe, central Asia, the Middle East, and much of Africa, but antibodies in humans and animals indicate an even wider distribution. Most human cases occur in rural areas among farmers or livestock handlers, or among medical personnel.

Transmission: Tickborne. Hares, hedgehogs, bats, and birds are the probable vertebrate reservoirs; ticks of the genus *Hyalomma* are arthropod reservoirs. Ticks are infected either transovarially or transstadially when immature stages feed upon infected animals. Other genera of ticks, including *Dermacentor, Rhipicephalus,* and *Boophilus,* may be vectors, and domestic sheep, goats, and cattle can amplify the virus during outbreaks. Humans are infected from bite of an infected tick or when infective fluids from a crushed tick enter broken skin. Infection may also result from contact with viremic animals, such as during butchering or skinning. Inter-human transmission may occur by exposure to blood and secretions of patients.

CONTROL AND PREVENTION

Individual/herd: An inactivated vaccine is available. Avoid tick-infested areas whenever possible. When necessary to enter areas known to harbor ticks, protective clothing should be worn and chemical repellents used, and the body should be inspected every 3-4 hours. Any attached ticks should be carefully removed to avoid crushing and to avoid leaving mouth parts in the wound. Hands should be protected with gloves or cloth when removing ticks. Patients should be isolated, and health-care personnel should exercise caution, wearing protective clothing, masks, and gloves. Any material contaminated with blood should be handled very carefully and disposed of by incineration or sterilized before washing.

Local/community: Although vector populations may be reduced by use of acaricides and host management, these means may be impractical. Public education regarding hazards of tick bite and means of personal protection.

National/international: None.

DISEASE: Eastern Equine Encephalitis (EEE)

AGENT
  RNA virus, genus *Alphavirus* (group A), family Togaviridae

RECOGNITION
  Syndrome: Human: Most commonly seen in persons under 15 and over 50 years of age. In adults, sudden onset of high fever, headache, vomiting, and lethargy, and progresses rapidly to include CNS signs, such as neck stiffness, convulsions, spasticity, delirium, tremors, stupor, and coma. In children, typically manifested by fever, headache, and vomiting for 1-2 days, apparent recovery, then fulminant encephalitis. Retardation or other permanent neurologic sequelae are frequent among survivors of all age groups.
  Animal: Equine infection is characterized by a biphasic febrile course, neurologic signs appearing during the second period of fever; permanent brain damage is common in animals that survive. Outbreaks also occur in commercially raised pheasants, chukars, bobwhite quail, ducks, turkeys, and emus.

  Incubation period: 7-10 days in humans, 18-24 hours in horses.

  Case fatality rate: About 65%-80% in humans, 75%-90% in horses.

  Confirmatory tests: Virus isolation from brain tissue or serologic tests (HI, CF, IFA, SN) of paired sera.

  Occurrence: Restricted to Americas: eastern and central United States and adjacent Canada, parts of Central and South America and Caribbean islands. Most epidemics occur between late August and the first killing frost, and generally begin 1-2 weeks after epidemics in horses. Cases are seen year-round in Florida and other hyperendemic areas.

Transmission: Mosquitoborne. In the eastern United States, mosquitoes of the genus *Culiseta* are major vectors. *Aedes* is important on the Atlantic coast and in the Southwest, where *Coquilletidia* may also be involved. In tropical America *Culex* and *Aedes* species are the main vectors, whereas other species of *Culex* maintain the virus in endemic foci. Birds, especially Passeriformes, are the reservoirs. The mosquitoes feed on infected birds, as well as horses and man, spreading infection. In pheasants the initial infection is mosquitoborne, but can be spread from bird to bird by pecking and cannibalism. Because humans and horses develop only low-level viremia, these species do not play a role in maintaining infection in nature. The term "equine" encephalitis refers only to the species from which the virus was first isolated.

CONTROL AND PREVENTION

Individual/herd: For humans, prevention of mosquito bites through use of protective clothing and chemical repellents, and installation of mosquito netting and screens to exclude mosquitoes from dwellings. A vaccine is available from U.S. Army Medical Research Institute for Infectious Disease, Ft. Detrick, Frederick, MD, and is recommended for researchers and other persons who are frequently and intensively exposed. Immune serum should be administered after accidental exposure to the agent. A multivalent inactivated vaccine is available for horses and birds.

Local/community: Education of public as to mode of spread and control; control of mosquitoes in area.

National/international: None.

DISEASE: Ebola Hemorrhagic Fever (EHF)

AGENT

RNA virus, genus *Filovirus,* family Filoviridae

RECOGNITION

Syndrome: Human: Clinically similar to Marburg disease. Sudden onset, the first signs being headache, fever, myalgia, and nausea, followed a few days later by development of a maculopapular rash, sore throat, diarrhea, and vomiting. Hemorrhage, ranging from mild to life-threatening, may begin early in the clinical course and usually takes the form of epistaxis, melena, hematemesis, and bloody diarrhea, and blood may seep from needle punctures. Death results from hemorrhage, shock, or renal and/or hepatic failure. In survivors of severe disease, convalescence is slow and often accompanied by desquamation of the skin. Subclinical infections and mild illness may occur.

Animal: Febrile illness in experimentally infected primates similar to humans.

Incubation period: 2-21 days.

Case fatality rate: 50%-90% in humans; 100% in experimentally infected primates.

Confirmatory tests: Virus isolation is very hazardous. Serologic tests include IFA, ELISA, and Western blot.

Occurrence: Major outbreaks with high fatality rates in humans occurred from 1976 to 1979 in Sudan and Zaire. Antibodies to EHF have been detected elsewhere in Africa, suggesting that subclinical infection also occurs. Fatal infection with an ebola-like virus occurred among monkeys in a research laboratory in Washington, D.C., in 1989. This virus was evidently imported in crab-eating monkeys from the Philippines, and has not been associated with human illness, although several animal handlers exposed to the monkeys developed antibodies.

Transmission: By direct contact with blood and other bodily fluids of affected patients; EHF virus persists in semen for many weeks after clinical recovery. Nosocomial outbreaks have resulted from use of contaminated syringes and needles. Spread by aerosol is also possible. No nonhuman reservoir or vector has been implicated.

CONTROL AND PREVENTION

Individual/herd: Infected persons should be kept in strict isolation and those involved in their care wear gloves, masks, and protective clothing. All excreta, sputum, blood, and other secretions should be sterilized by autoclaving before disposal, as should objects that come in contact with a patient or the patient's blood (laboratory glassware, etc.). Sexual intercourse with male survivors should be avoided until it is established that semen is free of virus. In case of accidental exposure via needle stick or other penetration of the skin, oral ribavirin should be administered. There is no vaccine.

Local/community: If an outbreak occurs, the public should be alerted to the communicability of EHF and the need for extreme caution when caring for patients. Handling of the deceased should be kept to a minimum and cremation is preferable to traditional burial.

National/international: None.

DISEASE: Encephalomyocarditis (EMC)

AGENT
RNA virus, genus *Cardiovirus,* family Picornaviridae

RECOGNITION
Syndrome: Human: Usually manifests as a brief fever and severe headache. May develop neck stiffness, abnormal reflexes, or paralysis. There is no myocardial involvement in humans, and recovery is complete and without sequelae in a few days. Most infections are subclinical.

Animal: A serious disease of young swine, and can cause death with no premonitory signs. In less acute cases, animals develop fever, anorexia, paralysis, hydropericarditis, and ascites. Meningitis and myocardial degeneration occur in fatal cases. Cattle may also be affected, with myocardial lesions. Also occurs in monkeys, which are at first sluggish and anoretic, progressing to paralysis and convulsions prior to death.

Incubation period: Unknown.

Case fatality rate: None in humans; 5%-50% in swine.

Confirmatory tests: For humans, virus isolation, or serologic tests (SN, HI) on paired sera. Animal infection confirmed by virus isolation.

Occurrence: Rare in humans. Virus has been isolated throughout the world. Human outbreaks have been recorded only in the Philippines, Germany, and the Netherlands, but in various regions up to 34% of children and 51% of adults have antibodies. Outbreaks in swine have occurred in the United States, Cuba, Panama, Australia, and New Zealand.

Transmission: Neither the reservoir nor the mode of transmission has been established. The virus is frequently isolated from rats, but it is also found in many other mammals and birds. Spread by food or water contaminated by droppings from infected animals is suspected, or by consumption of their meat or viscera.

CONTROL AND PREVENTION
Individual/herd: Because EMC is rare in humans, control measures are not considered practical. Although there is need for protection of swine, the lack of understanding of the epidemiology of EMC precludes the development of effective prevention.

Local/community: None.

National/international: None.

DISEASE: *Hantavirus* Pulmonary Syndrome (HPS)

AGENT
>   Muerto Canyon and other as yet unnamed viruses; RNA viruses, genus
>   *Hantavirus,* family Bunyaviridae

RECOGNITION
>   **Syndrome:** Human: A prodromal period of fever, achiness, and cough
>   is followed by sudden onset of acute respiratory distress. Headache
>   and abdominal pain, nausea, and vomiting also occur in early stages.
>   Bilateral pulmonary infiltrates, hypoxia, and hypotension develop as
>   the illness progresses. Most deaths have been associated with
>   respiratory failure, shock, and severe lactic acidosis. Survivors
>   recover without sequelae.
>   Animal: No clinical disease is known.
>
>   **Incubation period:** Unknown.
>   **Case fatality rate:** 60% of the first 55 cases reported.
>   **Confirmatory tests:** ELISA, PCR, and immunohistochemical staining
>   have been used.
>   **Occurrence:** A newly recognized manifestation of hantaviral infection
>   thus far only reported from the United States, with confirmed cases
>   in 15 states, most west of the Mississippi River (New Mexico,
>   Arizona, Colorado); only two cases have been reported from outside
>   the range of the deer mouse (Louisiana, Florida). Most have
>   occurred in spring and summer.
>   **Transmission:** Each strain of *Hantavirus* evidently has its own rodent
>   reservoir: Muerto Canyon virus, deer mouse; antigenically distinct
>   virus in Florida, cotton rat; virus in Louisiana, rodent unknown.
>   Apparently spread by inhalation of virus in aerosols from contami-
>   nated rodent feces or urine. All known cases were rural residents or
>   visited rural areas within 6 weeks of onset.

CONTROL AND PREVENTION
>   **Individual/herd:** In endemic areas, eliminate rodents from homes and
>   prevent them from entering. Pest control workers and persons
>   cleaning rodent-infested structures should wear protective clothing
>   (e.g. gloves, respirators, etc.) and avoid creating aerosols.
>   **Local/community:** Municipal rodent control.
>   **National/international:** None.

DISEASE: *Hantavirus* Renal Syndromes

AGENT
Hantaan, Seoul, and Puumala viruses; RNA viruses, genus *Hantavirus,* family Bunyaviridae

RECOGNITION
Syndrome: Human: Syndromes that primarily affect the kidneys range from severe—hemorrhagic fever with renal syndrome (HFRS), epidemic hemorrhagic fever (EHF), Korean hemorrhagic fever (KHF)—to mild—nephropathia epidemica (NE). Regardless of severity, almost all cases are characterized by sudden onset of high fever, chills, and pain in back, muscles, and abdomen. Hemorrhage and degree of renal impairment vary with the syndrome. In the severe forms, a petechial rash often occurs on the face and elsewhere on the body, and petechial hemorrhages develop on the soft palate and pharynx. As fever declines, hypotension begins, lasting from a few hours to a few days. Oliguria follows the hypotensive phase, and during this period hemorrhages, ranging from blood in urine and sputum to intracranial bleeding, may result from increased capillary fragility. The final stage is characterized by diuresis, which persists for a few days to several weeks. Recovery is slow but usually complete, although several months may be required to regain complete renal function. Most deaths caused by disseminated intravascular coagulation during the oliguric phase, but shock resulting from hypotension is also a significant cause. In the mild form, polyuria is common, and may follow an initial oliguria or anuria. Proteinuria and enlarged kidneys occur frequently. Overt hemorrhage develops in only about one-third of the cases (epistaxis being the most common manifestation), but hematuria is detected in up to 85%. The clinical course most often is uncomplicated and recovery rapid, although some renal impairment may persist for several months afterward.
Animal: Hantaviruses produce subclinical infections in rodents, which are the reservoir: striped field mouse for Hantaan virus, Norway rat for Seoul strain, and several European voles for Puumala virus.
Incubation period: 1-8 weeks, usually 2-3 weeks.
Case fatality rate: 5% or more for HFRS and KHF; less than 1% for NE.
Confirmatory tests: PCR can be used to detect hantaviruses in tissue, and serologic tests (IFA, SN, HI, ELISA, solid-phase RIA) are available.

Occurrence: Hantaviral renal syndromes occur in localized areas throughout much of Eurasia. Most cases are sporadic, but epidemics may occur, usually coincident with irruptions in rodent populations. Males 20-50 years of age, especially farmers and rural residents, are most often affected. Women are affected much less frequently and cases among children are rare. HFRS occurs over wide areas in the Far East, mostly in summer, but KHF cases peak in spring and autumn. NE occurs in Scandinavia and other parts of Europe and may occur in any month, but most epidemics have been in late summer, autumn, and early winter. Antibodies to the Seoul virus have been found in Norway rats in cities worldwide, including areas where no human hantaviral disease has been reported.

Transmission: Probably by inhalation of virus in aerosols from urine or feces of reservoir rodents. Human-to-human transmission has not been reported.

CONTROL AND PREVENTION

Individual/herd: Ribavirin may be used to treat patients. Excluding rodents from homes and avoiding contact with rodents whenever possible help to prevent infection.

Local/community: Rodent control in towns and villages.

National/international: None.

DISEASE: *Herpesvirus simiae* (B) Infection

AGENT

DNA virus, genus *Herpesvirus,* family Herpesviridae, closely related to the human herpes simplex virus.

RECOGNITION

Syndrome: Human: Initially, the wound site of cutaneous inoculation becomes hyperemic and painful and vesicles appear at the site. A regional lymphadenopathy develops, followed by sudden onset of fever and headache, with nausea, abdominal pain, and diarrhea; vesicles may also appear in the pharyngeal area. Signs of meningo-encephalitis develop, including vertigo, diaphragmatic spasm, photophobia, neck stiffness, and difficulty in swallowing. Flaccid paralysis of the lower extremities spreads to the upper extremities and thorax and leads to respiratory failure and death, usually within 5-28 days after onset. Most survivors have permanent neurologic sequelae.

Animal: Among nonhuman primates, *H. simiae* infection is similar to human herpes simplex infection. Small vesicles appear (generally in the mouth), ulcerate, then heal within a few days. The condition is benign and often goes unnoticed unless lesions appear on the lips, conjunctivae, or skin.

Incubation period: In humans, 3 days to 3 weeks.

Case fatality rate: 70%-85% in humans, none in monkeys.

Confirmatory tests: Virus isolation from the brain. Serologic test (SN) if patient survives.

Occurrence: Common in Asian monkeys of the genus *Macaca,* especially rhesus. A similar virus (SA-8) has been isolated from patas monkeys, African green monkeys, and baboons. Although rare in humans, veterinarians, animal care workers, and others having contact with Old World monkeys or monkey-cell cultures are at risk.

Transmission: Among monkeys, transmitted by direct contact, bites, scratches, and saliva-contaminated food or water. Humans are infected from monkey bites or when saliva from an infected monkey comes in contact with broken or abraded skin. The infection has also been acquired from conjunctival, nasal, or pharyngeal exposure to contaminated aerosols.

CONTROL AND PREVENTION

Individual/herd: Monkey handlers and others coming in contact with Old World monkeys should take precautions to prevent bites. Gloves, masks, and protective clothing should be worn. Any bite or scratch wound from a monkey or an object (e.g., cage wires, etc.) possibly contaminated with monkey secretions should be scrubbed immediately with soap and water and thoroughly disinfected with an iodine solution. Prompt treatment, either topical or parenteral, with acyclovir may be an effective prophylaxis. The animal should be observed for at least 2 weeks and its B-virus status determined. If vesicular lesions appear at the wound site, or if itching, numbness, or pain develops near the wound, immediate expert medical advice should be sought. No vaccine is available. Monkeys should not be housed in large groups, with no more than two per cage recommended. Recently imported monkeys should be quarantined for at least 6 weeks and any that have or develop herpetiform lesions should be destroyed. Rhesus monkeys should not be housed with any other species.

Local/community: None.

National/international: None.

DISEASE: Influenza

AGENT
RNA viruses, genus *Influenzavirus* (types A and B), family Orthomyxoviridae; type C is in a separate, unnamed genus.

RECOGNITION
Syndrome: Human: An acute respiratory disease. Signs of types A and B typically include fever, chills, headache and muscular aches, malaise, pharyngitis, and cough. Gastrointestinal signs, such as nausea, vomiting, and diarrhea, occur more in children than in adults. Type C is a milder illness, in which lacrimation, sneezing, and runny nose are more pronounced than in A and B; subclinical infection is frequent in type C. Generally most severe among the elderly and those with chronic, debilitating conditions, and other immunosuppressed persons, and it is among these groups that most deaths occur. May be complicated by pneumonia, both viral and bacterial. Reye syndrome, which affects the CNS and liver, may occur as a sequela in children who have taken aspirin during the illness. Recovery is usually complete in about a week.
Animal: Type A occurs most notably in swine, horses, and birds. In pigs, there is abrupt onset with inappetence, coughing, coryza, dyspnea, and fever. Recovery in uncomplicated cases is rapid, and subclinical infections occur. Type C also occurs in swine. In horses, signs include high fever, abundant nasal discharge, coughing, dyspnea, and depression lasting some 2-10 days, followed by 1-3 weeks of convalescence. Often more serious in colts than in mature horses. Avian influenza ("fowl plague") is most known for its effects on commercial poultry, and ranges from a subclinical or mild infection to severe disease with high mortality. Signs include anorexia, decreased egg production, coughing, sneezing, facial edema, coryza, and diarrhea. Other species from which influenza viruses have been isolated or antibodies detected include whales, fur seals, harbor seals, and dogs.
Incubation period: Human, 1-5 days; animal, 2-3 days.
Case fatality rate: Low in humans, swine, and adult horses, although in some human pandemics mortality has increased significantly. High in colts and seals, and may approach 100% in severe poultry outbreaks.
Confirmatory tests: Virus isolation from throat or nasal washings early in the illness. Serologic tests (HI, CF, SN) of paired sera.

Occurrence: Worldwide, usually in epidemics or pandemics, with high morbidity and generally low mortality, and sporadic cases. Type A causes most pandemics and annual epidemics, whereas type B outbreaks are less widespread and occur at less-frequent intervals. Sporadic cases and small clusters of infection are often attributable to type C. The attack rate during epidemics ranges 10%-30% in the general population, but in institutions, such as schools, nursing homes, etc., up to 70% of susceptible individuals may be affected. Generally occurs during the autumn and winter in temperate regions; in the tropics most cases occur during the rainy season, but sporadic outbreaks may occur in any month.

Transmission: Mainly by inhalation of aerosols and by direct contact with droplets. Among birds, also by the fecal-oral route. Type A is a zoonosis because there are instances, although few, of virus transmission between animals and humans. Several persons in contact with pigs have developed influenza with the same serotype as found in the swine, and marine biologists have been infected from seals. It is theorized that animal reservoirs provide a source of new strains that can affect humans, possibly by reassortment with existing human serotypes. In support of this hypothesis is the fact that the frequent changes in surface antigens that characterize type A serotypes do not occur in type B viruses, which do not occur in animals.

CONTROL AND PREVENTION

Individual/herd: Inactivated type A vaccines are highly effective when the serotypes in the vaccine match those currently circulating. For this reason, vaccines are reformulated annually to incorporate strains most likely to cause outbreaks. Because of the frequent changes in antigenic structure of type A viruses, vaccination is generally effective for only one season. Persons at high risk, e.g., the elderly, especially nursing home residents, immunosuppressed, and those with asthma or other respiratory problems, as well as health care workers and family members of people at high risk should be vaccinated. Avoid crowds during epidemics. Amantadine or rimantadine administered early in the illness can help alleviate symptoms and reduce the amount of virus in secretions. Inactivated vaccines are also available for horses and swine.

Local/community: Vaccination campaigns can help reduce the magnitude of epidemics.

National/international: None.

DISEASE: Japanese (B) Encephalitis (JBE)

AGENT
RNA virus, genus *Flavivirus* (group B), family Togaviridae

RECOGNITION
Syndrome: Human: Often subclinical, and mild systemic disease without neurologic signs may occur. Usually sudden onset of fever, headache, nuchal rigidity, prostration, and CNS signs. Sensory disturbances and convulsions often occur, with progression into coma in fatal cases. Highest fever is usually at 4-5 days, followed by gradual subsidence. Residual sequelae (motor, neurologic, and/or physiologic) are common in all ages, but especially so in children under 4 years.

Animal: Abortion and neonatal mortality in swine. Infected adult pigs have few signs beyond a brief fever; suckling pigs occasionally have encephalitis. Equine infection is usually subclinical; and morbidity low in cattle, sheep, and goats.

Incubation period: In humans, ≥4-14 days.

Case fatality rate: 20%-50% in humans; 50%-70% in swine; up to 25% in horses.

Confirmatory tests: Virus isolation from brain or from swine fetuses. Serologic tests used are HI, SN, and CF. A RIA is available for humans. The HI test can detect specific IgM antibodies, eliminating cross-reactions with SLE, WNF, or MVE antibodies.

Occurrence: Widespread in Asia, from Japan to India. In tropical areas, sporadic human cases occur all year, with epidemics in the rainy season. In temperate climates, epidemic outbreaks are seen in late summer and early autumn.

Transmission: Mosquitoborne. Infected swine are the primary means of virus amplification, although wild herons and egrets are also reservoirs. The virus may overwinter in frogs and snakes. *Culex tritaeniorhynchus* is the main vector in China and Japan, transmitting the virus to wild birds, swine, cattle, dogs, and humans.

CONTROL AND PREVENTION
Individual/herd: Prevention of mosquito bites through protective clothing, use of repellents, and avoidance of areas in which mosquitoes are active. A vaccine available from Connaught Laboratories is recommended for persons working with the virus, and for travelers to or residents of endemic areas if their risk of exposure is high. Inactivated and modified live vaccines are available for swine and horses.

Local/community: Mass vaccinations of swine are effective in reducing the prevalence of the virus. Mosquito control.

National/international: None.

DISEASE: Kyasanur Forest Disease (KFD)

AGENT

RNA virus, genus *Flavivirus* (group B), family Togaviridae; closely related to Omsk hemorrhagic fever

RECOGNITION

Syndrome: Human: Sudden onset, with fever, chills, headache, lower back and leg pain, insomnia, and anorexia. Diarrhea and vomiting are common. Fever usually abates after 1-1½ weeks, but many patients relapse after an afebrile period of 1-3 weeks. Neurologic signs, including neck stiffness, confusion, and tremors, often appear during the second phase of fever, which lasts for a few days to a week or more. Nasal and gastrointestinal bleeding may occur late in the course of fatal cases. Convalescence is usually slow.

Animal: Langurs and bonnet monkeys are severely affected. They are useful sentinels because mortality in monkeys indicates the virus is active and that a human outbreak is imminent. A biphasic disease occurs, characterized by initial viremia with erythrophagocytosis and thrombocytopenia, followed by encephalitis. Shortly before death there is a drop in blood pressure, bradycardia, epistaxis, diarrhea, and extensive hemorrhages.

Incubation period: About 8 days in humans.

Case fatality rate: 5%-10% in humans; high in nonhuman primates.

Confirmatory tests: Virus isolation, or serologic tests (CF, HI, SN, ELISA) on paired sera.

Occurrence: India only, mainly in the Kyasanur Forest. Reservoirs are probably rodents and shrews. Most cases occur in young male agricultural workers who go into the forest during the dry season (November to June). Epidemics cease when monsoon rains begin.

Transmission: Tickborne. KFD virus occurs in several species of forest rats, shrews, and mice, indicating a rodent reservoir. The main vector is *Haemaphysalis spinigera*, although KFD has been isolated from other *Haemaphysalis* and *Ixodes* species. Transovarial transmission maintains infection in the vectors. Humans become infected when bitten by the nymphal stage of *H. spinigera*.

CONTROL AND PREVENTION

Individual/herd: The usual tick-avoidance measures, i.e., protective clothing, chemical repellents, etc., are impractical among the population most affected. An inactivated vaccine has been developed, but a live attenuated vaccine is being developed that evidently will be more effective, providing 70%-100% protection for at least 18 months.

Local/community: None.

National/international: None.

DISEASE: Lassa Fever (LF)

AGENT

RNA virus, genus *Arenavirus,* family Arenaviridae

RECOGNITION

Syndrome: Human: The course is 1-4 weeks with gradual onset of malaise, headache, myalgia, general weakness, and fever. Pronounced pharyngitis, usually with small pharyngeal ulcers, and often edema of the face and neck. Thoracic pain, labored breathing, and coughing occur commonly, and abdominal pain, vomiting, and diarrhea may occur. Severe cases are characterized by hemorrhage from mucous membranes, encephalopathy, seizures, hypotension, and shock, and death is usually attributable to cardiac failure. More severe among pregnant women, causing abortion in over 80%; generally milder in children. Convalescence is slow and survivors may experience transient alopecia and ataxia; deafness, which follows 25% of illnesses, may be permanent. Subclinical infections probably outnumber clinical by at least 10 to 1.

Animal: Clinical signs do not occur in animals.

Incubation period: 1-3 weeks.

Case fatality rate: Probably 1%-2% of all infections; 15%-50% in hospitalized patients.

Confirmatory tests: Virus isolation. Serologic tests (ELISA, IFA).

Occurrence: Widespread in West Africa. Outbreaks have occurred in Nigeria, Liberia, and Sierra Leone, and antibodies detected in Guinea, the Central African Republic, Mali, Senegal, Cameroon, and Benin. Endemic in Sierra Leone, with community-acquired cases occurring in any month, whereas in Nigeria and Liberia LF has appeared during the dry season. Outbreaks in these two countries have been nosocomial (more than 1/3 of all LF cases), spreading from an index case.

Transmission: The reservoir is *Mastomys natalensis,* a rat widely distributed in sub-Saharan Africa. This rodent is both domestic and peridomestic, and in some areas of western Africa it is the most common rodent in dwellings. Some also hunt *M. natalensis* for food. LFV is spread horizontally among rats by contact with infectious excreta, and vertical transmission may occur. Community-acquired human infections result from direct or indirect contact with rodent urine or feces. Person-to-person transmission via contact with patient blood and other secretions is common, and airborne spread from persons with pulmonary infection may occur.

CONTROL AND PREVENTION

Individual/herd: Suspected LF patients should be maintained in strict isolation. Hospital personnel should wear protective clothing, including masks and gloves. Extreme care should be taken when handling blood or items contaminated with blood or other body fluids. All excreta, sputum, blood, and any object in contact with these or other secretions should be chemically disinfected, then autoclaved, incinerated, or boiled. Oral ribavirin should be administered to those with definite high-risk exposure, such as a needle stick; LF patients should be treated early with intravenous ribavirin. There is no vaccine.

Local/community: Control of *M. natalensis.*

National/international: Country of destination must be notified if an international traveler is exposed.

DISEASE: Louping III

AGENT

RNA virus, genus *Flavivirus* (group B), family Togaviridae; closely related to Russian spring-summer encephalitis

RECOGNITION

Syndrome: Human: Usually has a biphasic course, the first phase lasting up to 12 days and being characterized by fever, headache, malaise, and retro-orbital pain. These signs abate for about 5 days before onset of the second phase in which variable neurologic signs occur and the disease may be mistaken for meningoencephalitis or poliomyelitis. Convalescence is often prolonged.

Animal: In sheep, may be a biphasic febrile illness, although many recover after the first phase. If the virus invades the CNS, however, encephalomyelitis results, producing motor incoordination, tremors, a hopping gait, and, finally, prostration. Immunosuppressed animals are more likely to develop encephalomyelitis. Also seen occasionally in cattle, horses, and deer. Red grouse are severely affected, with high mortality occurring in chicks less than 2 months old.

Incubation period: Two to 8 days in humans; a few days to several weeks in animals.

Case fatality rate: Almost none in humans; in sheep, up to 50% with encephalomyelitis.

Confirmatory tests: For humans, virus isolation from blood (first phase) or CSF (second phase). In animals with encephalomyelitis, isolate virus from brain. Serologic tests (SN, CF, HI) useful.

Occurrence: Restricted to Ireland, Scotland, Wales, and northern England. Rare in humans; in sheep, outbreaks occur mainly in spring, early summer, and autumn.

Transmission: The vector is the tick *Ixodes ricinus,* and sheep are the main reservoir. Tick larvae and nymphs are infected when they feed on viremic sheep; the virus is transmitted transstadially to adult ticks. Inhalation by abattoir workers or accidental inoculation in the laboratory have been the main routes of human infection, perhaps because *I. ricinus* rarely bites humans.

CONTROL AND PREVENTION

Individual/herd: Tick control. An inactivated vaccine is available for sheep.

Local/community: None.

National/international: None.

DISEASE: Lymphocytic Choriomeningitis (LCM)

AGENT

RNA virus, genus *Arenavirus,* family Arenaviridae

RECOGNITION

Syndrome: Human: Generally mild, often has influenza-like signs, sometimes with orchitis and parotitis, and a course of only a few days. Occasionally, relapse occurs, and develop meningitis, or meningeal signs may begin initially. In these cases, LCM is characterized by nuchal rigidity, headache, fever, muscular pains, and malaise. Meningoencephalitis, with paralysis, somnolence, and coma, may occur in rare instances, as well as cases with hemorrhagic manifestations. Most patients, even those most severely affected, recover without sequelae, although convalescence is slow.

Animal: Usually no signs in naturally infected. Experimentally infected adult mice become immunosuppressed and have convulsions that are often fatal, but survivors recover fully and are no longer infected. When mice are infected as infants, however, growth is retarded and some die, but survivors develop a chronic infection with glomerulonephritis that persists lifelong.

Incubation period: Usually 1-2 weeks in humans, 2-3 weeks when initial meningitis; 5-6 days in experimentally infected mice.

Case fatality rate: Very low in humans and naturally infected rodents.

Confirmatory tests: Virus isolation from blood of febrile patients or CSF when meningitis. Serologic tests (CF, SN, IFA).

Occurrence: Widespread, LCM found in the Americas, Europe, and Asia. Although human LCM is not uncommon, it is probably underdiagnosed. Most cases are sporadic, but outbreaks may occur.

Transmission: Reservoir is the house mouse. Infected mice excrete LCM in urine, feces, and saliva; humans are infected from contaminated food, aerosols, mouse bites, or through breaks in the skin. Not transmitted from person to person.

CONTROL AND PREVENTION

Individual/herd: Eliminate mice from home and workplace, and thoroughly clean nest areas. Maintain surveillance to ensure that research mouse colonies are free from LCM.

Local/community: None.

National/international: None.

DISEASE: Marburg Disease

AGENT
RNA virus, genus *Filovirus,* family Filoviridae

RECOGNITION
Syndrome: Human: Similar to EHF. Sudden onset of fever, headache, prostration, muscle and joint aches, vomiting and diarrhea. A maculopapular rash and hemorrhagic signs such as gastrointestinal bleeding and epistaxis follow; conjunctivitis, jaundice, and renal involvement may also develop. Death may occur after about 7-8 days. Survivors have prolonged convalescence.

Animal: Only evidence from fatal experimental infections in rhesus, squirrel, and African green monkeys. Initial signs anorexia and weight loss; later may develop dyspnea, diarrhea, and bleeding from the rectum or vagina. Terminally, a sudden drop in body temperature occurs.

Incubation period: 4-9 days in humans, 2-6 days in experimentally infected monkeys.

Case fatality rate: About 25% in humans, usually fatal in experimentally infected monkeys that develop clinical illness.

Confirmatory tests: Serologic tests (IFA, ELISA, or Western blot). Virus isolation is extremely hazardous.

Occurrence: First recognized in 1967 in Marburg and Frankfurt, Germany, and in Belgrade, Yugoslavia, among laboratory personnel who had handled tissues from African green monkeys imported from Uganda. A few non-laboratory-associated cases have occurred in South Africa (although the index case originated in Zimbabwe) and Kenya.

Transmission: The reservoir is unknown; antibodies have not been found in wild green monkeys. Transmission to humans occurs by contact with infected blood, secretions, or tissues; in the initial outbreak, laboratory personnel exposed only to live monkeys were not infected. Nosocomial infections among contacts of patients have occurred, and airborne spread may occur. Sexual transmission via semen can occur many weeks after clinical recovery.

CONTROL AND PREVENTION
Individual/herd: Same as EHF.
Local/community: None.
National/international: None.

DISEASE: Monkeypox

AGENT
DNA virus, genus *Orthopoxvirus,* family Poxviridae

RECOGNITION
Syndrome: Human: Similar to smallpox, usually begins with fatigue, fever of 2-4 days' duration, headache, myalgia, pronounced lymphadenopathy of the neck and groin, and back pain. A generalized rash appears over the body and face, and lesions progress from macules to papules, vesicles, pustules, and scabs over approximately 10 days. Desquamation follows and lasts up to 3 weeks, leaving scars with initial hypopigmentation and later hyperpigmentation.

Animal: Severity varies with the species, anthropoid apes being more seriously affected than monkeys. Early signs include fever, anxiety, aggression, and anorexia. The cutaneous lesions are usually minor, the papules evolving into pustules containing a thick, purulent material, then umbilicating before desquamation. Most lesions appear on the buttocks, hands, and feet, but oral, pharyngeal, and tracheal eruptions also occur. A more serious form is characterized by pronounced facial edema, ulceration of mucous membranes, generalized lymphadenopathy, and respiratory distress. Death from asphyxia may result.

Incubation period: Human, 7-21 days; nonhuman primates, 3-4 days.

Case fatality rate: Human, about 10%-15%, low in nonhuman primates.

Confirmatory tests: Virus isolation from lesions. Serologic tests (RIA, immunodiffusion, ELISA).

Occurrence: Rainforest areas of western and central Africa. Human infections emerged in 1970 and have increased after smallpox vaccination was discontinued in 1980. Most cases have occurred in children.

Transmission: The reservoir evidently is squirrels. Both primates and humans can be infected by contact with infected animals, and airborne transmission is possible. Occasional human-to-human transmission has occurred.

CONTROL AND PREVENTION

Individual/herd: Patients should be isolated and health care workers should be vaccinated against smallpox. Care should be taken when working with infected animals; masks, gloves, and protective clothing should be worn.

Local/community: None.

National/international: None.

DISEASE: Murray Valley Encephalitis (MVE)

AGENT

RNA virus, genus *Flavivirus* (group B), family Togaviridae

RECOGNITION

Syndrome: Human: Similar to JBE, with children under 10 years of age and the elderly affected more frequently and more severely than other age groups. Signs include fever, headache, anorexia, irritability, myalgia, and vomiting. CNS effects include mental confusion, difficulty in swallowing, hyperactive reflexes, convulsions, and coma. Clinical course is about 2 weeks in both fatal and nonfatal cases. Neurologic or psychiatric sequelae are common among survivors. Subclinical infections are more common than overt encephalitis. Animal: Horses, cattle, dogs, and poultry may be infected, but do not develop clinical disease. Antibodies have been found in foxes, marsupials, and wild birds.

Incubation period: About 4-14 days.

Case fatality rate: 20%-60%.

Confirmatory tests: Virus isolation from CNS, serologic tests (HI, CF, SN), SN used to distinguish antibodies from other flaviviruses, especially Kunjin virus.

Occurrence: Widespread throughout Australia and New Guinea. Most outbreaks have occurred in the Murray-Darling River basin. Epidemics in summer and autumn in southern Australia are usually preceded by above normal rainfall during the spring in northern Australia.

Transmission: Mosquitoborne, but the cycle of infection is unclear. *Culex annulirostris* is considered the major vector. The virus may possibly circulate between birds and mosquitoes, but it is not known if domestic and wild mammals amplify the agent. Experimentally, many birds and mammals may be infected.

CONTROL AND PREVENTION

Individual/herd: Prevention of mosquito bites is the most effective means of preventing MVE. *C. annulirostris* is most active before dawn and after dusk. Use of protective clothing and repellents, avoidance of outdoor activities during periods of maximal vector activity, and excluding the insects from dwellings by installing screens and using mosquito netting are helpful. No vaccines are available.

Local/community: Mosquito vector control.

National/international: None.

DISEASE: Nairobi Sheep Disease (NSD)

AGENT

RNA virus, genus *Nairovirus* (ungrouped), family Bunyaviridae

RECOGNITION

Syndrome: Human: Usually subclinical. Some experience a transient influenza-like syndrome with a diphasic fever.

Animal: A hemorrhagic gastroenteritis occurs in sheep and goats. Usually subclinical among indigenous animals, whereas newly introduced susceptible animals become anoretic, have a mucopurulent nasal discharge and a fetid diarrhea which eventually becomes bloody. Pregnant animals frequently abort. Death may occur in 24 hours.

Case fatality rate: For humans, 0%. For sheep, 30%-90%; for goats, 0%-30%.

Incubation period: 4-15 days.

Confirmatory tests: Identify virus microscopically (FA) in mice or tissue culture infected from blood, spleen, or mesenteric node of patient. Detect antibody by IFA.

Occurrence: Endemic in East Africa, with serologic evidence of infection from Ethiopia to South Africa. Serologic evidence that human infection is common in endemic areas. Outbreaks in small ruminants occur when susceptible animals are moved into endemic areas.

Transmission: Tickborne. Viremia occurs during the febrile period. *Rhipicephalus appendiculatus* is the primary vector, but *Amblyomma* spp. have also been incriminated. The virus can survive in ticks for two years, and transovarial and transstadial transmission occur. The virus is maintained in a sheep-tick-sheep cycle. Transmission by blood transfusion from currently viremic persons can occur. Infection results in complete immunity.

CONTROL AND PREVENTION

Individual/herd: Prevent tick attachment by wearing protective clothing and using repellents in endemic areas. Remove attached ticks every few hours. Control ticks on animals by weekly dipping or spraying. An attenuated live virus vaccine is available for sheep and goats, but it is not very satisfactory. An experimental inactivated vaccine has provided excellent protection against laboratory challenge. Because of the mild disease, vaccination of humans is not indicated.

Local/community: Perform serologic screening of blood donors. Prevent spread of infected ticks from endemic areas by restricting animal movement.

National/international: None.

DISEASE: Newcastle Disease (ND)

AGENT

RNA virus, genus *Paramyxovirus,* family Paramyxoviridae

RECOGNITION

Syndrome: Human: Manifests primarily as conjunctivitis, usually unilateral, with congestion, lacrimation, pain, swelling of subconjunctival tissues, and pre-auricular lymphadenitis. Generally no systemic involvement, but persons exposed to aerosols develop an influenza-like illness of 3-4 days' duration. Recovery is complete in about a week. Subclinical infections also occur.

Animal: Among numerous bird species affected, chickens and turkeys are especially susceptible. Most common signs are respiratory, nervous, or both. Severity of outbreaks vary with the NDV strain; lentogenic strains are the least virulent, velogenic are the most, and mesogenic strains are intermediate. If the respiratory tract is affected, birds gasp and cough; neurologic signs include drooping wings, torticollis, circling, depression, anorexia, and paralysis. In laying flocks, egg production may cease. Viscerotropic syndrome is a more serious form, caused by some velogenic strains, characterized by sudden onset of watery, greenish diarrhea, tracheal discharge, and edema of the face and wattles; petechial hemorrhages occur in the mucosa of the proventriculus, and the intestinal mucosa becomes necrotic. Death often occurs in 1-3 days.

Incubation period: In humans, usually 1-2 days; 2-15 days in birds with respiratory or CNS disease, 2-4 days for viscerotropic.

Case fatality rate: None in humans. In poultry can range from none (with lentogenic strains) to 100% (in some outbreaks of velogenic viscerotropic disease).

Confirmatory tests: In humans, virus isolation is the only definitive test because a serologic response may not occur. In poultry, virus isolation early in an outbreak. Serologic tests include HI, SN, and ELISA.

Occurrence: Worldwide in wild birds, semidomestic, and domestic fowl in both epidemic and endemic forms, and is of major economic importance to poultry production. Human ND is rare, and usually occurs among laboratory personnel, poultry abattoir workers, and poultry vaccinators using live vaccines.

Transmission: Chickens are the main reservoir. NDV is spread from bird to bird mainly by aerosols, although NDV is also present in feces; the density of birds in commercial poultry farms facilitates transmission. Humans become infected when NDV contacts the eyes, as from aerosolized vaccines.

CONTROL AND PREVENTION

Individual/herd: Avian ND can be controlled by maintaining good hygiene on poultry farms, separating poultry houses, and vaccination. Human ND can be prevented by the use of goggles and masks when vaccinating poultry, and by using care to avoid aerosols when working with NDV in the laboratory.

Local/community: None.

National/international: Imported live birds of any species should be quarantined, and imports from countries where ND occurs should be prohibited.

DISEASE: Omsk Hemorrhagic Fever (OHF)

AGENT
RNA virus, genus *Flavivirus* (group B), family Togaviridae; closely related to Kyasanur Forest disease

RECOGNITION
Syndrome: Human: Sudden onset of fever, with headache and pain in legs and back. Diarrhea and vomiting follow, and bronchopneumonia often develops. CNS involvement is rare, but hemorrhage is seen in severe cases. Bleeding from the gums, nose, gastrointestinal tract, and uterus has been reported, and hematemesis and bloody stools may also occur. Leukopenia is common, and hypotension may develop even when hemorrhage is absent. The fever lasts about 5 days to 2 weeks, and may take a biphasic course, recurring after an afebrile period. Convalescence may be prolonged, and accompanied by alopecia.

Animal: Many small mammals are reservoirs of the virus, but the muskrat, an exotic species imported from North America to Russia in the 1920s and 1930s, is the only animal severely affected. In muskrats, OHF causes hemorrhages, marked viremia, and high mortality. The Siberian muskrat population was decimated by an epidemic in the mid-1940s, and subsequent outbreaks have prevented the species from ever recovering its earlier numbers. Infection in other mammals produces only subclinical or mild transitory illness.

Incubation period: 2-9 days in humans.

Case fatality rate: 1%-3% in humans; high in muskrats.

Confirmatory tests: Virus isolation from febrile patients, or serologic (SN, CF, HI) tests.

Occurrence: Throughout the forest steppes of western Siberia, with outbreaks occurring in the Omsk, Novosibirsk, Kurgan, and Tyumen regions.

Transmission: *Dermacentor pictus* ticks are both vectors and reservoirs, OHF virus being transmitted transovarially. It is unclear how muskrats become infected, inasmuch as they are not parasitized by ticks, but the European water vole is, and it shares the muskrats' large houses. Water voles may transmit the virus to muskrats via infected mites or some other means. Humans may be exposed while trapping and handling muskrats, or by drinking, or contact with, water contaminated by feces or urine of infected mammals. Humans, particularly agricultural workers, may be infected by tick bite.

CONTROL AND PREVENTION

Individual/herd: A highly effective vaccine is available for humans. However, because of adverse reactions associated with its use, and the low incidence and mortality rate of OHF, widespread use of the vaccine is not advisable. Individuals can take measures in tick-infested areas to prevent tick bites, such as wearing of long-sleeved shirts and long pants tucked into socks, use of repellents, and frequent inspection of the body to remove any ticks present.

Local/community: None.

National/international: None.

DISEASE: Pseudocowpox

AGENT

DNA virus, genus *Parapoxvirus,* family Poxviridae, closely related to BPS and contagious ecthyma

RECOGNITION

Syndrome: Human: Small, erythematous papules appear, usually on the hands, and over 4-6 weeks develop into firm nodules before resolving. There is no systemic involvement.

Animal: Papular lesions that umbilicate and pustulate appear on the udders and teats of dairy cows. Dark red scabs remain for about 2 weeks. In some cases lesions may persist longer, and often recur. Nursing calves may develop oral lesions.

Incubation period: Human, 5-7 days.

Case fatality rate: None.

Confirmatory tests: Electron microscopy of lesion fluid. Virus isolation from lesions.

Occurrence: Worldwide, but the prevalence is not well known. Many subclinical infections. Human infection mainly where milking is done by hand.

Transmission: Dairy cattle are the reservoir. Infection spreads within a herd by contamination of milking machines or the hands of milkers. Humans are infected by contact through skin abrasions.

CONTROL AND PREVENTION

Individual/herd: Good hygienic standards should be maintained in dairies, and infected cows milked last. Only treatment is topical ointment applied to teats. Acquired immunity is of short duration, and there is no vaccine.

Local/community: None.

National/international: None.

DISEASE: Rabies

AGENT

RNA virus, genus *Lyssavirus,* family Rhabdoviridae. Strain differences in virulence as well as reservoir host-related (i.e., bat, fox, etc. source) glycoprotein surface antigens.

RECOGNITION

Syndrome: Human: Onset is characterized by apprehension, headache, low-grade fever, malaise, and vague sensory changes, discomfort, and irritation in the area of a previous animal bite. Optic and auditory hyperesthesia develop. Paresis or paralysis follows, and spasmodic contractions of deglutitory muscles when attempting to swallow cause the patient to avoid liquids ("hydrophobia") and to stop swallowing saliva. Delirium and convulsions usually precede death from respiratory failure.

Animal: In dogs, rabies may occur as either a furious or paralytic ("dumb") form. The furious form begins with agitation, restlessness, and excitability. Aggression follows, with the dog attempting to bite objects, other animals, humans, and itself. Profuse salivation occurs, because spasms of deglutitory muscles prevent swallowing; the vocal cords are affected, altering the normal vocal sound. Terminally, convulsions and paralysis develop. Paralytic form begins with paralysis of the muscles of the head and neck, causing difficulty in swallowing. Paralysis of the extremities follows, then general paralysis and death. Cats usually develop the furious form, whereas cattle generally develop the paralytic form. In wild foxes, skunks, and raccoons, the furious form is more common than paralytic.

Incubation period: Variable, dependent on amount of virus received, site, and severity of bite wound. In humans, 5 days to a year or more, but usually 2-8 weeks; dogs, 10-60 days; cattle, 25-≥150 days; wild animals usually 10-180 days.

Case fatality rate: Almost 100% in all species.

Confirmatory tests: Direct FA (corneal impressions, lingual scrapings, or frozen skin sections from the nuchal area can be tested while the subject is alive). If human exposure, need test results within a day. Virus isolation from brain or salivary glands.

Occurrence: Worldwide, except for Australia, New Zealand, New Guinea, Japan, most of Oceania, some Caribbean islands, Uruguay, Great Britain, Ireland, the Netherlands, Norway, Sweden, Spain, and Portugal. In endemic regions, two cycles may occur: urban and sylvatic. Urban rabies, which accounts for most human cases, is transmitted by dogs; sylvatic rabies circulates among wild carnivores and bats, with some infection of dogs, cats, and livestock. World-wide, over 30,000 people die of rabies each year, most in developing nations.

Transmission: Most cases result from the bite of an infected animal; the virus is abundant in saliva. A few human cases have resulted from corneal transplants when rabies was the unsuspected cause of death of the donor. Airborne transmission may occur in bat caves.

CONTROL AND PREVENTION

Individual/herd: All dogs and cats should be vaccinated. In areas where vampire bats transmit rabies, valuable cattle and horses may be vaccinated. Although most vaccines are now inactivated, be sure any live (attenuated) vaccines are used only in the specific species intended because they may be virulent for others. Dogs and cats that have bitten a person should be quarantined and observed for at least 10 days; if signs of rabies appear the animal should be killed and its brain examined by FA microscopy. Wild animals that have bitten persons should be killed immediately and examined. If they have escaped, assume they are rabid. Any unvaccinated animal that is bitten by a rabid animal should be destroyed or quarantined for 6 months. In the event of a bite from a known or suspected rabid animal, immediate and thorough cleansing of the wound is essential. Flush with a strong stream of water and wash with soap or detergent, then a disinfectant, such as alcohol, tincture of iodine, or quaternary ammonium compounds, should be applied. The area around the wound should be infiltrated with antiserum, and suturing should be avoided or delayed to allow bleeding and drainage. For individuals without pre-exposure immunization, post-exposure prophylaxis consists of an injection of rabies immune globulin (RIG), half infiltrated around the wound site and half injected intramuscularly. This is followed by administration of vaccine, preferably human diploid cell vaccine (HDCV) in a 5-dose course. If the exposed person has had a full pre-exposure course of HDCV, RIG is not necessary and give only 2 doses of HDCV. Persons at risk, such as animal control personnel, veterinarians, field zoologists, etc., should receive pre-exposure prophylaxis and periodic boosters based on antibody response. HDCV is preferable, but is expensive and not generally available in all countries.

Local/community: Educate the public as to the need to vaccinate dogs and cats. Enforce animal control laws and eliminate stray animals. Avoid animals acting strangely and report them to animal control authorities. Control vampire bats. Oral vaccines are effective in free-ranging carnivore (e.g., fox, dog) populations.

National/international: Health certification and proof of vaccination should be required for importation of dogs. For rabies-free areas, enact and enforce laws requiring prolonged quarantine of dogs and other carnivores to be imported.

DISEASE: Rift Valley Fever (RVF)

AGENT
RNA virus, genus *Phlebovirus* (ungrouped), family Bunyaviridae

RECOGNITION
Syndrome: Human: Sudden onset of chills, muscular and back pain, headache, nausea, and fever lasting for a week or more. Most cases are mild and uncomplicated, with recovery complete in about 3 weeks. Of the severe forms there are three manifestations: hemorrhagic RVF, RVF with meningoencephalitis; and RVF with retinitis. Most fatalities occur among those with the hemorrhagic form, which begins with fever for 2-4 days, then progresses to jaundice and hemorrhages, including hematemesis, melena, hemorrhagic gingivitis, and dermal petechiae and purpura; hepatic necrosis may be found postmortem. The meningoencephalitic form follows the initial febrile period after 5-15 days, causing disorientation, hallucination, and vertigo, with meningitis and pleocytosis common. In the retinal form, patients experience loss of visual acuity 5-15 days after onset of fever, often with bilateral retinal lesions. Permanent loss of central vision is common among individuals with severe lesions.
Animal: Sheep, goats, cattle, and buffalo are most frequently affected. In some outbreaks, only lambs are affected, whereas in others, adults are affected. In newborn lambs the disease is rapid, without definite signs, and highly fatal. Pregnant ewes often abort; among nonpregnant adults, vomiting may be the only sign of illness. Cattle may abort, and often have a fever of short duration as well as anorexia, hypersalivation, and diarrhea. Dogs and cats may also be affected, with abortion in pregnant females.
Incubation period: In humans, 2-7 days; in animals, 1-2 days.
Case fatality rate: Human, about 3%; 18%-20% in ruminants. High mortality in puppies and kittens. May reach 95% among newborn lambs.
Confirmatory tests: Human infection in acute phase can be diagnosed by isolation of virus from blood. Serologic testing (SN, CF, HI, IFA, gel diffusion, and ELISA) of paired sera. Rapid diagnosis by seeding cell culture and performing FA test the next day.

Occurrence: Widespread throughout Africa, most south of the Sahara. Heavy rains in late summer and autumn, which allow the vector population to increase, are precursors to epidemics, although outbreaks also recorded in irrigated areas.

Transmission: Generally mosquitoborne. Species of at least six mosquito genera, including *Aedes* and *Culex,* transmit RVF virus, as do biting flies *Culicoides* and *Simulium,* which are mechanical vectors. The reservoir is unknown, but may be rodents or bats. Domestic sheep and cattle play a role in maintaining and amplifying the virus. Humans are highly susceptible, and usually are infected by contact with tissues of infected animals, e.g. veterinarians and persons slaughtering diseased livestock. Aerosol transmission is a factor in human infection. Because humans maintain a viremia for more than a week, they may be involved in virus amplification.

CONTROL AND PREVENTION

Individual/herd: Inactivated or modified live vaccines may be used to protect domestic animals. The modified live vaccine may cause abortion and it cannot be used in newborn animals. Because of the possibility of reversion to a virulent form, it should not be used in nonendemic areas. The risk of human infection during an outbreak can be lessened by carefully handling diseased or dead animals, and by use of protective clothing. An inactivated vaccine is available to protect individuals at high risk.

Local/community: Because domestic livestock are the main amplifiers of the virus, immunization programs may help prevent outbreaks. Butchering of diseased animals should be prohibited.

National/international: Restrict movement of animals from endemic areas.

DISEASE: Russian Spring-Summer Encephalitis (RSSE)

AGENT
RNA virus of genus *Flavivirus* (group B), Togaviridae; closely related to louping ill

RECOGNITION
Syndrome: Human: Early clinical signs resemble those of mosquitoborne encephalitides: sudden onset of severe headache, fever, nausea and vomiting, asthenia, hyperesthesia, and photophobia. Blurred or otherwise distorted vision, vertigo, delirium, and coma often follow. Flaccid paralysis of the upper extremities and back musculature and

epileptiform seizures distinguish RSSE from other similar diseases. The fever generally lasts 2-7 days, and survivors experience protracted convalescence and, often, residual paralysis. Death may occur 1-7 days after onset. Inapparent infections also occur.

Animal: Clinical disease rarely occurs in animals, although dogs and lambs are occasionally affected. The virus has also been isolated from rodents, goats, and cattle.

Incubation period: 8-20 days.

Case fatality rate: About 20%.

Confirmatory tests: Virus isolation from patients. Serologic tests are CF, HI, SN, and ELISA. Although these tests cannot differentiate RSSE from louping ill and other tickborne viral encephalitides, they do distinguish RSSE from other non-tickborne forms of encephalitis.

Occurrence: Mostly in wooded, rural areas of Asiatic regions of the former USSR. Seasonality is related to the periods when vector ticks are most active.

Transmission: From the bite of infected ticks, usually *Ixodes persulcatus*. There is no person-to-person transmission. Small mammals, mainly rodents and bats, are reservoirs and amplifiers of the virus, and larval ticks acquire the virus from these animals. RSSE virus is transmitted transstadially through the nymphal stages to adult ticks, both of which parasitize, and infect, domestic ruminants.

CONTROL AND PREVENTION

Individual/herd: As with other tickborne diseases, the wearing of protective clothing, chemical repellents, and frequent inspection of the body for ticks can help prevent bites. An inactivated vaccine is available for persons at high risk, such as forestry and agricultural workers.

Local/community: Education of public as to the dangers of RSSE and tick-avoidance methods.

National/international: None.

DISEASE: St. Louis Encephalitis (SLE)

AGENT

RNA virus, genus *Flavivirus* (group B), family Togaviridae

RECOGNITION

Syndrome: Human: Most infections are subclinical. There are three major clinical forms: febrile disease, aseptic meningitis, and encephalitis. The febrile course, which is the most common, is

usually not life threatening with fever and severe headache of several days' duration. Aseptic meningitis is characterized by sudden onset of fever, neck stiffness, and abnormal muscular flexion, although neurologic function is not impaired. In the encephalitic phase, fever of sudden onset accompanied by evidence of brain inflammation, such as a personality change, confusion, delirium, lethargy, paresis, or convulsions, is seen. This form occurs more often in patients over 60 years old.
Animal: Subclinical only.

Incubation period: Estimated to be 4-21 days.

Case fatality rate: 5%-10% in humans, higher among those over 50 years of age.

Confirmatory tests: Serologic testing (CF, SN, HI) of paired sera is the only reliable means of diagnosis.

Occurrence: Americas from Canada to Argentina. Occurring mainly in late summer and early autumn, most years SLE ranks either first or second among causes of arboviral encephalitides in the United States. It is endemic and sporadic in the western United States, with epidemics occurring only rarely. In the East, however, outbreaks are more frequent, and also occur in Canada and Mexico. Occasional cases occur in the Caribbean and Central and South America, but epidemics have not been recorded in these areas.

Transmission: Mosquitoes of the genus *Culex* transmit the virus from infected birds, which serve as the reservoir, to humans. Peridomestic birds, such as house sparrows and pigeons, and domestic fowl, amplify and maintain the virus; migratory birds spread it from area to area. Humans are accidental hosts and have no role in the natural cycle of SLE, nor do most wild or domestic mammals, in which viremia is mild and transitory. Bats may maintain the virus during the winter in temperate climates.

CONTROL AND PREVENTION

Individual/herd: Prevent mosquito bites through protective clothing and use of repellents. Prevent mosquitoes from entering dwellings by screening windows and doors. No vaccine is available.

Local/community: Mosquito control.

National/international: None.

DISEASE: Sicilian Sandfly Fever

AGENT
RNA virus, genus *Phlebovirus* (group PHL), family Bunyaviridae

RECOGNITION

Syndrome: Human: Sudden onset of high fever, muscular aches, headache, sore throat, retro-orbital pain, and conjunctivitis lasting 3-5 days.

Animal: Unknown.

Incubation period: Usually 3-4 days.

Case fatality rate: None.

Confirmatory tests: Serologic detection of specific IgM, or virus isolation.

Occurrence: In Mediterranean and other areas of Europe, Asia, and Africa where the vector occurs. Usually occurs between April and October, particularly in troops and tourists from outside endemic areas.

Transmission: By the bite of an infected sandfly, *Phlebotomus papatasi*. Gerbils may be reservoir.

CONTROL AND PREVENTION

Individual/herd: Prevent sandfly bites by use of screens on windows, mosquito netting, etc., and avoid areas, particularly at night, where vector may be active. Applications of insecticides to living areas are also helpful.

Local/community: Mass control of sandfly populations.

National/international: None.

DISEASE: Tanapox

AGENT

Unnamed DNA virus, family Poxviridae; related to Yaba virus

RECOGNITION

Syndrome: Human: Characterized by fever of 3-4 days' duration, possibly with headache, backache, and prostration, followed by eruption of one or two papules on the face, arms, neck, or trunk. Pustules do not form, but the lesions may umbilicate. No permanent damage to the skin.

Animal: In macaques, lesions may be single or multiple and occur on the face, chest, and perianal areas. They are raised, firm, circular areas that become umbilicated and covered with a central scab. May be up to 8 weeks before the most severe lesions resolve. Infections in African green monkeys are subclinical.

Incubation period: Unknown for humans; 4-5 days for monkeys.

Case fatality rate: None.

Confirmatory tests: Virus isolation from lesions.

Occurrence: Kenya. Humans in contact with infected monkeys are at risk.

Transmission: African green monkeys are the reservoir. In primate centers, other species may become infected by direct or indirect contact; airborne transmission is possible. Human epidemics may have involved an arthropod vector.

CONTROL AND PREVENTION

Individual/herd: In research facilities, African and Asian monkeys should be separated and good hygiene practiced. Monkeys can be vaccinated against tanapox. Animal care workers should use caution when handling monkeys and seek medical attention for any cuts or abrasions. Smallpox vaccination is not protective.

Local/community: None.

National/international: None.

DISEASE: Venezuelan Equine Encephalitis (VEE)

AGENT

RNA virus, genus *Alphavirus* (group A), family Togaviridae, endemic and epidemic strains

RECOGNITION

Syndrome: Human: A range of clinical signs from nonspecific fever to influenza-like signs to encephalitis, but is usually a mild to severe respiratory infection. Usually rapid onset of fever, malaise, chills, retro-orbital and muscular pain, headache, nausea, vomiting, and diarrhea. Acute illness lasts 1-4 days or more, and length of convalescence is proportional to the duration of fever. Recovery is rapid and complete when febrile course is short, but patients experience profound weakness with prolonged fever, and convalescence may take several weeks. Permanent sequelae seldom develop. Encephalitis similar to other mosquitoborne encephalitides is more often seen in children. Meningitis is rare.

Animal: VEE produces clinical signs only in the Equidae, although many vertebrate species have been infected with VEE virus. In some equines the disease is mild, with fever of a few days' duration, anorexia, and depression. Viremia may be low-titer, and affected animals recover without sequelae. The encephalomyelitic form, however, is more typical and more severe, producing a viremia of high titer. It has a sudden onset of high fever, depression, anorexia and weight loss, grinding of teeth, and diarrhea or constipation. Neurologic signs, including imbalance, stupor, falling, excitation, circling, and convulsions, are frequent.

Incubation period: 1-6 days for humans; 1-3 for equines.

Case fatality rate: Usually 0.2%-1% in humans, but may be higher in absence of adequate medical care. Up to 80% in equines.

Confirmatory tests: Direct isolation of virus from blood or nasopharyngeal washings during the first 72 hours of illness; serologic testing of paired sera, or detection of specific IgM.

Occurrence: Americas only. Endemic from the southern United States through the Caribbean and Central America, to northern South America. Outbreaks occur mainly in northern and western South America, but have spread through Central America into the United States.

Transmission: Mosquitoborne. Endemic serotypes are maintained by a rodent-mosquito cycle, and humans are exposed only when they enter foci of the virus, such as swampy areas within rain forests. *Culex, Aedes, Mansonia, Psorophora, Haemagogus, Sabethes,* and *Anopheles* mosquitoes may be infected with these virus types, whereas the main reservoirs are rodents. Marsupials may also be involved, and one subtype is maintained in birds. In the virus type that causes human epidemics, horses function as the major amplifiers. *Psorophora, Aedes, Mansonia,* and *Anopheles* are the vectors in epidemic disease, as well as biting flies *Culicoides* and *Simulium.*

CONTROL AND PREVENTION

Individual/herd: Use of protective clothing and repellents to prevent mosquito bites, avoidance of areas in which mosquitoes are active. A live attenuated vaccine, available from USAMRIID, should be used to protect individuals at high risk. Horses may also be immunized.

Local/community: Mass immunization of horses and prevent movement from affected areas to non-affected areas. Institute mosquito vector control programs.

National/international: None.

DISEASE: Vesicular Stomatitis (VS)

AGENT

RNA virus, Indiana (3 subtypes) and New Jersey serotypes, genus *Vesiculovirus,* family Rhabdoviridae

RECOGNITION

Syndrome: Human: Sudden onset of fever, headache, retro-orbital pain, and muscle aches. Vesicles may appear in the mouth or pharynx, or on the hands, and gastrointestinal signs, including nausea, vomiting, and diarrhea, sometimes occur. Most cases are mild and of short duration.

Animal: Initially similar to foot-and-mouth disease (FMD does not affect horses), with fever followed by papules and vesicles developing in the mouth, on udders, in interdigital spaces, and on the coronary band; there may also be an increase in salivation. Animals usually recover in about a week. Infections are usually subclinical.

Incubation period: 1-2 days in humans, 2-4 days in animals.

Case fatality rate: None in humans, low in animals.

Confirmatory tests: Serologic tests (CF, SN) of paired sera. Virus isolation from lesions.

Occurrence: Western Hemisphere only; endemic in tropical and semitropical forests, particularly in Central and South America. Sporadic outbreaks occur in temperate regions (north and south) of the hemisphere. Some epidemiologic differences (host, locality) between the serotypes. Most human cases have been laboratory acquired, but high antibody prevalence exists in some endemic areas. Occurs in cattle, horses, swine, and less often, sheep. Wild animals, such as bats, carnivores, and rodents, may be infected.

Transmission: Mechanisms not completely known, but VSV may circulate between arboreal and semiarboreal wild animals and arthropods; VSV has been isolated from *Aedes* mosquitoes, and sandflies of the genus *Lutzomyia* can transmit VSV vertically. When teat lesions are present, can directly transmit from an infected cow during milking. VSV is also found in saliva, and contamination of a preexisting wound with saliva can also transmit. Humans are infected by inhalation of aerosols or through breaks in the skin, both in the laboratory and by direct contact with infected animals.

CONTROL AND PREVENTION

Individual/herd: Wear gloves and protective clothing when handling infected animals, practice good hygiene, and seek medical attention for cuts or abrasions. Prevent contact between diseased and healthy animals; natural immunity does not persist, and no cross-protection between strains. There is no vaccine for humans.

Local/community: None.

National/international: None.

DISEASE: Viral Hepatitis Type A (HA)

AGENT

Hepatitis A virus (HAV); RNA virus, genus *Enterovirus,* family Picornaviridae

RECOGNITION

Syndrome: Human: Sudden onset of fever, malaise, anorexia, and nausea. Dark urine and jaundice may also develop. Generally more serious in adults, often subclinical in children.

Animal: Nonhuman primates are susceptible to HA infection, although many are subclinical. Clinical manifestations are variable, and can range from mild respiratory involvement to nonspecific gastrointestinal signs. Anorexia and persistent diarrhea may occur.

Incubation period: Human, 15-50 days; 3-4 weeks in nonhuman primates.

Case fatality rate: <1.0% in humans.

Confirmatory tests: Serologic testing to detect IgM anti-HAV in paired sera.

Occurrence: Worldwide, most commonly among older children and young adults, and may be sporadic or epidemic. In many developing nations, adults are immune because of prior infection. Humans and nonhuman primates are reservoirs.

Transmission: Shed in feces, with the highest concentrations occurring late in incubation period and early in illness. Among humans, transmission is primarily person-to-person, usually by the fecal-oral route, and is facilitated by poor hygiene. Infected food handlers are often the cause of outbreaks, and infections are common at day-care centers with diapered children. Intravenous drug users are frequently infected, as are sexual and other intimate contacts of acutely ill. Contaminated water or food also may be sources. Clams, oysters, and other filter-feeders from contaminated waters are often a source. Nonhuman primates are infected via ingestion of contaminated food or water or coprophagy; humans may become infected from exposure to infected primates when hygienic precautions are not observed.

CONTROL AND PREVENTION

Individual/herd: Food handlers should practice careful hygiene and wash hands frequently. Travelers to endemic areas who may be at high risk should receive pre-exposure IG. While in endemic areas, avoid drinking unbottled water or beverages with ice and eating uncooked shellfish or uncooked fruits or vegetables. Care in handling nonhuman primates is important to avoid contact with excreta.

Local/community: Public education campaigns should be conducted to alert people to the mode of spread of the virus and to emphasize the importance of good hygiene, especially thorough hand washing and the sanitary disposal of feces. Proper sewage and water treatment systems should be provided.

National/international: None.

DISEASE: Viral Hepatitis Type B (HB)

AGENT

Hepatitis B virus (HBV); DNA virus, genus *Hepadnavirus,* family Hepadnaviridae

RECOGNITION

Syndrome: Human: Insidious onset of anorexia, malaise, and gastrointestinal signs, frequently progressing to jaundice. Mild fever, arthralgias, and skin rashes may also occur. Severity is variable, from subclinical to fulminant life threatening. Chronic infections can develop, particularly if infected in infancy or early childhood; a long-term carrier state, often progressing to cirrhosis, may result. Is a major cause of primary hepatocellular carcinoma, and may be responsible for up to 80% of cases worldwide.

Animal: Nonhuman primates are susceptible to infection, as antibodies have been detected in several species, but clinical disease is rare. Infections in cynomolgus monkeys caused anorexia, lethargy, and hepatomegaly, and infected chimpanzees also developed jaundice.

Incubation period: In humans, 45-180 days, average 120 days. Over 180 days in chimpanzees.

Case fatality rate: About 1.4% of reported human cases.

Confirmatory tests: RIA or ELISA testing for HBV surface antigen (HBsAg) or other markers.

Occurrence: Worldwide, and variably endemic. In the United States, western Europe, and Australia, HB is of low endemicity. In these areas, infection usually contracted in young adulthood, and less than 1% of the population are chronically infected. Intravenous drug addicts, homosexual men, heterosexuals with multiple partners, and health care personnel who have frequent and routine exposure to blood and other body fluids are at greatest risk. In China, Southeast Asia, Africa, Oceania, the Middle East, and the Amazon Basin, HB is highly endemic. Most HB in these countries is acquired at birth or during childhood, and 8%-15% of the population are carriers. In moderately endemic areas, 2%-7% of the population have chronic infections. High prevalence rates of HB antibodies have been found in some species of nonhuman primates.

Transmission: In humans, mainly by percutaneous or permucosal contact with infective body fluids. Contaminated needles and syringes contribute to spread among drug addicts, and is also transmitted by sexual activity. In highly endemic areas, perinatal infection is frequent.

CONTROL AND PREVENTION

Individual/herd: Vaccines are available and should be administered to individuals at high risk. Pregnant women should be screened for HBsAg, and newborn infants of those testing positive should receive HB immunoglobulin (HBIG). Persons exposed via percutaneous or permucosal contact should receive HBIG and vaccine. Blood donated to blood banks should be tested for HBsAg. Gloves should be worn when handling infected animals or when there is likelihood of skin contact with infectious material.

Local/community: In hyperendemic and moderately endemic areas, vaccinate infants and children.

National/international: None.

DISEASE: Viral Hepatitis Type C (HC)

AGENT
Hepatitis C virus (HCV); unclassified RNA virus, possibly a flavivirus

RECOGNITION

Syndrome: Human: Insidious onset of anorexia, gastrointestinal discomfort, nausea, and vomiting; jaundice develops less frequently than in HB. Severity is variable, from subclinical to fulminating, although rarely life threatening. Chronic HC develops in about 50% of patients but does not usually progress to cirrhosis; clinical improvement is often seen within 2-3 years.

Animal: Chimpanzees may be infected with HCV, and typical liver lesions produced, but clinical and biochemical changes may not occur.

Incubation period: In humans, usually about 6-9 weeks.

Case fatality rate: Low.

Confirmatory tests: Serologic testing. Most with chronic HC have antibodies, but there may be a long period after onset of acute disease before detectable antibodies develop.

Occurrence: Worldwide. In the United States, causes 20%-40% of community-acquired acute viral hepatitis and about 90% of post-transfusion hepatitis. Groups at high risk include transfusion recipients, users of illicit parenteral drugs, dialysis patients, health care workers who have frequent contact with blood and persons who have had hepatitis in the past, and household and sexual contacts of infected persons. Spontaneous HC infections have not been reported in nonhuman hosts.

Transmission: Percutaneous exposure to blood or plasma from an infected person, either by direct contact (e.g., transfusion) or by contaminated needles and syringes, is most common. Exposure by person-to-person contact and sexual activity also may occur.

CONTROL AND PREVENTION

Individual/herd: Similar to HB. Because of the lack of a sensitive test for HCV antibodies, blood banks should discard any donated units with elevated liver enzyme levels. The value of administration of prophylactic IG to persons exposed to HC has not been established. Interferon may be useful in treating patients with chronic disease. No vaccine is available. Gloves should be worn when handling infected chimpanzees and when there is likelihood of skin contact with infectious material.

Local/community: None.

National/international: None.

DISEASE: Viral Hepatitis Type D (HD)

AGENT

Hepatitis delta virus (HDV), a defective RNA virus that requires the presence of HBV to replicate

RECOGNITION

Syndrome: Human: Always occurs either concurrently with acute HB, or superimposed upon an existing chronic HB infection. Clinical signs are similar to HB, and are usually of abrupt onset. Usually more severe in superinfections than in co-infections, and often leads to chronic HD.

Animal: Clinical signs develop when infect HBV-infected chimpanzees.

Incubation period: Uncertain in humans; 2-10 weeks in chimpanzees.

Case fatality rate: Similar to HB.

Confirmatory tests: Serologic testing (RIA, ELISA).

Occurrence: Worldwide, mostly among populations with high HB prevalence. Epidemics have occurred in Brazil, Venezuela, Colombia, and the Central African Republic. In the United States, groups at highest risk are hemophiliacs and others receiving blood or blood derivatives, users of parenteral street drugs, health care workers who have frequent contact with blood or infected persons, and male homosexuals. Spontaneous HD infection has not been reported in nonhuman hosts.

Transmission: Same as HB.

CONTROL AND PREVENTION

Individual/herd: Same as HB. HDV cannot occur in the absence of HB. No vaccine is available for HD, and neither IG nor HBIG protects against HDV superinfection. Gloves should be worn when handling infected animals or when there is likelihood of skin contact with infectious material.

Local/community: In endemic areas, vaccination of infants and children against HB will also reduce occurrence of HD.

National/international: None.

DISEASE: Viral Hepatitis Type E (HE)

AGENT

Not yet completely characterized, but serologically distinct from other hepatitis viruses.

RECOGNITION

Syndrome: Human: Similar to HA, with sudden onset of fever, malaise, anorexia, and nausea; dark urine and jaundice are often present. Chronicity does not develop.

Animal: Clinical signs develop in experimentally infected chimpanzees, cynomolgus macaques, owl monkeys, tamarins, and marmosets. Natural infections may occur.

Incubation period: 15-64 days, usually 26-42 days in humans.

Case fatality rate: Generally less than 1%, except may reach 20% among pregnant women in the third trimester.

Confirmatory tests: Diagnosis by serologically excluding other hepatitis viruses, especially HA.

Occurrence: Epidemics have occurred in Asia, North and East Africa, and Mexico. Not endemic in the United States or western Europe, as cases in these countries have been limited to travelers returning from endemic areas. Young to middle-aged adults, especially men, are most often affected. Children and the elderly seldom affected.

Transmission: Fecal-oral route, with contaminated water the source of most epidemics. Poor hygiene can also result in person-to-person transmission.

CONTROL AND PREVENTION
Individual/herd: In endemic areas, avoid drinking unbottled water or beverages with ice and eating uncooked shellfish or uncooked fruits or vegetables. Avoid fecal-oral exposure. No vaccine is available.

Local/community: Proper sewage disposal. Chlorinate public water supplies.

National/international: None.

DISEASE: Wesselsbron Disease (WSL)

AGENT
RNA virus, genus *Flavivirus* (group B), family Togaviridae

RECOGNITION
Syndrome: Human: Most infections are subclinical. Illness may be very mild, but the usual signs include fever, headache, and pain in muscles and joints; a rash and cutaneous hypersensitivity sometimes occur. Although the fever is usually only 2-3 days, muscular pain may continue for an extended period. Recovery is often complete after 4-5 days.

Animal: Similar to RVF, affects mainly sheep. Animals of all ages are susceptible, and neonatal mortality may be high. In addition, causes abortion and death among pregnant ewes, although nonpregnant females have only fever. In fatal cases the liver is affected, with areas of necrotic foci. Only fever produced in cattle, horses, and swine. Nevertheless, in some endemic areas up to 50% of cattle have antibodies, and abortions and fetal abnormalities have been attributed to WSL.

Incubation period: In humans, usually 2-4 days; in sheep, 1-4 days.

Case fatality rate: Low in humans; in sheep, high in newborn lambs and pregnant ewes.

Confirmatory tests: For humans, isolation of virus during febrile state or serologic testing of paired sera. For sheep, virus isolation from necropsy specimens.

Occurrence: Widespread throughout Africa, a disease of the late summer and autumn, particularly in low-lying, humid areas. In

South Africa, prevalence of antibodies in ruminants may reach 50%. Subclinical human infection common in endemic areas.

Transmission: Species of *Aedes* mosquitoes are vectors. The complete cycle is not well-established, although sheep and cattle develop a high-titer viremia for 3-4 days which can amplify the virus for mosquito infection. Rodents and birds may be reservoirs. Disease may occur among persons who handle infected tissue.

CONTROL AND PREVENTION

Individual/herd: Nonpregnant sheep and lambs over 6 months old may be immunized with an attenuated live vaccine. Veterinarians or others in contact with infected animals should wear gloves and protective clothing and take precautions to prevent aerosols.

Local/community: Mass immunization of sheep, and control of vector mosquitoes.

National/international: None.

DISEASE: Western Equine Encephalitis (WEE)

AGENT

RNA virus, genus *Alphavirus* (group A), family Togaviridae

RECOGNITION

Syndrome: Human: In adults, sudden onset with fever, headache, neck and back stiffness, lethargy, vision disturbances, and vertigo; mental confusion is common. In children, neurologic signs are preceded by fever, headache, and malaise; convulsions, vomiting, and neck stiffness often follow, and flaccid and spastic paralyses are more frequent than in adults. Fever persists for 7-10 days. Adults usually recover without permanent sequelae, but children often have mental retardation, spastic paralysis, and recurrent convulsions.

Animal: Of the species susceptible to infection, only horses and emus develop clinical illness, although not all affected animals will develop encephalitis. Neurologic signs, e.g., restlessness, unsteady gait, lack of coordination, and somnolence, appear after fever and viremia have ceased. Neurologic sequelae, usually abnormal reflexes, are common among animals that survive.

Incubation period: ≥5-10 days in humans, 1-3 weeks in horses.

Case fatality rate: In humans, 3%-14%; in horses, usually 20%-30%, but can be as high as 50%.

Confirmatory tests: Virus isolation from brain tissue, or serologic tests (CF, HI, SN, or FA) on paired sera.

Occurrence: Usually appears in summer, most cases occurring in young adults and children under 1 year of age, in the Americas from Canada to Argentina; rarer in humans than in horses. Equine cases occur almost every year in the western United States. In hyperendemic areas, serologic evidence of infection among horses is high.

Transmission: Mosquitoborne. Wild birds, especially Passeriformes, are reservoirs, and develop a viremia that can infect mosquitoes. In the western United States, mosquitoes of the genus *Culex* are the usual vectors, and *Aedes* is involved in some areas. The infection is maintained by transmission from a viremic to a susceptible wild bird, which constitutes the endemic and amplifying link in the circulation of the virus. Snakes possibly may play a role in maintaining the virus through the winter. Both man and horses are accidental hosts and are not involved in the basic cycle.

CONTROL AND PREVENTION
Individual/herd: Same as EEE.
Local/community: Same as EEE.
National/international: None.

DISEASE: West Nile Fever (WNF)

AGENT
RNA virus, genus *Flavivirus* (group B), family Togaviridae

RECOGNITION
Syndrome: Human: Ranges in severity from subclinical to a febrile course of short duration to encephalitis, with more serious illness in elderly persons than in children. Most common signs include sudden onset of fever, headache, enlarged lymph nodes, and a maculopapular rash on the trunk, though ocular, muscular, and joint pain may also occur. Duration typically is about 3-5 days, generally followed by rapid and complete recovery. Convalescence is sometimes prolonged and accompanied by profound weakness. Myocarditis, meningitis, and encephalitis are occasional complications.

Animal: Most infections are subclinical. Horses may occasionally develop meningoencephalitis. No other domestic mammal clinically affected. Peridomestic birds, such as pigeons, turtledoves, and crows may be affected, as may some wild birds.

Incubation period: Human, 3-6 days.

Case fatality rate: Negligible in humans; up to 25% in horses, and high in experimentally infected crows.

Confirmatory tests: Virus isolation during acute phase, or serologic testing (SN) of paired sera.

Occurrence: Occurs in summer, is both endemic and epidemic. Widely distributed throughout Africa, Asia, and Europe where the virus has been isolated from humans, other mammals, birds, and arthropods. Endemic in the Nile Delta, epidemics occur in Israel, and occurs sporadically in South Africa. Human prevalence of infection in Egypt may exceed 60%.

Transmission: Mosquitoborne. Birds are the reservoir, developing a persistent, high-titer viremia that allows infection of *Culex* mosquitoes. Humans, sheep, and cattle, are accidental hosts that do not develop viremia sufficient to infect vectors.

CONTROL AND PREVENTION

Individual/herd: Prevent mosquito bites with protective clothing and use of repellents. No vaccine is available.

Local/community: Vector control is difficult because the species of mosquito that transmits the infection to humans is not well-established in all areas affected. *Culex* mosquitoes transmit infection bird-to-bird, but may not infect humans. Another vector that connects the wild cycle with human outbreaks is likely, and control of this latter vector is important.

National/international: None.

DISEASE: Yabapox

AGENT

Unclassified DNA virus, family Poxviridae, related to Tanapox

RECOGNITION

Syndrome: Human: Pseudotumors up to 2 cm in diameter develop on the hands and feet, accompanied by regional lymphadenopathy and fever. Resolution is spontaneous within a few weeks.

Animal: Can infect rhesus monkeys, baboons, and macaques. Pseudotumors, which propagate via the lymphatic system to form multiple nodules, appear mainly on the extremities and face. They resolve spontaneously within about 6 weeks.

Incubation period: In human volunteers, 5-7 days; 4 months in a laboratory-acquired case. 3-4 weeks in experimentally infected monkeys.

Case fatality rate: None.

Confirmatory tests: Serologic detection by FA.

Occurrence: Outbreaks have occurred in primate centers, the first in Yaba, Nigeria.

Transmission: Unknown, although arthropod vectors are possible, and one primate outbreak was traced to use of a contaminated tattoo needle. Human infection resulted from a laboratory accident.

CONTROL AND PREVENTION

Individual/herd: In primate centers, good hygiene should be practiced. Separate healthy from infected animals. Disinfect contaminated equipment. Animal care workers should use caution when handling monkeys, and seek medical attention for any cuts or abrasions. Smallpox vaccination is not protective.

Local/community: None.

National/international: None.

DISEASE: Yellow Fever (YF)

AGENT

RNA virus, genus *Flavivirus* (group B), family Togaviridae

RECOGNITION

Syndrome: Human: Subclinical to severe, life-threatening disease of short duration. Mild cases may be indeterminate. Typically, begins with sudden onset of high fever, headache, chills, backache, muscle pain, prostration, nausea, and vomiting. Fever may subside after 3-4 days, then return in the second phase of illness, during which hepatic and renal involvement and hemorrhage may occur. Nasal and oral bleeding, hematemesis ("black vomit"), and melena occur. The name derives from the jaundice that often results from liver impairment. Most deaths occur between days 3 and 7, with prognosis improving if survive at least 10 days.

Animal: Nonhuman primates may be affected, with varying degrees of severity among species. Monkeys in the Americas are more severely affected and have a higher mortality rate than those in Africa, a possible factor being YF has long been endemic in Africa whereas it is more recent in Neotropical regions. The clinical course in primates is similar to that in humans.

Incubation period: In humans, 3-6 days.

Case fatality rate: In endemic regions, often less than 5%, but in nonindigenous groups and in epidemics fatalities may exceed 50%.

Confirmatory tests: Virus isolation during the first few days of illness is most reliable. Viral antigen can be detected in serum by ELISA testing. Serologic tests include HI, SN, CF, and IFA. Cross-reactions, however, can occur with other flaviviruses, and antibodies developed after vaccination are indistinguishable from those produced as a result of infection.

Occurrence: Restricted to Africa and the Americas. In Africa, both urban and sylvatic cycles of infection occur. The urban cycle occurs mainly in savannah areas, particularly those bordering rain forests, such as in Burkina Faso and Nigeria. Sylvatic YF occurs from the Sahara east to Ethiopia and Somalia and south as far as Angola and Zaire. In the Americas, urban YF no longer exists, because of successful urban mosquito eradication programs, but the sylvatic cycle continues in forests of northern South America. Most human cases occur in the Amazon Basin, the plains of southeastern Colombia, and eastern Bolivia and Peru.

Transmission: Mosquitoborne. In Africa, green monkeys, patas monkeys, leaf-eating monkeys, and baboons are infected from *Aedes africanus. Ae. bromeliae, Ae. simpsoni,* and other species of *Aedes* can transfer the virus from monkeys to humans. In the New World, *Ae. aegypti* was the vector for the urban form. Today, the sylvatic cycle is maintained by howler monkeys and spider monkeys, both of which usually die when affected with YF, as well as the more resistant capuchins, owl monkeys, marmosets, and squirrel monkeys. The vectors are *Ae. leucocelaenus, Ae. fulvus, Sabethes chloropterus,* and *Hemagogus* spp., all canopy-dwelling species that usually come in contact with humans only during logging or other tree-felling operations.

CONTROL AND PREVENTION

Individual/herd: Vaccinate travelers to endemic areas. Vaccinate family members and other contacts of YF patients.

Local/community: For urban YF, mass vaccination campaigns, mosquito control. For sylvan YF, vaccinate people living near or entering affected forests and avoid those areas for one week post-vaccination.

National/international: If YF in a human is discovered in a nonendemic area, the WHO and adjacent countries must be notified immediately, as specified in the International Health Regulations. YF among nonhuman vertebrates in newly discovered or reactivated foci must also be reported. Monkeys and other nonhuman primates arriving in YF-free areas from areas where YF occurs must be quarantined for 7 days. Proof of vaccination against YF is required by many countries for travelers who have come from or through areas where YF occurs.

INDEX

Boldface numbers represent primary information.

Printed in the United States
31216LVS00004B/1-39